Social Determinants of Health

PHE1SDH

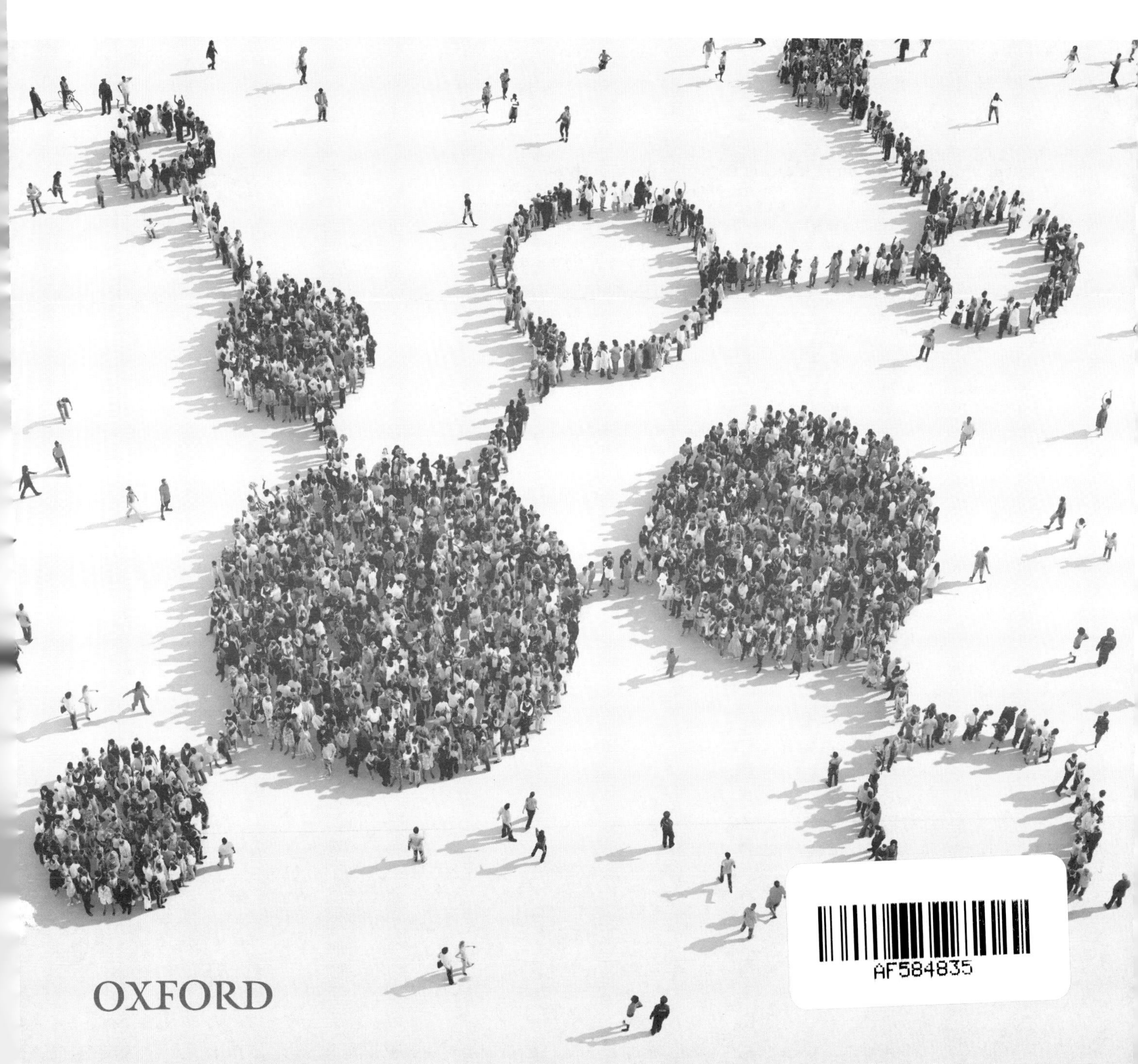

OXFORD

OXFORD
UNIVERSITY PRESS
Oxford University Press is a department of the University of Oxford.

It furthers the University's objective of excellence in research, scholarship, and education by publishing worldwide. Oxford is a registered trademark of Oxford University Press in the UK and in certain other countries.
Published in Australia by
Oxford University Press
253 Normanby Road, South Melbourne, Victoria 3205, Australia

First published 2018

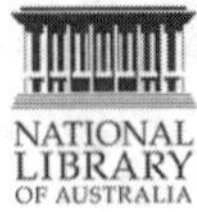

A catalogue record for this book is available from the National Library of Australia

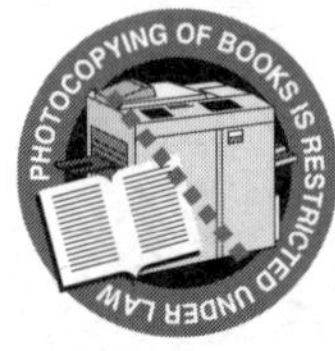

Typeset by Kerry Cooke, eggplant communications
Printed and bound in Australia by Ligare Book Printers, Pty Ltd

About This Publication

The following Oxford University Press textbooks have been used in this publication:

- Davidson, A. 2015, *Social Determinants of Health: A Comparative Approach*, Oxford University Press, Don Mills, Canada.
- Germov, J. 2013, *Second Opinion*, 5th Edn, Oxford University Press, Melbourne.
- Liamputtong, P., Fanany, and R., Verrinder, G. 2012, *Health, Illness and Wellbeing*, Oxford University Press, Melbourne.

Pagination, running headers and footers, and cross-references

The pages from the source books have not been altered, except as follows:

- The first page of each chapter/reading gives the reading number for this custom publication, rather than the chapter number from the original publication.
- A shaded strip along the bottom of each page gives information specific to this publication—the page number for this publication, the topic number and name, the reading number and name, and the name/s of the author/s of the reading.

The running headers come from the original publications and contain the page numbers from the original publications. Any cross-references within the chapters refer to the text of the original publications.

Contents

Health, illness, and well-being: An introduction

Pranee Liamputtong, Rebecca Fanany, and Glenda Verrinder

TOPICS COVERED

This chapter covers the following topics:

- an introduction to health, illness, well-being, and disease
- cultural understanding of health, illness, and well-being
- determinants of health
- biological determinants
- environmental determinants
- social determinants of health
- gender, ethnicity, and social class
- health inequality

KEY TERMS

Biological determinants
Culture
Determinants of health
Disease
Environmental determinants
Ethnicity
Gender
Health
Illness
Social class
Social determinants
Well-being

Introduction

Health There is no definite meaning of health. Its meaning can be different depending on individuals, social groups, and cultures and can differ at different times. However, the World Health Organization (1978, p. 2) defines health as 'a state of complete physical, mental and social well-being and not merely the absence of disease or infirmity'.

The concept of **health** has different meanings to different people (Jirojwong & Liamputtong 2009). Each individual has a different perception and experience of health, illness, and well-being. For some people, health may mean being active and fit. For others, health means having a balance in their lives, being productive or able to fulfil their responsibilities (Blaxter 2004; Levin & Browner 2005; Taylor 2008a; Jirojwong & Liamputtong 2009; AIHW 2010a). Additionally, members of one cultural group may see health, illness, and well-being differently.

In Australia, the notion that health is of primary importance is pervasive. This is reflected in the fact that health and illness are featured in all kinds of media. Often, there are reports or stories about health issues, health-related behaviours and experiences, the importance of fitness and health, new medical and scientific discoveries, healthcare services and government policies (Taylor 2008a; Germov & Freij 2009).

There are many things that can determine our health, illness, and well-being. These range from societal influences to individual aspects such as genetic makeup as well as the healthcare to which we have access. These are referred to as 'the determinants of health' since they 'determine how likely we are to stay healthy or become ill' (AIHW 2010a, p. 63; see section below on determinants of health). According to the Australian Institute of Health and Welfare (AIHW) (2010a, p. 63), the health, illness, and well-being of an individual comprise many aspects: 'They result from complex interplay between societal, environmental, socioeconomic, biological and lifestyle factors.'

This chapter will take you through several important concepts. First, the meaning of health, illness, well-being, and disease is introduced. Then these meanings are discussed within a cultural context. The determinants of health are then introduced. Last, the relationships between health determinants are discussed, in particular the intersection of gender, ethnicity, and social class.

Conceptualising health

According to Keleher and MacDougall (2009), it is impossible to find a universal definition of health which can be applied to all individuals, locations, and time. The meanings of health are 'embedded in the unique individual, family, social and cultural contexts in which the term is used'. Hence, health is 'socially and culturally constructed' (Taylor 2008a, p. 5). The AIHW (2010a, p. 3) defines health as an essential component of well-being. It is about how we 'feel and function'. Health is not simply about the non-existence of injury or illness but about degrees of wellness and illness in health. Health is situated within broad social and cultural contexts. The state of health of individuals in the society also contributes to the social and economic well-being of that particular society. The following quotes suggest that health is defined differently according to the contexts within which the definition is located.

> Health is a personal and social state of balance and well-being in which a woman feels strong, active, creative, wise and worthwhile: where her body's vital power of functioning and healing is intact; where her diverse capacities and rhythms are valued; where she may decide and choose, express herself and move about freely. (Centre for Health Education, Training and Nutrition Awareness 2011)
>
> Health is a social, economic and political issue and above all a fundamental human right. Inequality, poverty, exploitation, violence and injustice are at the root of ill-health and the deaths of poor and marginalised people. (People's Health Movement 2011, p. 2)
>
> Health is 'a sustainable state of wellbeing, within sustainable ecosystems, within a sustainable biosphere'. (Honari 1993, p. 23)

Keleher and MacDougall (2009, pp. 5–6) outline different perspectives which can be used to conceptualise health. Several perspectives are relevant to this textbook. The lay or cultural perspective suggests that health is understood and interpreted differently by individuals depending on their experiences, life situations, and cultural backgrounds. The biological perspective examines the role of genes and risk factors as well as their interactions with other health determinants (see later section on these determinants). Closely related to the biological approach is the biomedical perspective. Within this approach, health and illness are perceived in terms of a person's 'medically defined pathology'.

The behavioural perspective advocates that superior quality of life results from having good health, which is founded on risk factors and lifestyle behaviours. Health education is often the response to improving these determinants. The health promotion approach includes all of these perspectives and in addition pays attention to the powerful impact of a 'place' or location in determining health. Hence, we see projects such as 'Healthy Schools', 'Healthy Workplace', and 'Healthy Cities' (Baum 2008, p. 13). Research suggests that disadvantaged individuals such as poor people may have poorer health because they reside in places which are damaging to health (Macintyre & Ellaway 2000; Baum 2008). The influence of location on health can be clearly seen in remote indigenous communities in Australia and other parts of the world where important health facilities such as healthy food, clean water, good sewerage system, suitable accommodation, and access to healthcare are insufficient or absent (Baum 2008). This also applies to poor people living in slums in many parts of the globe.

The Ottawa Charter for Health Promotion (WHO 1986) is considered the formal beginning of the new public health, which has its focus on the social causes of illness and disease, health equity, and social justice (Baum 2008). It suggests that social inequalities and health are situated within the complex connection between social, economic, political, and environmental determinants (see also the section below in this chapter). As such, health is perceived as 'a complex outcome' which is influenced by factors including genetic, environmental, economic, social, and political circumstances (Baum 2008, p. 16). This perspective is the focus of this book.

Disease, illness, health, and well-being

Disease A condition adversely affecting health that has measurable (clinical) symptoms.

Illness A condition adversely affecting health as perceived by the individual in question.

When an individual experiences ill symptoms, two terms tend to be used to describe the sickness: 'disease' and 'illness'. The term **disease** refers to as 'medically defined pathology' (Blaxter 2004, p. 20). It is a malfunctioning of biological mechanisms (Jirojwong & Liamputtong 2009). The word incorporates 'a set of signs and symptoms and medically diagnosed pathological abnormalities' (Baum 2008, p. 4). On the other hand, **illness** involves the subjective experience of ill health of an individual (Blaxter 2004; Baum 2008; Taylor 2008a). Primarily, it is about how a person lives through the disease (Baum 2008). Often, it involves personal, social, and cultural reactions to a disease. Illnesses can disrupt people's lives, which may lead individuals to seek medical care. An ailing person may have to rely on others for their basic needs in daily living (Spector 2009; Suwankhong 2011).

Health, when situated within a biomedical framework of biological determinants, can be seen as 'the absence of disease or pathology' in a person (Taylor 2008a, p. 10). It suggests that if the person does not have a disease, he or she is healthy. Taylor (2008a, p. 10) contends that this view implies two main assumptions. First, there are two opposite states of being: an individual is either healthy or ill. In this view, health and illness are seen as uniform and permanent concepts. Second, it implies that having good health is the norm and being ill is deviant. Thus, illness connotes 'abnormality, deficiency or impairment' (see also Scambler 2003; Blaxter 2004). As Blaxter (2004, p. 7) contends, 'the objective observation of a lack of "normality" meets a very ancient and universal tendency to see the sick person as in some way morally tainted or bewitched. Possibly, they are responsible for their own condition.'

The concept of health as the absence of disease has been perceived as being 'too narrow' (Taylor 2008a, p. 11). Health should be seen as a more credible and holistic condition (Blaxter 2004; Levin & Browner 2005; Taylor 2008a). This is reflected in the definition of health proposed by the World Health Organization (WHO 1978, p. 2), which advocates that health is 'a state of complete physical, mental and social well-being and not merely the absence of disease or infirmity'. This definition suggests that it is not only the biological functioning of individuals that determines the state of their health, but also their social and psychological conditions. These components do not function separately but interact with each other in complicated processes (Taylor 2008a; see the section below on determinants of health).

This view of health is also reflected in the mental health area. There has been an attempt to define mental health in a way that moves beyond the focus on biological factors (Baum 2008). The Victorian Health Promotion Foundation (VicHealth 1999, p. 4) developed the following positive definition: 'Mental health is the embodiment of social, emotional and spiritual well-being. Mental health provides individuals with the vitality necessary for active living, to achieve goals and to interact with one another in ways that are respectful and just.'

Well-being A positive conceptualisation of health: feeling healthy, happy, or doing well in life. It can be completely separated from the objectively measured health or disease status of an individual.

The WHO definition of health also incorporates the concept of **well-being**. This concept is seen as more expansive than that of health because it signifies an individual's sense of general contentment with life (Eckersley 2001; Taylor 2008a).

Well-being is used in a subjective sense in that there is nothing wrong, and can be completely separated from the objectively measured health or disease status of an individual (Jirojwong & Liamputtong 2009). People may possess a sense of personal well-being even when they are in very deprived situations, for example during stressful life events or confronted with acute or chronic disease. In a way, according to Jones and Creedy (2008), it could be said that well-being symbolises the opposite of illness.

Stop and Think

- What does health mean to you?
- What does illness mean to you?
- What does well-being mean to you?
- How do you know if someone is healthy or not?

Stop and Think

Sophie is a 78-year-old woman who has experienced a range of symptoms in the last few years. She suffers from severe tinnitus (ringing in the ear) in both ears. She has also suffered from hearing loss in one ear. Additionally, she has high blood pressure which is being controlled by prescribed medication. Although she is slower with everyday activities and often has aches and pains, she still eats and sleeps well. She is poor but she has good support from her children. She thinks what she has been experiencing is part of growing old. She does not think she is ill.

- What do you think about Sophie's idea of her health?
- In your view, should Sophie's conditions be categorised as illness? Discuss.

Health, illness, well-being, and culture

All human beings have to deal with good health, illness, disease, sickness, and death. In all human groups, no matter how small or large, whether technologically primitive or advanced, there exists a set of beliefs about the nature of health and illness, its cause and cures, and its relations to other aspects of life. These are conditions that shape an aspect of social experience and cultural knowledge. As such, concepts of health, illness, and well-being are likely to reflect a marked cultural influence (Mackenzie et al. 2003; Helman 2007; Jones & Creedy 2008). What is seen as health or illness in one location, or by the members of one group, is not always perceived the same way in another (Jones & Creedy 2008). Because health and illness are socially constructed, different **cultures** would have different perceptions of health and illness. It has been shown that cultural understandings of health and illness operate as an important aspect in determining the health and illness of individuals (Julian 2009).

Culture A system of shared ideas, attitudes, and practices that defines the social system of its members.

While health is well understood by most people in mainstream Australian society, within Indigenous Australian cultures there is no one single word that stands for health (O'Connor-Fleming

& Parker 2001). Concepts of health and well-being entail 'relationship with family, community and connectedness with traditional land or country rather than referring to an individual as a separate entity' (Taylor 2008a, p. 6). These collective approaches of health are held by many Indigenous people (Levin & Browner 2005). In the Indigenous context, the concept of 'well-being' has a broader meaning than 'health' since it embraces the wider relationship and connection of people with their environment and community (O'Connor-Fleming & Parker 2001; Taylor 2008a).

For Thai people, being in good health is understood as being normal and strong, and free of illness and disease. In the Thai worldview, this understanding symbolises the characteristics of people's capability and is related to traditional understanding of *me ar-kaan crop sam-sib-song pra-garn* (having the complete 32 components of the body) in order to fulfil a person's normal routine such as eating, sleeping, and working (Suwankhong 2011). Thai people also have their own cultural knowledge about causes of good health and illness which has been part of the culture for centuries. These include *kam* (bad karma), loss of soul, imbalance of bodily elements, and supernatural beings (Muecke 1979; Liamputtong 2007; Lundberg & Kerdonfag 2010).

Hmong people, including the Hmong ethnic community in Australia, have a number of beliefs concerning supernatural beings that can cause illness and death to humans. Although they believe the primary cause of such misfortune is the loss of soul (see Case Study 1.1), they also see that some illnesses are due to natural or organic factors. The Hmong are conscious of the influence of natural forces on a person's good health or illness. When a woman has just given birth, her body is believed to be in a state of disequilibrium with nature. She is therefore prohibited from participating in daily work for 30 days. During this period, she needs to rest and be mindful of 'cold' and 'wrong' food. Hot food, mainly chicken cooked with herbal medicines, is consumed for the entire period of 30 days. Failure to do this is believed to result in ill health later in life (Liamputtong Rice 2000).

Traditional healers, referred to as shamans, are an important part of Hmong life (Cha 2003; Symonds 2004; Liamputtong 2009a). In Australia, there is at least one shaman in each state, and there are at least four shamans in Melbourne. The rituals of a shaman are mainly concerned with fertility, protection, and curing (Cha 2003; Culhane-Pera et al. 2004; Liamputtong 2009a). The majority of Hmong in Australia continue to seek help from their traditional healers despite the availability of care within the Australian healthcare system. This is most obvious when the Hmong are confronted with severe illnesses and health-related issues which are seen to be closely related to the Hmong cosmos (such as in the case of childhood illnesses, burns, bone fractures, infertility, and childbirth).

Case Study 1.1 Childbirth and soul loss

The Story of Mai

This case study is from Pranee's research with women from the Hmong ethnic community in Melbourne (see Liamputtong Rice et al. 1994; Liamputtong 2010a). Mai was 34 years old, married, and had six children. Four children were born in a refugee camp in Thailand and two in Australia. Five of her children were born naturally. However, when Mai had her last child she was advised that she needed a caesarean operation since the baby was in a transverse lie.

Mai refused the operation and insisted that she could give birth naturally. She was told that if she attempted a vaginal birth the baby might not survive. Because of the concern about the survival of her baby, Mai agreed to a caesarean. However, the caesarean was done under a general anaesthetic and she was alone in the operating theatre as her husband was not allowed to stay with her. Since the birth of her last child Mai had been physically unwell. She had seen a number of specialists about her health, but they could find nothing wrong with her.

Mai believed that while she was unconscious under the general anaesthetic, one of her souls, which takes care of her well-being, left her body and was unable to re-enter. Because she was moved out of the operating theatre and regained consciousness in a recovery room, she believed that her soul was left in the operating theatre. She strongly believed that the departure of this soul was the main cause of her ill health because she had frequent bad dreams in the next ten months, occurring two or three times a week. Each time, after the dream, she felt very ill and experienced bad pains. In her dreams, she wandered to faraway places. She did not know where she was going since she had never seen those places before. It was as if she just had to keep walking and there was no ending. Mai believed this was the sign that her lost soul was wandering in another world.

In order to regain her health, she believed that she must undergo a soul-calling ceremony and that this must be performed at the theatre in which the caesarean was done, where the soul would still be waiting to be called back. Pranee asked her if she had considered a soul-calling ceremony at the operating theatre but she thought this would not be possible as the hospital staff would not understand her customs and would refuse the request since the ceremony involves taking a live chicken into the theatre and burning an incense stick there. Her husband commented that since he was not able to accompany his wife into the operating theatre, it would be impossible to be granted permission to perform a ceremony that is alien to Western healthcare providers. Because Mai was unable to perform a soul-calling ceremony at the operating theatre, the family believed that the soul had left her body for a lengthy period and transformed into another living thing. As a consequence, her health continued to deteriorate.

Concerned about Mai's well-being, Pranee and her colleagues discussed the possibility of taking Mai back to the hospital to perform the ceremony. They contacted one of the hospital staff. Through this person, the deputy CEO of the hospital agreed to the request. Her positive response was that 'the hospital is more than happy to do anything for the woman if this can help her'. She left the name of a person to contact for making the arrangements.

Pranee approached the operating theatre manager to arrange the ceremony. She was told the theatre would be quite busy during the week so she suggested that Mai have it done on the weekend. Since the date was not important, Mai agreed to have the ceremony performed on a Sunday morning. At eight o'clock one Sunday morning, Mai, her husband, and a shaman met Pranee and her bi-cultural research assistant at the ground floor of the hospital with the essential ingredients including a live chicken in a cardboard box. They reached the theatre where the charge nurses were expecting them. The nurses were very helpful and supportive. They showed Mai where she was put to sleep and where she regained consciousness. They also showed her the path along which she was carried to the operating theatre because they wanted to ensure that the ceremony was performed appropriately. At 8.30 a.m. the shaman performed a soul-calling ritual in the operating theatre. There, it took him about 20 minutes to persuade Mai's soul to come home with her. However, to ensure the soul would not be confused with the body and where it belonged, the shaman performed the same ritual at the spot where Mai regained consciousness in the recovery room. This took him only 10 minutes. Then they all went back to Mai's house to perform another ceremony. This was to welcome the soul back to its home.

Stop and Think

» Could this situation have been prevented? In your view, how could it be prevented?

The positive aspect of this ceremony was the agreement of the hospital to allow Mai and her family to perform a soul-calling ceremony in the operating theatre in addition to the concerns about her well-being by hospital staff. This illustrates how mainstream health services can provide culturally sensitive care to consumers from different cultural backgrounds, if informed of these cultural beliefs and practices.

» If you are a healthcare provider where Mai gave birth, how would you respond to her case? What would you do to accommodate for cultural differences among your clients?

Cross-cultural studies have shown that people's experience of health can be usefully organised under the following categories:

- feeling vital, full of energy
- having good social relationships
- experiencing a sense of control over one's life and living conditions
- being able to do things one enjoys
- having a sense of purpose in life
- experiencing connectedness to 'community' (Labonte 1997, p. 15).

This positive cross-cultural perspective on health enables us to plan different healthcare systems from the current dominance of the focus in Australia on illness care.

Determinants of health

Situated within the new public health perspective, the health, illness, and well-being of individual persons, groups, and communities are determined by a diverse range of complex individual, social, cultural, environmental, and economic factors and healthcare systems (AIHW 2010a). This is referred to as the determinants of health (Marmot & Wilkinson 1999; Taylor 2008a). Conceptually, the focus of this perspective is on factors that could influence and determine the health of people, instead of on the state and outcomes of their health. It also underscores the prevention of ill health, rather than the measurement of illness (Keleher & Murphy 2004; Taylor 2008a).

Case Study 1.2 Samantha

Samantha, a 3-year-old child, was born into a poor family and lived in a remote part of the country. One day, while running around in the street with her older brother, she was pierced by a nail that was discarded on the ground. Her mother bandaged the wound for her. Several days later, the wound became infected. Samantha began to feel pain in her groin and had fever. Her mother tried to manage her pain and fever with whatever she could within her capacity. However, Samantha became very unwell and this prompted her mother to take her to a hospital, which was many kilometres away. Tragically, Samantha died a few days after being admitted to the hospital (adapted from Werner 1997).

Stop and Think

- What do you think contributed to Samantha's tragic death?
- Could her death have been prevented? How?
- Who or what should be blamed for her death?
- Would her death have occurred if she had been born into a better-off family and lived in an urban area like Melbourne or Perth?

Determinants of health A range of individual, social, economic, environmental, and cultural conditions that have the potential to contribute to or detract from the health of individuals, communities, or whole populations.

The **determinants of health** are characteristics or factors which can bring about a change in the health and illness of individuals and populations, for better or worse (Reidpath 2004; Taylor 2008a). Determinants of health include biological and genetic factors; health behaviours (such as risky lifestyles, abuse of alcohol, and cigarette smoking); socio-cultural and socio-economic factors (such as gender, ethnicity, education, income, and occupation); and environment factors (such as housing, social support, social connection, geographical position, and climate). Resources and systems also have effects on the health and well-being of individuals and populations. These include access to health services, healthcare policy, and the healthcare system (Najman 2001; AIHW 2010a).

Essentially, these determinants are connected with conditions that can either improve or hinder individuals' possibilities of having and sustaining good health. Some conditions have a direct impact on the health and illness of individuals, for example direct contact with heat or asbestos in their environment, cigarette smoking, or lack of physical activities. Other conditions have an indirect impact on individuals. They can increase or reduce the influences of other factors, for example when people are poor and cannot access suitable healthcare (Cashmore 2001). These conditions can interact and function in complex ways. For instance, when people do not have good health, they may not be able to work or take exercise. And this in turn will have further impact on their health (Taylor 2008a).

According to the AIHW (2010a, p. 64), health determinants can be perceived as 'a web of causes', but they can also be described as part of broad causal pathways that can influence health. Figure 1.1 presents a conceptual framework that shows

Figure 1.1 Determinants of health

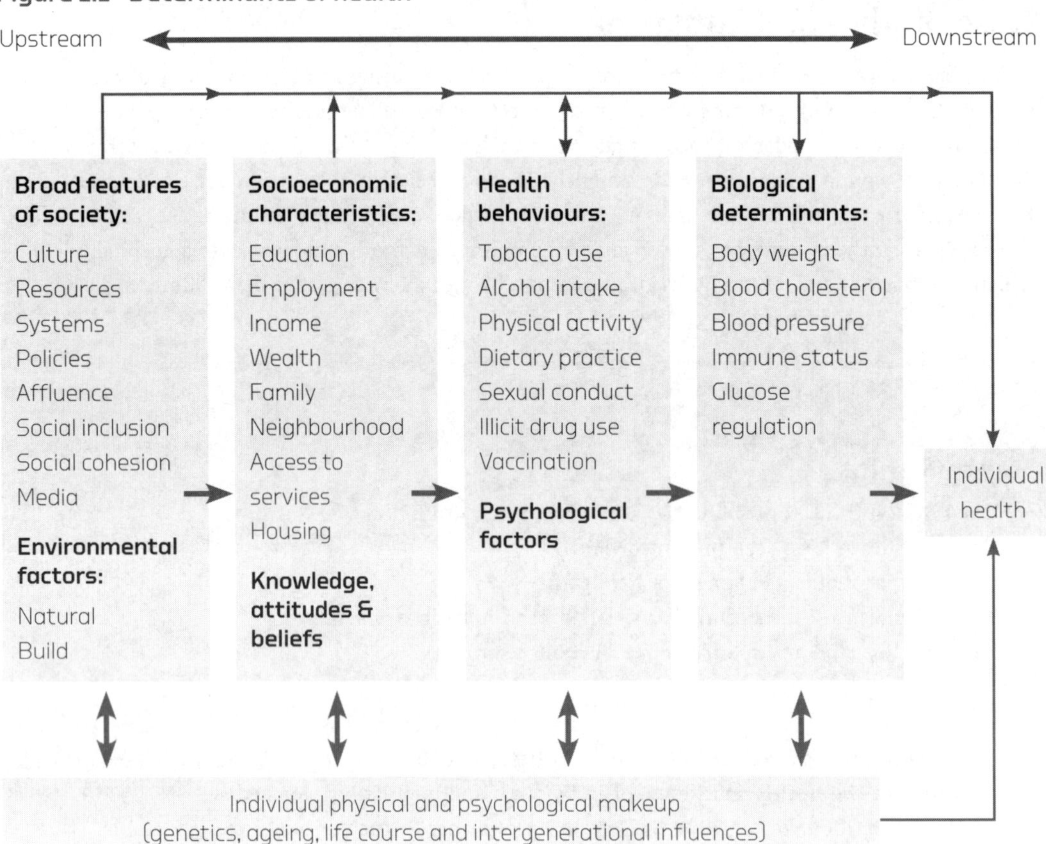

Source: Adapted from AIHW 2010a, p. 64

the complex relationships of health determinants. The determinants are divided into four main categories. The direction of influence moves from left to right: from the 'upstream' factors (such as culture, resources, and affluence) to more 'downstream' or direct influences (such as body weight and blood pressure). The figure illustrates how one broad category (the broad features of society and environmental factors) can determine the nature of another main group (individuals' socio-economic characteristics such as their level of education and employment). Both these broad categories in turn have an impact on individuals' health behaviours, their psychological state and safety. These can then affect biomedical components, such as body weight and blood pressure, which would have further health effects through different pathways. Along the different paths and states, these various factors interact with the genetic composition of the individuals. It should also be noted that the direction of these influences can occur in reverse. For instance, an individual's health can also have an impact on his or her levels of physical activity, employment status, and wealth.

Health-promoting conditions can also be divided into four main categories from the upstream factors such as ecosystem viability, equitable public policies, and convivial communities, through to health-promoting mediating structures, for example caring relationships, and service to others, through to health lifestyles such as town planning to promote physical fitness and on to community-managed health services (Labonte 1997). It is argued that equitable public policies, for example, do much to promote healthy lifestyle choices.

The intersections of biological, environmental, and social determinants of health

As discussed in the previous section, health determinants interact in a complex way; it is important to examine some of the relationships between the three major determinants of health that play an important part in the health, illness, and well-being of individuals: biological, environmental, and social determinants.

Biological determinants

The **biological determinants** of health and disease indicate a diverse range of 'heterogeneous, intra-individual factors' which push, intervene, or mitigate the passage of an individual towards health or disease (Swinburn & Cameron-Smith 2009, p. 248). Fundamentally, genes play a crucial role in underlying biological differences between individuals, but genes also interact with other social and environmental components that influence health and disease (see examples below) (Bortz 2005; Swinburn & Cameron-Smith 2009). According to Swinburn and Cameron-Smith (2009, p. 248), 'the genetic and physiological systems within the body are dynamic, complex, and highly interconnected, with whole systems balancing and competing against each other' to achieve homeostasis. This is very similar to the complex processes of the social and environmental system outside the physical body of the individual.

Biological determinants The inner physiological aspect of health and disease. Genes play a crucial role in underlying biological differences between individuals.

This can be seen in the case of HIV. HIV is dispersed in three ways: through sexual intercourse, blood transfusions (also through the use of needles and syringes), and from mother to child (Vaughan 2009). While everyone can be infected with HIV, there are biological factors that increase an individual's susceptibility to infection. For instance, if an individual has another sexually transmitted infection (STI) such as *Chlamydia* or gonorrhoea, the risk of becoming infected with HIV during sex is higher. If someone has a blood disorder (which indicates that they need regular blood transfusions), that person is also at higher risk of contracting HIV. If a woman who is infected with HIV has health problems during pregnancy and also breastfeeds her baby, there is a greater chance that the infection will be transmitted to the baby. According to Vaughan (2009, p. 176), the risk of HIV infection is also connected with the behaviours of individuals, for instance having multiple sexual partners and having sex without a condom. Sharing equipment used for injecting drugs is also a high-risk behaviour among certain groups of people. Hence, although the biological factors are important, a focus on biological risk factors only will not stop the spread of HIV epidemic in populations (Vaughan 2009).

Three biological determinants that play a part in health and illness are race, sex, and age. However, these three are also intertwined with social and environmental determinants. Sometimes it can be difficult to differentiate between biological or other social or environmental conditions that determine people's health and illness.

Age is a clear biological determinant of the health of human beings (Miller 2009; West & Bergman 2009). According to Keleher and Joss (2009, p. 370), genes may have some impact on the causation of disease. However, for many diseases the causes are environmental. For example, cognitive functioning decline among older people is not only the result of being old but may also be affected by lack of exercise, illness (such as depression), behaviours (such as the use of medications), psychological components (such as lack of confidence, motivation, and low expectations), and social aspects (such as isolation and loneliness). Some aspects of race and gender will be covered under the social determinants of health in a section below.

Environmental determinants

Environmental determinants Physical environmental factors such as climate and location, which can affect the health of people.

The important connection between the **environment** in which individuals live and their health and well-being has long been observed (Hancock 1985; WHO 1986; McMichael 1993, 2001; Nicholson & Stephenson 2009; Griffith et al. 2010). Historically, environmental dangers to people's health tended to be related to issues of underdevelopment such as inadequate water quality, the absence of sanitation, and poor housing. Although these traditional threats have been managed successfully in the more affluent areas within the developed countries, there are still problems among socially disadvantaged and vulnerable groups of developed nations, and also in the poorer countries of the globe (Nicholson & Stephenson 2009). This can be seen clearly in the environmental threats some indigenous people have to deal with in Australia and elsewhere. Nowadays, we see 'modern' threats, which have emerged because of overconsumption and overdevelopment in developed nations (WHO 1997a). These modern threats, including climate change, have now become global hazards (McMichael 1993, 2001; Eisenberg et al. 2007; Baum 2008; Nicholson & Stephenson 2009). Australia is one developed nation that is highly susceptible to the impacts of climate changes (Diamond 2004; Garnaut 2008; Kennedy et al. 2010).

Global climate changes can impact on many aspects of human life and health (Goldsworthy et al. 2009). Thermal extremes, such as heatwaves, can cause difficulty for many people, in particular the very young, very old, very poor, and very sick (Baum 2008; Goldsworthy et al. 2009; Nicholson & Stephenson 2009; Talbot & Verrinder 2009). In 1959, a fourfold increase from the normal mortality was the result of a long period of heatwave in Melbourne (McMichael 1993). Climate change and global warming are also directly connected with the dispersion of infectious disease vectors and pests as well as with reduced food production (Nicholson & Stephenson 2009; Talbot & Verrinder 2009). And this of course will affect people from poor areas and nations more than those from rich areas and locations with better resources (Hancock 1994; Baum 2008). Poor people who live in poor nations are disproportionately burdened by environmental problems and their related health impacts (Hancock 1994; Agyeman & Evans 2002; Baum 2008).

Mythbuster

Consider whether you see the following as questionable. What does this tell you about your own values?

- Your government wishes to develop a plan for a more sustainable environment for the city and country as a whole. But this necessitates commitment and a huge budget, which means more tax levies on local people. This has created anger among some people, particularly those with high incomes.
- There has been an extensive drought in your country for a number of years. The government has developed a plan to save more water and this means certain cuts in the use of water in some sectors of the country, particularly farmers. Those who are affected blame people who live in the city for an unequal access to water.

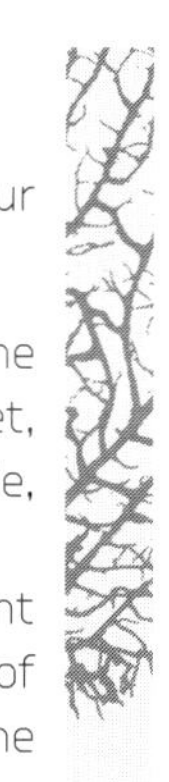

The World Health Organization (1997a, p. 198) puts it clearly: 'Impoverished populations...are at greater risk from degraded environmental conditions. The cumulative effects of inadequate and hazardous shelter, overcrowding, lack of water supply and sanitation, unsafe food, air and water pollution and high accident rates impact heavily on the health of these vulnerable groups.'

Increasingly and globally, we have witnessed more environmental hazards and the health impacts of climate change resulting from human behaviours. Severe drought, flooding, storms, and extreme temperatures have become very common in recent years (Nicholson & Stephenson 2009, p. 122; Verrinder 2011). This is what we have recently experienced in Australia—the Black Saturday bushfires in Victoria in February 2009, the widespread floods in Queensland, New South Wales, and Victoria in January 2011, the Yasi cyclone in north Queensland, and the Carlos cyclone in Darwin in February 2011.

Social determinants

Not all illnesses are caused by biological and environmental agents. The health and well-being of individuals is also influenced by a number of **social determinants**. According to Lawn (2008, p. 36), there are a number of factors, including social, cultural, economic, and political, which can impact health. This position goes beyond the restricted view of biological and genetic aspects of health (Marmot & Wilkinson 1999; Kelly et al. 2007; Keleher & MacDougall 2009). Social determinants of health are also seen as determinants that are 'attributable to the structure and functioning of society' (Reidpath 2004, p. 22). For example, transportation can be seen as one social determinant of health since it can impact on individuals' physical activities, and this in turn can influence their nutritional intake and cardiovascular condition. Social expectations regarding sexual behaviours are also social determinants of health as they can influence individuals' approaches to risky sexual conducts, and this can lead to marginalisation, stigma, and discrimination (Reidpath 2004).

Social determinants
A number of factors, including social, cultural, economic, and political, which can impact on the health of individuals.

Important social determinants of health are related to the positions of social life including gender, ethnicity, and social class (Reidpath 2004).

Stop and Think

» Have you ever looked at the homeless men who sleep on the local park bench with a blanket to cover their bodies, while their possessions are kept in some plastic bags next to them? When they wake, they tend to talk to themselves and do not seem to care about others around them. Have you ever thought about how they came to be like this? Have you been curious enough about what type of journey they have been through in their lives and what it would have been like for them before this misfortune, such as when they were somebody's son, father, husband, or colleague?

To develop an understanding of the life of these men necessitates some understanding of the social determinants of health (adapted from Lawn 2008, p. 36).

Gender Socially and culturally constructed categories reflecting what it means to be 'masculine' and 'feminine' and associated expectations of roles and behaviours of men and women.

Ethnicity Refers to a shared cultural background which is a characteristic of a group within a society.

Social class The position of a person in a system of structured inequality; it is grounded in unequal distribution of income, wealth, status, and power.

Gender is understood as a social construct, referring to the distinguishing characteristics of being female or male. Gender can be seen as the full range of personality traits, attitudes, feelings, values, behaviours, and activities that 'society ascribes to the two sexes on a differential basis' (Keleher & MacDougall 2009, p. 56). It is different from sex, which is a 'biological construct premised upon biological characteristics enabling sexual reproduction' (Krieger 2003, p. 653). **Ethnicity** refers to 'a shared cultural background'; it is a characteristic of a group within a society (Julian 2009, p. 177). Ethnicity includes other dimensions than biological determinants (which are referred to as race). These are social, cultural, and economic factors. Ethnicity is now accepted as the more appropriate determinant of health than race (Jones & Creedy 2008; Swinburn & Cameron-Smith 2009). **Social class** (also termed socio-economic status or SES) refers to the position of a person in 'a system of structured inequality' which is grounded in the unequal distribution of income, wealth, status, and power (Germov 2009, p. 86). Income, poverty, and wealth are closely connected with health; people who live in poverty are likely to have worse health status than those who are better-off (Marmot & Wilkinson 1999; Reidpath 2004; Baum 2008; Germov 2009). The Australian Institute of Health and Welfare (AIHW 2006a, p. 232) states that 'people who are poorer or socioeconomically disadvantaged in other ways generally live shorter lives and suffer more illness and reduced quality of life than those who are well-off'.

None of these social determinants exists in isolation (Reidpath 2004). They intersect in a way that can create inequalities in health among people. For example, women from a low socio-economic background are likely to be in poorer health than those from a higher social class (Baum 2008; Germov 2009). Men from ethnic minority groups and lower social classes are also likely to be disadvantaged in terms of health and well-being in comparison to white Anglo-Celtic men with a higher income (Jones & Creedy 2008; Julian 2009). We have witnessed examples of such relationships. Saggers and colleagues (2011) suggest that the most influential indicator of health inequalities is life expectancy at birth. From 2005 to 2007, the life expectancy of Indigenous males was 67.2 years and 72.9 for Indigenous females. They live 11.5 and 9.7 years less than their non-Indigenous counterparts (ABS 2009b, p. 7). Indigenous Australians also fare worse in health issues. For example, they are three times more likely than non-Indigenous Australians to suffer heart attacks, more than twice as likely to die from them and, even if admitted to hospital, likely to receive different treatment from their non-Indigenous counterparts (Mathur et al. 2006). The health inequalities of Indigenous Australians are the consequences of 'poorer socio-economic status, long-standing marginalisation from mainstream society and healthcare and, in many instances, geographical location and isolation' (Taylor 2008a, p. 18; see also Genat & Cripps 2009; Gray & Saggers 2009; MacDonald 2010; Saggers et al. 2011).

We have also seen that there are a number of circumstances and conditions which have created basic inequalities that not only contribute to the ill health of people, but also establish a recurrence of adverse physical and mental health consequences for many individuals and groups within the current socio-cultural, economic, and political contexts around the globe including in Australia (Lawn 2008). As such, there exists health inequality among populations. Health inequality, according to Kawachi and colleagues (2002, p. 647), is a term that is employed 'to designate the differences, variations, and disparities in the health achievements of individuals and groups'. Inequalities are the consequence of inequitable societies and are addressed through social justice. As such, it has been suggested that social justice approaches to health are crucial for any healthcare system that aims to fulfil individuals' rights to good health (Marmot 2000; Keleher & MacDougall 2009; Wilkinson & Pickett 2009).

Stop and Think

» Consider the following examples. What do they tell you about our society and our own values?

- Rachel is an old woman who has been widowed for more than ten years. She has little education and has always been poor. She does not have her own house to live in and has been renting a house in a suburb in Sydney. Recently, she was told to leave the house because the owner wishes to renovate it and increase the rent. Rachel does not have another place to move into and it has been very difficult to find rental accommodation in Sydney.
- Due to some difficulties in his life, Jack has become an alcoholic. He has been drinking heavily recently and as a result he was asked to leave his job. He is separated from his wife and two young children, and has been living on his own in a small flat. Because of his drinking problem and the difficulty he has caused to his family, his colleagues and social network do not wish to have anything to do with him. Virtually, he has lost all of his social support.

Summary

Health, illness, and well-being are inevitable aspects of our lives and have always played a part in the life of all human beings. However, the concepts of health, illness, and well-being are socially and culturally constructed because individuals and cultures see them differently. Diverse factors can have an impact on the health, illness, and well-being of individuals, groups, and populations. These are known as determinants of health and include biological, environmental, social, cultural, and economic determinants. These determinants can affect how healthy or sick an individual can be. Additionally, within the social determinants of health, there are three crucial social structures that can affect the health and well-being of people: gender, ethnicity, and social class. These three factors do not operate in isolation, but rather interrelate to the extent that they create inequality in health among people.

Tutorial exercises

1. Form a group of five with your peers in the class. Each of you needs to write down as many definitions of health as you can. Then compare your answers with your peers in the group. Are there similarities in your definitions? Are they different? Discuss the similarities and differences that you have noted in the group and how they have come about.
2. After finishing this chapter, have a tour around the university campus and take note of any determinants that can make you healthy or ill. What have you noticed?
3. It has been suggested that women live longer and men die sooner. What is your view about this suggestion? Is it true? What would be the determinants of this difference?
4. As a group, watch the documentary *The Shape of Water* (2006) (available online: www.theshapeofwatermovie.com). Discuss the possible determinants that can create inequalities and social justice in different groups of people.

Further reading

Annandale, E., & Hunt, K. (eds) (2000). *Gender inequalities and health*. Buckingham, UK: Open University Press.

Australian Institute of Health and Welfare (2010a). *Australia's health 2010*. Canberra: AIHW. <www.aihw.gov.au>.

Baum, F. (2008). *The new public health: An Australian perspective*, 2nd edn. Melbourne: Oxford University Press.

Bergholt, K. (2008). *Wellbeing: A cultural history of healthy living*, translated by Jane Dewhurst. Cambridge: Polity Press.

Blaxter, M. (2004). *Health*. Cambridge: Polity Press.

Cockerham, W.C. (2007). *Social causes of health and disease*. Cambridge: Polity Press.

Fadiman, A. (1997). *The spirit catches you and you fall down: A Hmong child, her American doctors, and the collision of two cultures*. New York: Farrar, Straus & Giroux.

Germov, J. (ed.) (2009). *Second opinion: An introduction to health sociology*, 4th edn. Melbourne: Oxford University Press.

Keleher, H., & MacDougall, C. (eds) (2009). *Understanding health: A determinants approach*, 2nd edn. Melbourne: Oxford University Press.

Kennedy, D., Stocker, L., & Burke, G. (2010). Australian local government action on climate change adaptation: Some critical reflections to assist decision-making. *Local Environment*, 15(9–10), 805–16.

MacDonald, J.J. (2010). Health equity and the social determinants of health in Australia. *Social Alternatives*, 29(2), 34–40.

Marmot, M., & Wilkinson, R.G. (eds) (2006). *Social determinants of health*, 2nd edn. Oxford: Oxford University Press.

Robertson, S. (2007). *Understanding men and health: Masculinities, identity and well-being*. Berkshire: Open University Press/McGraw Hill.

Taylor, S. (2008a). The concept of health. In S. Taylor, M. Foster & J. Fleming (eds), *Healthcare practice in Australia*. Melbourne: Oxford University Press, 3–21.

Thackrah, R., & Scott, K. (eds) (2011). *Indigenous Australian health and cultures: An introduction for health professionals*. Sydney: Pearson.

Websites

<www.unep.org>

This is the website of the United Nations Environment Program (UNEP). It gives a number of resources regarding environmental issues, for example urban issues, waste, water quality, sanitation, air quality, climate change, and ozone depletion.

<www.who.int/social_determinants/en>

This is the website of the World Health Organization's Commission on Social Determinants of Health. It is a good source of discussions on social determinants and provides crucial background papers and reports as well as examples of actions in relation to social determinants.

<http://phmovement.org/cms>

The website of the People's Health Movement (PHM) provides discussions about health and inequalities in health. It contains information about health networks and activists who have their concerns about the inequalities and inequities in health.

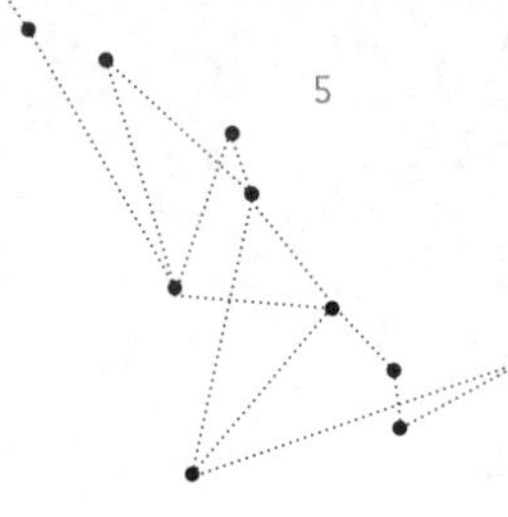

READING 2

IMAGINING HEALTH PROBLEMS AS SOCIAL ISSUES

John Germov

Overview

- What is sociology and how can it be used to understand health and illness?
- What social patterns of health and illness exist?
- What is the social model of health and how does it differ from the medical model?

THE FOREST THROUGH THE TREES

We live in a health-obsessed age. We are bombarded with messages from health authorities, health professionals, and fitness gurus to 'do this' and 'not to do that'. Everywhere we turn we are urged to take individual responsibility for our health. Our personal experience of illness means that we tend to view it in an individualistic way—as a product of bad luck, poor lifestyle, or genetic fate. As individuals we all want quick and effective cures when we are unwell and thus we turn to medicine. Yet this is only part of the story. Even the highly individualised and very personal act of suicide occurs within a social context. For example, Australian men have a suicide rate over triple that of women (AIHW 2012). In fact, the social patterning of suicide was first highlighted in the late nineteenth century by the sociologist Émile Durkheim (1858–1917). While Durkheim (1897/1951) acknowledged individual reasons for a person committing suicide, he found that suicide rates varied between countries and between different social groups within a country. By studying such social patterns, health sociology exposes the 'forest through the trees'—how individual health problems can be part of a social patterning of illness that has social origins and requires social solutions.

Key terms

agency
biological determinism
biomedicine/biomedical model
Cartesian dualism
class (or social class)
epidemiology/social epidemiology
eugenics
lifestyle choices/factors
new public health
public health/public health infrastructure
reductionism
social construction/constructionism
social Darwinism
social institutions
social model of health
social structure
sociological imagination
state
structure–agency debate
victim-blaming

Introduction: the social origins of health and illness

This chapter introduces you to the sociological perspective and how it can be used to understand a wide range of health issues. Health sociology focuses on the social patterns of health and illness—such as the different health statuses between women and men, the poor and the wealthy, or the Indigenous and non-Indigenous populations—and seeks social rather than biological or psychological explanations. It provides a second opinion to the conventional medical view of illness derived from biological and psychological explanations, by exploring the social origins of health and illness—the living and working conditions that fundamentally shape why some groups of people get sicker and die sooner than others.

The social origins of health and illness can clearly be seen when we compare the life expectancy figures of various countries. As we all know, life expectancy in the least developed countries is significantly lower than that in industrially developed and comparatively wealthy countries such as Australia, Sweden, Germany, and Japan. For example, the average life expectancy at birth of people living in the least developed countries of the world is around 20 years less than that for developed countries such as Australia, which has an average life expectancy of 82 years (AIHW 2012; UNDP 2013). As Table 1.1 shows, though, life expectancy varies among developed countries as well. Therefore, the living conditions of the country in which you live can have a significant influence on your chances of enjoying a long and healthy life.

Australian life expectancy is one of the highest in the world, second only to Japan. This is not due to any biological advantage in the Australian gene pool, but is rather a reflection of our distinctive living and working conditions. We can make such a case for two basic reasons. First, life expectancy can change in a short period of time, and in fact it did increase for most countries during the twentieth century. For example, Australian life expectancy has increased by more than 25 years since 1910 (AIHW 2012), which is too short a time frame for any genetic improvement to occur in a given population. Second, data compiled over decades of immigration show that the health of migrants comes to reflect that of their host country over time, rather than their country of origin. The longer migrants live in their new country, the more their health mirrors that of the local population (Marmot 1999).

While the average Australian life expectancy figure is comparatively high, it is important to distinguish between different social groups within Australia. Life expectancy figures are crude indicators of population health and actually mask significant health inequalities among social groups within a country. For example, in Australia those in the lowest socio-economic group have the highest rates of illness and premature death, use preventive services less, and have higher rates of illness-related behaviours such as smoking (AIHW 2012). Furthermore, as Table 1.1 shows, life expectancy for Indigenous Australians is around 12 years less than the national average. In fact, the current life expectancy of Indigenous Australians is closer to that of Australians born in the early twentieth century (AIHW 2012). The indigenous population of New Zealand, the Māori, also have a lower life expectancy—around 7.3 years less than the national average (Statistics New Zealand 2013).

TABLE 1.1 LIFE EXPECTANCY AT BIRTH, 2010

COUNTRY	LIFE EXPECTANCY	
	Men	*Women*
Australia	79.5	84.0
Indigenous Australians (2005–07)	67.0	73.0
Canada (2008)	78.5	82.7
France	78.0	84.7
Germany	78.0	83.0
Italy (2009)	79.4	83.8
Japan	79.6	86.4
New Zealand (2010–12)	79.3	83.0
Maori (2010–12)	72.8	76.5
Russian Federation	63.0	74.9
Sweden	79.5	83.5
UK	78.6	82.6
US	76.2	81.1

Source: Adapted from OECD 2013; AIHW 2010; Statistics New Zealand 2013

Introducing the sociological imagination: a template for doing sociological analysis

What is distinctive about the sociological perspective? In what ways does it uncover the social structure that we often take for granted? How is sociological analysis done? The American sociologist Charles Wright Mills (1916–62) answered such questions by using the expression **sociological imagination** to describe the distinctive feature of the sociological perspective. The sociological imagination is 'a quality of mind that seems most dramatically to promise an understanding of the intimate realities of ourselves in connection with larger social realities' (Mills 1959, p. 15). According to Mills, the essential aspect of thinking sociologically, or seeing the world through a sociological imagination, is making a link between 'private troubles' and 'public issues'.

SOCIOLOGICAL IMAGINATION
A term coined by Charles Wright Mills to describe the sociological approach to analysing issues. We see the world through a sociological imagination, or think sociologically, when we make a link between personal troubles and public issues.

As individuals, we may experience personal troubles without realising they are shared by other people as well. If certain problems are shared by groups of people, they may have a common cause and be best dealt with through collective action. As Mills (1959, p. 226) states, 'many personal troubles cannot be solved merely as troubles, but must be understood in terms of public issues ... public issues must be revealed by relating them to personal troubles'. The Australian sociologist Evan Willis (1993; 2011) suggests that the sociological imagination consists of four interrelated parts:

1 *historical factors*: how the past influences the present;
2 *cultural factors*: how culture impacts on our lives;
3 *structural factors*: how particular forms of social organisation affect our lives;
4 *critical factors*: how we can improve our social environment.

This four-part sociological imagination template is an effective way to understand how to think and analyse in a sociological way.

Figure 1.1 represents the sociological imagination template as a diagram that is easy to remember. Any time you want to analyse a topic sociologically, picture this diagram in your mind.

FIGURE 1.1 THE SOCIOLOGICAL IMAGINATION TEMPLATE

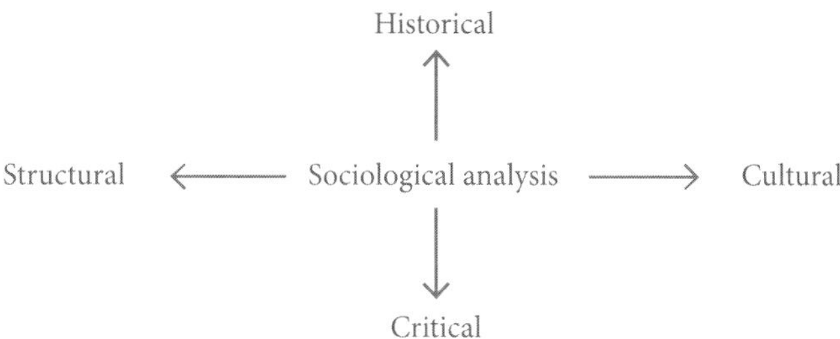

Sociological analysis involves applying these four aspects to the issues or problems under investigation. For example, a sociological analysis of why manual labourers have a shorter life expectancy would examine how and why the work done by manual labourers affects their health, by examining:

1. *historical factors*: to understand why manual workplaces are so dangerous;
2. *cultural factors*: such as the cultural value of individual responsibility;
3. *structural factors*: such as the way work is organised, the role of managerial authority, the rights of workers, and the role of the state;
4. *critical factors*: such as alternatives to the status quo (increasing the effectiveness of occupational health and safety legislation, for instance).

By using the four parts of the sociological imagination template, you begin to 'do' sociological analysis. It is worth highlighting at this point that the template simplifies the process of sociological analysis. When analysing particular topics, it is more than likely that you will find that the parts overlap, making them less clear-cut than the template implies. It is also probable that for some topics, parts of the template will be more relevant and prominent than others—this is all to be expected. The benefit of the template is that it serves as a reminder of the sorts of issues and questions a budding sociologist should be asking.

SOCIAL STRUCTURE
The recurring patterns of social interaction through which people are related to each other, such as social institutions and social groups.

SOCIAL INSTITUTIONS
Formal structures within society—such as health care, government, education, religion, and the media—that are organised to address identified social needs.

IS SOCIETY TO BLAME? INTRODUCING THE STRUCTURE–AGENCY DEBATE

As individuals we are brought up to believe that we control our own destiny, especially our health. It is simply up to each individual to 'do what they wanna do and be what they wanna be'. This belief ignores the considerable influence of society. Sociology makes us aware that we are social animals and are very much the product of our environment, from the way we dress to the way we interact with one another. We are all influenced by the **social structure**, such as our cultural customs and our **social institutions**. The idea of social structure serves to remind us of the social or human-created aspects of life, in contrast to purely random events or products of nature (López & Scott 2000).

Understanding the structure of society enables us to examine the social influences on our personal behaviour and our interactions with others. Yet to what extent are we products of society? How much **agency** do we have over our lives? Are we solely responsible for our actions or is society to blame? These questions represent a key debate in sociology, often referred to as the **structure–agency debate**. There is no simple resolution to this debate, but it is helpful to view structure and agency as interdependent; that is, that humans shape and are simultaneously shaped by society. In this sense, structure and agency are not 'either/or' propositions in the form of a choice between constraint and freedom, but are part of the interdependent processes of social life. Therefore, the social structure should not automatically be viewed in a negative way, as only serving to constrain human freedom, since in many ways the social structure enables us to live, by providing health care, welfare, education, and work. As Mills maintained, an individual 'contributes, however minutely, to the shaping of this society and to the course of its history, even as he is made by society and by its historical push and shove' (1959, p. 6). Mills was clearly a product of the 'historical push and shove' of his social structure, as he uses the masculine 'he' to refer to both men and women—a usage now seen as dated and sexist.

AGENCY
The ability of people, individually and collectively, to influence their own lives and the society in which they live.

STRUCTURE–AGENCY DEBATE
A key debate in sociology over the extent to which human behaviour is determined by social structure.

Peter Berger long ago warned against depicting people as 'puppets jumping about on the ends of their invisible strings' (1966, p. 140). If we use the 'all the world's a stage and we are mere actors' analogy, we could liken life to a theatre in which we all play our assigned roles (father, mother, child, labourer, teacher, student, and so on). Whether it is how we are dressed as we walk down the street or how we present ourselves at a funeral, customs and traditions dictate expected modes of behaviour. In this sense we are all actors on a stage. Yet, we have the scope consciously to participate in what we do. We can make choices about whether simply to act, or whether to modify or change our roles and even the stage on which we live our lives.

Although we are born into a world not of our making, and in countless ways our actions and thoughts are shaped by our social environment, we are not simply 'puppets on strings'. Humans are sentient beings—we are self-aware and thus have the capacity to think and act individually and collectively to change the society into which we are born. Structure and agency may be in tension, but they are interdependent; that is, one cannot exist without the other. Sociology is the study of the relationship between the individual and society; it examines how human behaviour both shapes and is shaped by society, or how 'we create society at the same time as we are created by it' (Giddens 1986, p. 11).

Social medicine and public health

Recognition of the social origins of health and illness actually occurred prior to the formal development of sociology as an academic discipline, and can be traced to the mid-nineteenth century, with the development of 'social medicine' (coined by Jules Guérin in 1848) or what more commonly became known as **public health** (sometimes referred to as social health, community medicine, or preventive medicine). At this time, infectious diseases such as cholera, typhus, smallpox, diphtheria, and tuberculosis were major killers for which there were no cures and little understanding of how they were transmitted. During the nineteenth century, a number of people such as René Villermé (1782–1863), Rudolph Virchow (1821–1902), John Snow (1813–58), Edwin Chadwick (1800–90), and Friedrich Engels (1820–95) established clear links between infectious diseases and poverty (Rosen 1972; Porter 1997).

PUBLIC HEALTH/ PUBLIC HEALTH INFRASTRUCTURE
Public policies and infrastructure to prevent the onset and transmission of disease among the population, with a particular focus on sanitation and hygiene such as clean air, water and food, and immunisation. Public health infrastructure refers specifically to the buildings, installations, and equipment necessary to ensure healthy living conditions for the population.

Engels, Karl Marx's collaborator and patron, made a strong case for the links between disease and poor living and working conditions as an outcome of capitalist exploitation in *The Condition of the Working Class in England* (1845/1958). He used the case of 'black lung', a preventable lung disease among miners, to make the point that:

> the illness does not occur in those mines which are adequately ventilated. Many examples could be given of miners who moved from well-ventilated to badly ventilated mines and caught the disease. It is solely due to the colliery owners' greed for profit that this illness exists at all. If the coalowners would pay to have ventilation shafts installed the problem would not exist. (1845/1958, p. 281)

CLASS (OR SOCIAL CLASS)
A position in a system of structured inequality based on the unequal distribution of power, wealth, income, and status. People who share a class position typically share similar **life chances**.

Engels also noted the differences in the death rates between labourers and professionals, claiming that the squalid living conditions of the working **class** were primarily responsible for the disparity, stating that 'filth and stagnant pools in the working class quarters of the great cities have the most deleterious effects upon the health of the inhabitants' (1845/1958, p. 110).

In 1854, a cholera epidemic took place in Soho, London. John Snow, a medical doctor, documented cases on a city map and investigated all of the 93 deaths that had occurred within a well-defined geographical area. After interviewing residents he was able to establish that people infected with cholera had sourced their water from the same public water pump in Broad Street. Snow came to the conclusion that the water from the pump was the source of cholera, and at his insistence, the pump's handle was removed and the epidemic ceased (Snow 1855/1936; Rosen 1972; Porter 1997; McLeod 2000). This case is famous for being one of the earliest examples of the use of **epidemiology** to understand and prevent the spread of disease.

EPIDEMIOLOGY/ SOCIAL EPIDEMIOLOGY
The statistical study of patterns of disease in the population. Originally focused on epidemics, or infectious diseases, it now covers non-infectious conditions such as stroke and cancer. Social epidemiology is a sub-field aligned with sociology that focuses on the social determinants of illness.

Virchow, often remembered in medical circles for his study of cellular biology, also made a clear case for the social basis of medicine, highlighting its preventive role when he claimed:

> Medicine is a social science, and politics nothing but medicine on a grand scale … if medicine is really to accomplish its great task, it must intervene in political and social life … The improvement of medicine would eventually prolong human life, but improvement of social conditions could achieve this result even more rapidly and successfully. (cited in Rosen 1972, p. 39 and Porter 1997, p. 415)

STATE
A collection of institutions, including the parliament (government and opposition political parties), the public-sector bureaucracy, the judiciary, the military, and the police.

Virchow was a significant advocate for public health care and argued that the **state** should act to redistribute social resources, particularly to improve access to adequate nutrition. Therefore, social medicine and the public health movement grew from recognition that the social environment played a significant role in the spread of disease (Rosen 1972; Porter 1997). In other words, the infectious diseases that afflicted individuals had social origins that necessitated social reforms to prevent their onset (see Rosen 1972 and 1993 and Waitzkin 2000 for informative histories of social medicine; Porter 1997 for a very readable history of medicine in general; Bloom 2002 for a history of medical sociology; and White 2001 for access to early writings on health sociology).

In the UK, Chadwick was a key figure in the development of the first *Public Health Act* (1848), which was based on his 'sanitary idea'—that disease could be prevented through improved waste disposal and sewerage systems. In particular, he focused on removing cesspools of decomposing organic matter from densely populated areas, as well as the introduction of high-pressure flushing sewers, and food hygiene laws to protect against food adulteration. Public health legislation in Australia was first introduced in Victoria in 1854, largely mirroring the British Act, with other colonies following suit (Reynolds 1995; Lawson & Bauman 2001). By the early twentieth century, public health had become part of the nation-building project in Australia, as efforts aimed at facilitating a fit, strong, and patriotic 'race' of Australians mixed with ideas about **social Darwinism** and **eugenics** that were prevalent at the time (see Powles 1988; Crotty et al. 2000). In Australia and elsewhere, public health approaches were resisted by many doctors who viewed them as unscientific and as potentially undermining the need for medical services (Porter 1997; Waitzkin 2000). Such views had some popularity given the dominant laissez-faire political philosophy of the time, which supported only minor state intervention in economic and public affairs. Nonetheless, investment in public health was made, perhaps because infectious disease knew no class barriers (that is, it was worth spending money on the poor to prevent the spread of disease to the rich).

Despite the influence of social medicine and the success of public health measures, health care would develop in an entirely different direction. The insights of social medicine would be cast aside for almost a century as the new science of **biomedicine** gained ascendancy.

SOCIAL DARWINISM
The incorrect application of Charles Darwin's theory of animal evolution to explain social inequality by transferring his idea of 'survival of the fittest' among animals to 'explain' human inequality.

EUGENICS
The study of human heredity based on the unproven assumption that selective breeding could improve the intellectual, physical, and cultural traits of a population.

BIOMEDICINE/ BIOMEDICAL MODEL
The conventional approach to medicine in Western societies, based on the diagnosis and explanation of illness as a malfunction of the body's biological mechanisms. This approach underpins most health professions and health services, which focus on treating individuals, and generally ignores the social origins of illness and its prevention.

The rise of the biomedical model

In 1878, Louis Pasteur (1822–96) developed the germ theory of disease, whereby illness was caused by germs infecting organs of the human body: a model of disease that became the foundation of modern medicine. Robert Koch (1843–1910) refined this idea via the doctrine of 'specific aetiology' (meaning specific cause of disease) through 'Koch's postulates': a set of criteria for proving that specific bacteria caused a specific disease (Dubos 1959; Capra 1982). The central idea was that specific micro-organisms caused disease by entering the human body through air, water, food, and insect bites (Porter 1997). This mono-causal model of disease, which came to be known as the medical or biomedical model, became the dominant medical paradigm by the early twentieth century. While early discoveries led to the identification of many infectious diseases, there were few effective cures, though.

One of the earliest applications of the scientific understanding of infectious disease was the promotion of hygiene and sterilisation procedures, particularly in surgical practice, to prevent infection through the transmission of bacteria (Capra 1982). Until the early twentieth century, it had been common practice to operate on patients without a concern for hygiene or the proper cleaning and sterilisation of equipment, resulting in high rates of post-operative infection and death.

The biomedical model is based on the assumption that each disease or ailment has a specific cause that physically affects the human body in a uniform and predictable way, meaning that universal 'cures' for people are theoretically possible. It involves a mechanical view of the body as a machine made up of interrelated parts, such as the skeleton and circulatory system. The role of the doctor is akin to that of a body mechanic identifying and repairing the broken parts (Capra 1982). Throughout the twentieth century, medical research, training, and practice increasingly focused on attempts to identify and eliminate specific diseases in individuals, and thus moved away from the perspective of social medicine and its focus on the social origins of disease (Najman 1980).

Before the development of medical science, quasi-religious views of health and illness were dominant, whereby illness was connected with sin, penance, and evil spirits; the body and soul were conceived as a sacred entity beyond the power of human intervention. Therefore, the 'body as machine' metaphor represented a significant turning point away from religious notions towards a secular view of the human body. The influence of scientific discoveries—particularly through autopsies that linked diseased organs with symptoms observed before death, as well as Pasteur's germ theory—eventually endorsed a belief in the separation of body and soul. In philosophical circles, this view came to be known as mind–body dualism and is sometimes referred to as **Cartesian dualism** after the philosopher René Descartes (1590–1650). Descartes, famous for the saying 'I think therefore I am', suggested that although the mind and body interacted with one another, they were separate entities. Therefore, the brain was part of the physical body whereas the mind (the basis of individuality) existed in the spiritual realm and was apparent evidence of a God-given soul. Such a distinction provided the philosophical justification for secular interventions on the physical body in the form of medical therapies. Since the body was merely a vessel for the immortal soul or spirit, medicine could rightly practise on the body while religion could focus on the soul (Capra 1982; Porter 1997). The assumption of mind–body dualism underpinned the biomedical model, whereby disease was seen as located in the physical body, and thus, the mind, or mental state of a person, was considered unimportant.

CARTESIAN DUALISM
A belief that the mind and body are separate entities, also called mind–body dualism and named after the philosopher René Descartes. This assumption underpins medical approaches that view disease in physical terms and thus ignore the psychological and subjective aspects of illness.

The limits of biomedicine

While the biomedical model represented a significant advance in understanding disease and resulted in beneficial treatments, it has come under significant criticism from both within medicine and from a range of social and behavioural disciplines such as sociology and psychology. The major criticism is that the biomedical model underestimates the complexity of health and illness, particularly by neglecting social and psychological factors (Powles 1973).

The idea of specific aetiology in fact only applies to a limited range of infectious diseases. As early as the 1950s, René Dubos (1959, p. 102) argued that 'most disease states are the indirect outcome of a constellation of circumstances rather than the direct result of single determinant factors'. Furthermore, Dubos noted that not all people exposed to an infectious disease contracted it. For example, we may all come into contact with someone suffering from a contagious condition such as the flu, but only a few of us will get sick. Therefore, disease causation is more complex than the biomedical model implies and is likely to involve multiple factors such as physical condition, nutrition, and stress, which affect an individual's susceptibility to illness (Dubos 1959).

The biomedical model, underpinned by mind–body dualism and a focus on repairing the 'broken' parts of the machine-like body, can lead to the objectification of patients. Since disease is viewed only in physical terms, as something that can be objectively observed, treating 'it' takes primacy over all other considerations, and patients may become objectified as 'diseased bodies' or 'cases', rather than treated as unique individuals with particular needs. This form of criticism often underpins claims of doctors' poor interpersonal and communication skills. Such a situation is also related to what Fritjov Capra (1982) calls 'medical scientism'; that is, a reverence for scientific methods of measurement and observation as the most superior form of knowledge about understanding and treating disease. Therefore, patients' thoughts, feelings, and subjective experiences of illness are considered 'unscientific' and are mostly dismissed.

A further criticism of biomedicine is its **reductionism**. The development of medical science has led to an increasing focus on smaller and smaller features of human biology for the cause and cure of disease—from organs to cells to molecules and most recently to genes. By reducing its focus on disease to the biological, cellular, molecular, and genetic levels, medicine has ignored or downplayed the social and psychological aspects of illness, so that the experience of disease is treated as if it occurred in a social vacuum. Not only does this marginalise the importance of social support networks, but it also ignores the role played by social factors such as poverty, poor working conditions, and discrimination in affecting an individual's physical and mental health.

REDUCTIONISM
The belief that all illnesses can be explained and treated by reducing them to biological and pathological factors.

A related outcome of reductionism has been an ever-growing number of medical specialists, such as cardiologists (heart specialists) and ophthalmologists (eye specialists), based on the assumption that each body part and function can be treated almost in isolation from the others. Such an approach has fuelled the search for 'magic bullet' cures, resulting in huge expenditure on medical drugs, technology, and surgery. It has also led to a curative and interventionist bias in medical care, often at the expense of prevention and non-medical alternatives.

Reductionism can also lead to **biological determinism**, a form of social Darwinism that assumes people's biology causes or determines their inferior social, economic, and health status. Biological determinism underpins most elitist, racist, and sexist beliefs. For example, some people argue that the poor are poor because they are born lazy and stupid. Such views have often been used to justify slavery and exploitation of blacks, women, children, and workers; it is a very convenient 'explanation', particularly when those at the top of the social ladder espouse it. When people argue that social or health inequalities are biologically determined, the implication is that little can or should be done to change them.

BIOLOGICAL DETERMINISM
An unproven belief that individual and group behaviour and social status are an inevitable result of biology.

A final criticism of the biomedical model is its tendency towards **victim-blaming** (Ryan 1971) by locating the cause and cure of disease as solely within the individual. As Capra states, '[i]nstead of asking why an illness occurs, and trying to remove the conditions that lead to it, medical researchers try to understand the biological mechanisms through which the disease operates, so that they can then interfere with them' (1982, p. 150). Therefore, the individual body becomes the focus of intervention, and health and illness become primarily viewed as individual responsibilities. A preoccupation with treating the individual has the potential to legitimate a victim-blaming approach to illness, either in the form of genetic fatalism (your poor health is the result of poor genetics) or as an outcome of poor **lifestyle choices**. By ignoring the social context of health and illness and locating primary responsibility for illness within the individual, there is little acknowledgment of social responsibility; that is, the need to ensure healthy living and working environments.

VICTIM-BLAMING
The process whereby social inequality is explained in terms of individuals being solely responsible for what happens to them in relation to the choices they make and their assumed psychological, cultural, and/or biological inferiority.

LIFESTYLE CHOICES/FACTORS
The decisions people make that are likely to impact on their health such as those relating to diet, exercise, smoking, alcohol, and other drugs. The term implies that people are solely responsible for choosing and changing their lifestyle.

The critique of the biomedical model above has necessarily been a generalisation and does not imply that all doctors work from within the confines of this model. In fact, many of the criticisms of the model have come from those within the medical profession itself. While it is now widely accepted that the causes of illness are multifactorial, it is still fair to claim that the biomedical model remains the dominant influence over medical training and practice to this day.

Rediscovering the social origins of health and illness

Thomas McKeown (1976; 1979; 1988), a doctor and epidemiologist, was one of the earliest authors to expose the exaggerated role of medical treatment in improving population health. McKeown argued that the medical profession and governments had overestimated the influence of medical discoveries on improvements in life expectancy during the twentieth century. McKeown (1976; 1979) found that mortality (death) from most infectious diseases had declined before the development of effective medical treatments, meaning that improvements in life expectancy were not substantially due to medical intervention. Similar findings have been reported in the US (McKinlay & McKinlay 1977) and Australia (Gordon 1976; Lawson 1991). Figure 1.2 provides a graphic example of this, showing the declining rate of tuberculosis for Australia—which occurred before effective medical treatment. The same trend occurred in the UK and the US in the period given. Graphs for most infectious diseases tell a similar story (aside from smallpox and polio), indicating that the contribution of medicine to population-level improvements in life expectancy appears to have been smaller than is commonly assumed.

FIGURE 1.2 DECLINE IN THE NUMBER OF TUBERCULOSIS AND TYPHOID DEATHS IN AUSTRALIA

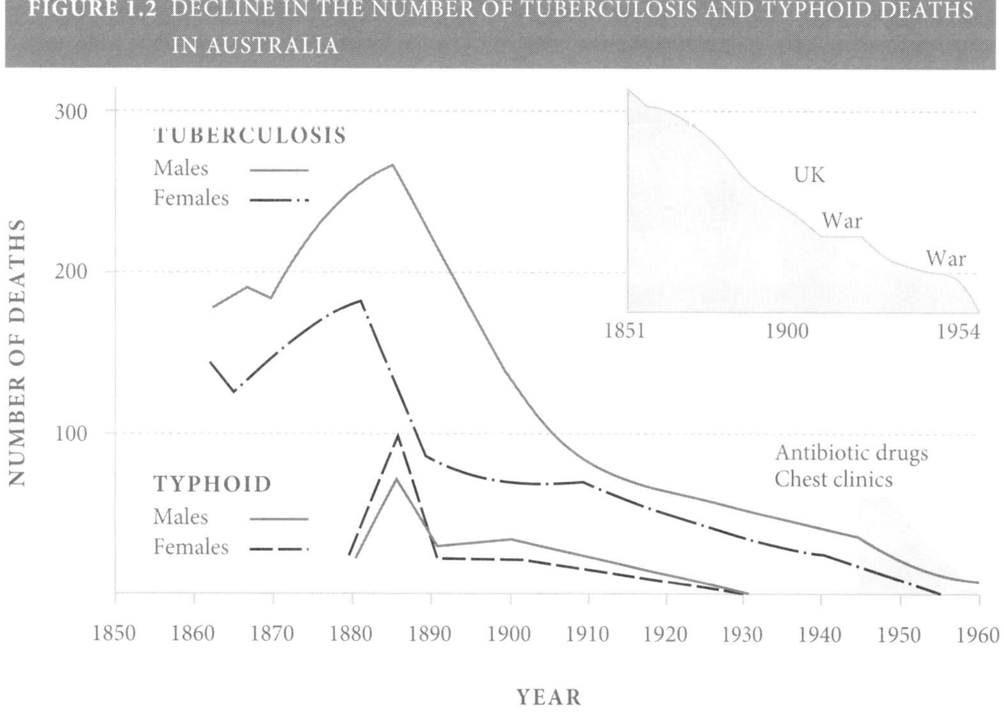

Source: Gordon 1976, after graph by H. Silverstone, Department of Social and Preventive Medicine, University of Queensland; data from O. Lancaster and colleagues

McKeown (1979) suggests that the major reason for the increase in life expectancy throughout the twentieth century was not due to medical treatments, but rather to rising living standards, particularly improved nutrition, which increased people's resistance to infectious disease. While McKeown's work highlighted the importance of social, non-medical interventions for improving population health, Simon Szreter (1988, p. 37) provides a more complex argument. He suggests that rather than the '"invisible" hand of rising living standards', it was the state's redistribution of economic resources that increased life expectancy through improved working conditions and a range of public health measures such as better public housing, food regulation, education, and sanitation reforms.

While the exact contributions of public health measures, rising living standards, and medicine to improving population health is impossible to determine, the significance of McKeown's work and subsequent findings has been to highlight the importance of addressing the social origins of health and illness. As McKeown states, 'improvement in health is likely to come ... from modification of the conditions which lead to disease, rather than from intervention in the mechanism of disease after it has occurred' (1979, p. 198).

It is important to note that McKeown himself was not anti-medicine, but wanted to reform medical practice so that it focused on prevention of what he saw were the new threats to health: 'personal behaviour', as evidenced through smoking, alcohol consumption, drug taking, poor diet, and lack of exercise. Therefore, he still viewed health care in individualistic terms, by focusing preventive efforts at the level of modifying the behaviour of individuals (see Box 1.1).

There is no denying the significant role medicine has played in the treatment of illness, particularly in trauma medicine, palliative care, and general surgery, as well as the prevention of illness through immunisation. The primary expertise of doctors lies in combating disease and attempting to treat individuals once they are ill. Yet as we have seen, this is only part of the story and has tended to obscure the social origins of health and illness.

BOX 1.1
DOING HEALTH SOCIOLOGY: FROM RISK-TAKING TO RISK-IMPOSING LIFESTYLE FACTORS

While the notion of 'lifestyle diseases' or 'diseases of affluence' is a clear indication of the social origins of illness, most disease prevention efforts have aimed to reform the individual, rather than pursue wider social reform (often ignoring the fact that diseases of affluence tend to affect the least affluent much more). By solely targeting risk-taking individuals, there has been a tendency toward victim-blaming: ignoring the social determinants that give rise to risk-taking in the first place, such as stressful work environments, the marketing efforts of corporations, and peer group pressure. As Michael Marmot (1999, p. 1) incisively puts it, there is a need to understand the 'causes of the causes'. In other words, rather than just focusing on risk-taking individuals, there is also a need to address 'risk-imposing factors' and 'illness-generating social conditions' (Waitzkin 1983; Ratcliffe et al. 1984)—the social, cultural, economic, and political features of society that create unhealthy products, habits, and lifestyles.

The World Health Organization (WHO) effectively acknowledged this limitation of biomedicine in 1946, when it included in its constitution the now-famous holistic definition of health as 'a state of complete physical, mental and social well-being and not merely the absence of disease or infirmity' (WHO 1946). This often-quoted definition implies that a range of biological, psychological, and social factors influence health. Furthermore, health is conceptualised as 'not merely the absence of disease', but rather in the positive sense of

SOCIAL MODEL OF HEALTH
Focuses on social determinants of health such as the social production, distribution, and construction of health and illness, and the social organisation of health care. It directs attention to the prevention of illness through community participation and social reforms that address living and working conditions.

'well-being'. While this definition has been criticised for its utopian and vague notion of 'complete well-being', it is of symbolic importance because it highlights the need for a broader approach to health than the biomedical model alone can deliver.

The widespread recognition of the biomedical model's limitations, from those within and outside the medical profession, has led to the development of a variety of multifactorial models, such as the biopsychosocial model (Engel 1977; 1980; Cooper et al. 1996), the web of causation model (MacMahon & Pugh 1970), and the ecological model (Hancock 1985). While these models represent a significant advance on the biomedical model in acknowledging the multiple determinants of health, to greater and lesser degrees they remain focused on health interventions aimed at the individual, particularly through lifestyle/behaviour modification and health education. What is required is an explicitly **social model of health** in order to propose effective health interventions at the population and community levels (Waitzkin 1983; Ashton & Seymour 1988; Baum 2008).

The social model of health

NEW PUBLIC HEALTH
A social model of health linking 'traditional' public health concerns about physical aspects of the environment (clean air and water, safe food, occupational safety), with concerns about the behavioural, social, and economic factors that affect people's health.

The social model of health, sometimes referred to as the **new public health** approach, focuses attention on the societal level of health determinants and health intervention. The two terms are used interchangeably by some authors, but have different disciplinary origins, with the new public health approach arising from the health sciences (particularly public health), and the social model drawn primarily from the field of health sociology. Some new public health approaches arising from the health sciences have been criticised by sociologists for an over-reliance on individualistic solutions in practice (see Lupton 1995; Petersen & Lupton 1996). Yet there are significant examples of sociologically informed approaches that can make it problematical to draw distinctions between the two terms (see especially Beaglehole & Bonita 1997; Baggott 2000; Baum 2008). A recent further development has been the promotion of an ecological public health model (see Rayner & Lang 2012), which suggests a greater need to address the complex interrelatedness of humans and their (natural and social) environment. For our purposes we will use the term 'social model of health', as it better reflects the unique theories, research methods, and modes of analysis of health sociology discussed in this book.

The social model of health has been used as a general umbrella term to refer to approaches that focus on the social determinants of health and illness (see Broom 1991; Gillespie & Gerhardt 1995). As Dorothy Broom (1991, p. 52) states: 'the social model locates people in social contexts, conceptualises the physical environment as socially organised, and understands ill health as a process of interaction between people and their environments.' It is one of the aims of this book to map out in more detail what a social model of health entails. Table 1.2 contrasts the key features of the biomedical model with the social model to highlight the different focuses, assumptions, benefits, and limitations of each. It is important to emphasise that the social model does not deny the existence of biological or psychological aspects of disease that manifest in individuals, or deny the need for medical treatment. Instead, it highlights that health and illness occur in a social context and that effective health interventions, particularly preventive efforts, need to move beyond the medical treatment of individuals. In exposing the social origins of illness, it necessarily implies that a greater balance between individual and social interventions is required, since the vast majority of health funding continues to be directed towards medical intervention. Therefore, the social model is not intended as a replacement for the biomedical model, but rather coexists alongside it.

The social model assumes that health is a social responsibility by examining the social determinants of individuals' health status and health-related behaviour. While the biomedical model concentrates on treating disease and risk-taking among individuals, the social model focuses on societal factors that are risk-imposing or illness-inducing (for example, toxic pollution, stressful work, discrimination, and peer pressure), and in particular highlights the health inequalities suffered by different social groups based on class, gender, ethnicity, and occupation, to name a few. What should be clear from the comparison offered in Table 1.2 is that health issues have a number of dimensions.

TABLE 1.2 A COMPARISON OF BIOMEDICAL AND SOCIAL MODELS OF HEALTH: KEY CHARACTERISTICS

	BIOMEDICAL MODEL	SOCIAL MODEL
Focus	• Individual focus: acute treatment of ill individuals • Clinical services, health education, immunisation	• Societal focus: living and working conditions that affect health • Public health infrastructure and legislation, social services, community action, equity/access issues
Assumptions	• Health and illness are objective biological states • Individual responsibility for health	• Health and illness are social constructions • Social responsibility for health
Key indicators of illness	• Individual pathology • Hereditary factors, sex, age • Risk-taking factors	• Social inequality • Social groups: class, gender, 'race', ethnicity, age, occupation, unemployment • Risk-imposing factors
Causes of illness	• Gene defects and micro-organisms (viruses, bacteria) • Trauma (accidents) • Behaviour/lifestyle	• Political/economic factors: distribution of wealth/income/power, poverty, level of social services • Employment factors: employment and educational opportunities, stressful and dangerous work • Cultural and structural factors
Intervention	• Cure individuals via surgery and pharmaceuticals • Behaviour modification (non-smoking, exercise, diet) • Health education and immunisation	• Public policy • State intervention to alleviate health and social inequalities • Community participation, advocacy, and political lobbying
Goals	• Cure disease, limit disability, and reduce risk factors to prevent disease in individuals	• Prevent illness and reduce health inequalities to aim for an equality of health outcomes
Benefits	• Addresses disease and disability of individuals	• Addresses the social determinants of health and illness
Criticisms	• Disease focus leads to lack of preventive efforts • Reductionist: ignores the complexity of health and illness • Fails to take into account social origins of health and illness • Medical opinions can reinforce victim-blaming	• Utopian goal of equality leads to unfeasible prescriptions for social change • Overemphasis on the harmful side effects of biomedicine • Proposed solutions can be complex and difficult to implement in the short-term • Sociological opinions can underestimate individual responsibility and psychological factors

The social model logically implies that any attempts to improve the overall health of the community need to address overall living and working conditions such as poverty, employment opportunities, workplace health and safety, and cultural differences. The social model gives equal priority to the prevention of illness along with the treatment of illness, and aims to alleviate health inequalities. Such issues necessitate community participation and state interventions—including social services and public policies (such as workplace safety and pollution controls)—which lie outside the strict confines of the health system or individuals' control. It must be acknowledged that this makes the interventions proposed by advocates of the social model more complex and difficult to achieve, given their broad thrust, long-term implications, and need for intersectoral collaboration.

THE THREE MAIN DIMENSIONS OF THE SOCIAL MODEL OF HEALTH

The social model arose as a critique of the limitations and misapplications of the biomedical model. Sociological research and theorising, which underpins the social model of health, have comprised three main dimensions that are reflected in the structure of this book:

1 *The social production and distribution of health and illness* highlights that many illnesses are socially produced. For example, illnesses arising from exposure to hazardous work practices are often beyond an individual's control and therefore need to be addressed at a societal level, such as through occupational health and safety legislation. Furthermore, there is an unequal social distribution of health, whereby some social groups suffer higher rates of morbidity and mortality. Therefore, a focus on the social production and distribution of health examines the role that living and working conditions can play in causing and alleviating illness.
2 *The social construction of health and illness* refers to how definitions of health and illness can vary between cultures and change over time—what is considered a disease in one culture or time period may be considered normal and healthy elsewhere and at other times. For example, homosexuality was once considered a psychiatric disorder despite the lack of scientific evidence of pathology. It is no longer medically defined as a disorder. This is an example of how cultural beliefs, social practices, and social institutions shape, or construct, the ways in which health and illness are understood. Notions of health and illness are not necessarily objective facts, but can be **social constructions** that reflect the culture, politics, and morality of a particular society at a given point in time.
3 *The social organisation of health care* concerns the way a particular society organises, funds, and utilises its health services. A central focus of study has been the dominant role of the medical profession, which has significantly shaped health policy and health funding to benefit its own interests, largely to the detriment of preventive approaches and nursing, allied, and alternative health practitioners. Unequal relationships between the health professions can prevent the efficient use of health resources and the optimal delivery of health care to patients.

SOCIAL CONSTRUCTION/ CONSTRUCTIONISM: The socially created characteristics of human life, based on the idea that people actively construct reality, meaning it is neither 'natural' nor inevitable. Therefore, notions of normality/abnormality, right/wrong, and health/illness are subjective human creations that should not be taken for granted.

Conclusion

> Question: What do you get when you cross a sociologist with a member of the Mafia?
> Answer: An offer you can't understand.
>
> (GIDDENS 1996, p. 1)

A common accusation made of sociology is that it is just common sense dressed up in unnecessary jargon. The subject matter of sociology is familiar, and as members of society it is easy to think we should all be experts on the subject. This familiarity can breed suspicion and sometimes contempt. All disciplines have specialist concepts to help classify their subject matter and sociology is no different. Sociological concepts, such as those you have been introduced to in this chapter, are used to impose a sense of intellectual order on the complexities of social life; they are a form of academic shorthand to summarise a complex idea in a word or phrase.

As this chapter has shown, to understand the complexity of health and illness we need to move beyond biomedical approaches and incorporate a social model of health. Sociology enables us to understand the links between our individual experiences and the social context in which we live, work, and play. With a sociological imagination, seeing health problems as social issues can be a healthy way of opening up debate on a range of topics previously unimagined.

SUMMARY OF MAIN POINTS

- Much of health sociology has arisen as a critique of the dominance of the medical profession and its biomedical model.
- Health sociology examines social patterns of health and illness, particularly various forms of health inequality, and seeks to explain them by examining the influence of society. When groups of people experience similar health problems, there are likely to be social origins that require social action to address them.
- The sociological imagination, or sociological analysis, involves four interrelated features—historical, cultural, structural, and critical—which can be applied to understand health problems as social issues.
- Health sociology challenges individualistic and biological explanations of health and illness through a social model of health that involves three key dimensions: the social production and distribution of health, the social construction of health, and the social organisation of health care.

SOCIOLOGICAL REFLECTION

A SOCIOLOGICAL AUTOBIOGRAPHY

Apply the four parts of the sociological imagination template to explain the person you have become. In other words, write a short sociological autobiography by briefly noting the various things that have influenced you directly or indirectly in terms of your beliefs, interests, and behaviour.

- Historical factors: how has your family background or key past events and experiences shaped the person you are?
- Cultural factors: what role have cultural background, traditions, and belief systems played in forming your opinions and influencing your behaviour?
- Structural factors: how have various social institutions influenced you?
- Critical factors: have your values and opinions about what you consider important changed over time? Why or why not?

Complete another sociological reflection, this time applying the sociological imagination template to a health problem of interest to you. Briefly note any key points that come to mind under the four parts of the template. What insights can you derive by adopting a sociological imagination?

DISCUSSION QUESTIONS

1 How can illness have social origins? Give examples in your answer.
2 What are the advantages and limitations of the biomedical model?
3 What have been some of the consequences of the dominance of biomedical explanations for our understanding of health and illness?
4 Why did the insights of social medicine/public health approaches have such a limited influence over the development of modern medicine?
5 What are the three key dimensions of the social model of health? Provide examples of each in your answer. What are the advantages and limitations of the model?
6 In 1946, the World Health Organization defined health as 'a state of complete physical, mental and social well-being and not merely the absence of disease or infirmity'. Why might some groups regard this definition as 'radical' and utopian? Who might these groups consist of? What do you think of the definition?

FURTHER INVESTIGATION

1 The influence of the biomedical model is waning—the future belongs to public health. Discuss.
2 Illness is simply a matter of bad luck, bad judgment, or bad genetics. Critically analyse this statement by applying a sociological imagination to explore the social origins of illness.

FURTHER READING

Australian Institute of Health and Welfare (AIHW) 2012, *Australia's Health 2012*, AIHW, Canberra: <www.aihw.gov.au/publication-detail/?id=10737422172>.

Blaxter, M. 2010, *Health*, 2nd edn, Polity Press, Cambridge.

Cockerman, W.C. 2013, *Social Causes of Health and Disease*, 2nd edn, Polity Press, Cambridge.

Gabe, J. & Monaghan, L. 2013, *Key Concepts in Medical Sociology*, 2nd edn, Sage, London.

Nettleton, S. 2013, *The Sociology of Health and Illness*, 3rd edn, Polity Press, Cambridge.

Rayner, G. & Lang, T. 2012, *Ecological Public Health: Reshaping the Conditions for Good Health*, Routledge, Oxford.

Sointu, E. 2012, *Theorizing Complementary and Alternative Medicines: Wellbeing, Self, Gender*, Palgrave Macmillan, Houndmills.

Willis, E. 2011, *The Sociological Quest: An Introduction to the Study of Social Life*, 5th edn, Allen & Unwin, Sydney.

Wright, K. 2011, *The Rise of the Therapeutic Society: Psychological Knowledge & the Contradictions of Cultural Change*, New Academia Publishing, Washington, DC.

WEB RESOURCES

American Sociological Association: Medical Sociology: <www2.asanet.org/medicalsociology>.

Australian Institute of Health and Welfare (AIHW): <www.aihw.gov.au>.

British Sociological Association: Medical Sociology (MedSoc) Study Group: < www.britsoc.co.uk/medsoc>.

Public Health Association of Australia (PHAA): <www.phaa.net.au>.

World Health Organization (WHO): Social Determinants of Health: <www.who.int/social_determinants/en>.

DOCUMENTARIES/FILMS

The Trouble with Medicine (1993): Six 55-minute episodes

A documentary series dealing with various challenges and limitations relating to biomedicine. ABC TV, BBC TV & Thirteen-WNET.

REFERENCES

Ashton, J. & Seymour, H. 1988, *The New Public Health: The Liverpool Experience*, Open University Press, Milton Keynes.

Australian Institute of Health and Welfare (AIHW) 2010, *Australia's Health 2010*, AIHW, Canberra.

Australian Institute of Health and Welfare (AIHW) 2012, *Australia's Health 2012*, AIHW, Canberra: <www.aihw.gov.au/publication-detail/?id=10737422172>.

Baggott, R. 2000, *Public Health: Policy and Politics*, Palgrave, Basingstoke.

Baum, F. 2008, *The New Public Health*, 3rd edn, Oxford University Press, Melbourne.

Beaglehole, R. & Bonita, R. 1997, *Public Health at the Crossroads*, Cambridge University Press, Cambridge.

Berger, P.L. 1966, *Invitation to Sociology: A Humanistic Perspective*, Penguin, Harmondsworth.

Bloom, S. 2002, *The Word as Scalpel: A History of Medical Sociology*, Oxford University Press, New York.

Broom, D. 1991, *Damned if We Do: Contradictions in Women's Health Care*, Allen & Unwin, Sydney.

Capra, F. 1982, *The Turning Point: Science, Society and the Rising Culture*, Simon & Schuster, New York.

Cooper, N., Stevenson, C. & Hale, G. (eds) 1996, *Integrating Perspectives on Health*, Open University Press, Buckingham.

Crotty, M., Germov, J. & Rodwell, G. (eds) 2000, '"A race for a place": eugenics, Darwinism and social thought and practice in Australia', *Proceedings of the History & Sociology of Eugenics Conference*, University of Newcastle, 27–28 April, Faculty of Arts and Social Science, University of Newcastle, Newcastle.

Dubos, R. 1959, *Mirage of Health: Utopias, Progress, and Biological Change*, Harper & Row, New York.

Durkheim, E. 1897/1951, *Suicide: A Study in Sociology*, Free Press, Glencoe.

Engel, G.L. 1977, 'The need for a new medical model: a challenge for biomedicine', *Science*, vol. 196, no. 4286, pp. 129–36.

Engel, G.L. 1980, 'The clinical application of the biopsychosocial model', *American Journal of Psychiatry*, vol. 137, no. 5, pp. 535–44.

Engels, F. 1845/1958, *The Condition of the Working Class in England*, trans. W.O. Henderson & W.H. Chaloner, Basil Blackwell, Oxford.

Giddens, A. 1986, *Sociology: A Brief but Critical Introduction*, 2nd edn, Macmillan, London.

Giddens, A. 1996, *In Defence of Sociology: Essays, Interpretations and Rejoinders*, Polity Press, Cambridge.

Gillespie, R. & Gerhardt, C. 1995, 'Social dimensions of sickness and disability', in G. Moon & R. Gillespie (eds), *Society and Health: An Introduction to Social Science for Health Professionals*, Routledge, London, pp. 79–94.

Gordon, D. 1976, *Health, Sickness and Society: Theoretical Concepts in Social and Preventive Medicine*, University of Queensland Press, Brisbane.

Guérin, J. 1848, 'Medicine sociale', *Gazette Medicale de Paris*, No. 11, 11 de mars.

Hancock, T. 1985, 'The mandala of health: a model of the human ecosystem', *Family and Community Health*, November, vol. 8, no. 1, pp. 1–10.

Lawson, J.S. 1991, *Public Health Australia: An Introduction*, McGraw-Hill, Sydney.

Lawson, J.S. & Bauman, A.E. 2001, *Public Health Australia: An Introduction*, McGraw-Hill, Sydney.

López, J. & Scott, J. 2000, *Social Structure*, Open University Press, Buckingham.

Lupton, D. 1995, *The Imperative of Health: Public Health and the Regulated Body*, Sage, London.

MacMahon, B. & Pugh, T.F. 1970, *Epidemiological Principles and Methods*, Little Brown, Boston.

Marmot, M.G. 1999, 'Introduction', in M. Marmot & R.G. Wilkinson (eds), *Social Determinants of Health*, Oxford University Press, Oxford.

McKeown, T. 1976, *The Role of Medicine: Dream, Mirage or Nemesis?*, Nuffield Hospital Trust, London.

McKeown, T. 1979, *The Role of Medicine: Dream, Mirage or Nemesis?*, 2nd edn, Basil Blackwell, Oxford.

McKeown, T. 1988, *The Origins of Human Disease*, Basil Blackwell, Oxford.

McKinlay, J.B. & McKinlay, S.M. 1977, 'The questionable effect of medical measures on the decline of mortality in the United States in the twentieth century', *Milbank Memorial Fund Quarterly*, vol. 55, no. 3, pp. 405–28.

McLeod, K.S. 2000, 'Our sense of Snow: the myth of John Snow in medical geography', *Social Science & Medicine*, vol. 50, no. 7, pp. 923–35.

Mills, C.W. 1959, *The Sociological Imagination*, Oxford University Press, New York.

Najman, J. 1980, 'Theories of disease causation and the concept of general susceptibility: a review', *Social Science & Medicine*, vol. 14A, no. 3, pp. 231–7.

OECD 2013, 'Life expectancy at birth', in *OECD Factbook 2013*, OECD Publishing, Paris: <www.oecd-ilibrary.org/economics/oecd-factbook-2013/life-expectancy-at-birth_factbook-2013-table244-en>.

Petersen, A. & Lupton, D. 1996, *The New Public Health: Health and Self in the Age of Risk*, Allen & Unwin, Sydney, and Sage, London.

Porter, R. 1997, *The Greatest Benefit to Mankind: A Medical History of Humanity from Antiquity to the Present*, HarperCollins, London.

Powles, J. 1973, 'On the limitation of modern medicine', *Science, Medicine and Man*, vol. 1, no. 1, pp. 1–30.

Powles, J. 1988, 'Professional hygienists and the health of a nation', in R. MacLeod (ed.), *The Commonwealth of Science: ANZAAS and the Scientific Enterprise in Australasia 1888–1988*, Oxford University Press, Melbourne, pp. 292–307.

Ratcliffe, J., Wallack, L., Fagnani, F. & Rodwin, V. 1984, 'Perspectives on prevention: health promotion vs health protection', in J. de Kervasdoue, J.R. Kimberley & G. Rodwin (eds), *The End of an Illusion: The Future of Health Policy in Western Industrialized Nations*, University of California Press, Berkeley, CA, pp. 56–84.

Rayner, G. & Lang, T. 2012, *Ecological Public Health: Reshaping the Conditions for Good Health*, Routledge, Oxford.

Reynolds, C. 1995, *Public Health Law in Australia*, Federation Press, Leichhardt.

Rosen, G. 1972, 'The evolution of social medicine', in H.E. Freeman, S. Levine & L.G. Reeder (eds), *Handbook of Medical Sociology*, 2nd edn, Prentice Hall, Englewood Cliffs, NJ, pp. 30–60.

Rosen, G. 1993, *A History of Public Health*, Johns Hopkins University Press, New York.

Ryan, W. 1971, *Blaming the Victim*, Vintage, New York.

Snow, J. 1855/1936, *On the Mode of Communication of Cholera* [reprinted as *Snow on Cholera*], Hafner, New York.

Statistics New Zealand 2013, *New Zealand Period Life Tables: 2010–12*: <www.stats.govt.nz/browse_for_stats/health/life_expectancy/NZLifeTables_HOTP10-12.aspx>.

Szreter S. 1988, 'The importance of social intervention in Britain's mortality decline c. 1850–1914: a re-interpretation of the role of public health', *Society for the Social History of Medicine*, vol. 1, no. 1, pp. 1–37.

United Nations Development Programme (UNDP) 2013, *Human Development Report 2012: The Rise of the South: Human Progress in a Diverse World*, UNDP, New York.

Waitzkin, H. 1983, *The Second Sickness: Contradictions of Capitalist Health Care*, Free Press, New York.

Waitzkin, H. 2000, *The Second Sickness: Contradictions of Capitalist Health Care*, 2nd edn, Rowman & Littlefield, Lanham.

White, K. (ed.) 2001, *The Early Sociology of Health and Illness*, 6 vols, Routledge, London.

World Health Organization (WHO) 1946, *Constitution of the World Health Organization*, WHO, Geneva.

Willis, E. 1993, *The Sociological Quest: An Introduction to the Study of Social Life*, Allen & Unwin, Sydney.

Willis, E. 2011, *The Sociological Quest: An Introduction to the Study of Social Life*, 5th edn, Allen & Unwin, Sydney.

READING 3

Health as a social construct

Claire Henderson-Wilson

TOPICS COVERED

This chapter covers the following topics:

- social and cultural constructions of health, illness, and well-being
- social model of health
- health sociology
- social skeleton: health, illness, and structure agency model
- ecological models
- social ecological model

KEY TERMS

Biomedical model of health
Gender
Health sociology
Social class
Social construction of health
Social ecological model
Social model of health
Social Skeleton: health, illness and structure agency model

Introduction

> The concept of health is...complex and dynamic. Its meanings are embedded in the unique individual, family, social and cultural contexts in which the term is used; as such, it is said to be socially and culturally *constructed*. (Taylor 2008a, p. 5)

Social construction of health Refers to a range of social forces that combine to create and modify the experience of health, such as social groups, social institutions, and the wider culture.

As Taylor (2008a) suggests, different people ascribe different meanings to health, so for some people 'health' may mean being free from disease and for others it may mean maintaining balance between the mind, body, and spirit. This is referred to as the **social construction of health** as it involves a range of social forces (i.e. social groups, social institutions, and the wider culture) that combine to create and modify the experience of health (Brown 1995). Constructions of 'health', 'illness', and 'well-being' have moved beyond traditional biomedical interpretations that focused on an individual's medically defined pathology (Keleher & MacDougall 2009) to an awareness of how they are influenced by social and cultural contexts and determinants.

The first section of this chapter will define and discuss the social model of health, using relevant examples; it will explore how valuable this model is for understanding the social construction of health, illness, and well-being. The next section will discuss how health sociology can aid an understanding of health, illness, and well-being. Drawing on Germov's (2005) Social skeleton: Health, illness and structure agency model, the chapter will explore how social groups, social institutions, and the wider culture influence perceptions of health, illness, and well-being. Finally, it will discuss how ecological models can be used to explore social constructions of health, illness, and well-being, using Bronfenbrenner's social ecology model.

Social model of health

> The social model locates people in social contexts and conceptualises the physical environment as socially organised, and understands ill health as a process of interaction between people and environments. (Broom 1991, p. 52)

Biomedical model of health Suggests that illness results from a malfunction of the body (i.e. germs or disease) and that each disease affects the body in a predictable way.

Social model of health Suggests that health is influenced by a dynamic set of social structures and aims to identify the factors within a society that inhibit the health of individuals.

For much of the 20th century, the 'biomedical model' dominated understanding of health, illness, and well-being. This model suggests that illness results from a malfunction of the body (i.e. germs or disease) and that each disease affects the body in a predictable way (Germov 2009). However, the quote from Broom above indicates that illness is much more than just a 'mono-causal model of disease' (Germov 2009, p. 10), and this is the main focus of this chapter, which will demonstrate how our constructs of health, illness, and well-being are shaped by social and cultural context.

By moving beyond the limitations of the **biomedical model of health**, which draws on biochemical explanations of health and illness, the **social model of health** can be useful in understanding how perceptions of health, illness, and well-being comprise a dynamic interaction of social structures (Germov 2005; Yuill 2010). The social model aims to identify the factors within a society that inhibit the health of individuals (Moon & Gillespie 1995). It acknowledges that infectious pathogens can affect health, but the focus is more on how these pathogens are not distributed randomly or shared equally among the population (Broom 1991). Therefore, the social model of health aims to address health inequities by directing attention towards the prevention of illness via social reforms that concentrate on living conditions (Jirojwong & Liamputtong 2009). Essentially, 'the social model gives equal priority to the prevention of illness along with the treatment of illness and aims to alleviate health inequalities' (Germov 2005, p. 17).

According to Yuill (2010), there are six key features of the social model of health:

1. Individual health is enabled or inhibited by social context.
2. The body is simultaneously social, psychological, and biological.
3. Health is cultural.
4. Biomedicine and medical science is something—but not everything.
5. Health is political.
6. Other voices matter.

Consideration of these features allows the social model of health to provide deeper understanding of health, illness, and well-being.

In terms of the first feature, perceptions of health and illness are often thought to be based on personal choices. For example, someone may choose to smoke cigarettes or eat foods high in saturated fat. Yuill (2010) contends that while personal choices can influence health, it is vital to consider the social context in which people find themselves and how this affects their ability to exercise control over their health. This is supported by Wilkinson and Marmot (2003), who argue that people who have more control over their lives tend to be healthier than those who do not. They cite examples of people who experience stress and a lack of control over their home and work life (i.e. social contexts) and how this can lead to poor mental and physical health and eventually premature death.

Second, Yuill (2010) proposes that bodies are made up of more than just biology and anatomy; they are based on relationships involving social, cultural, psychological, biological, and individual processes. For example, one of these processes concerns identity, whereby people develop a sense of identity through their pursuit of a certain body shape. When people experience chronic illness, their self-identity may be challenged or questioned. Martin and Peterson (2010, p. 580) support this contention and propose that when people experience illness, 'this implies a threat to the individual's inner and social being by the biological component of their own body'.

The third feature proposed by Yuill (2010) suggests that perceptions and assumptions of health and illness vary by culture. In Western cultures, people tend to see slenderness as equating to healthiness, particularly for women, whereas in other cultures larger women are seen as healthy (Parson 1990). Additionally, Blaxter (2004) points out that in countries like China, India, and some African nations, herbal therapies are often prescribed to people experiencing illness along with Western biomedical treatments. Furthermore, Germov (2005) states that Vietnamese people believe that emotional and physical illnesses are a result of the imbalance in the forces of *am* and *duong* (commonly translated as hot and cold). From these examples, it is clear that culture influences how people construct and perceive health and illness.

The fourth feature of the social model of health acknowledges that the biomedical model has merits that should not be ignored by social scientists. Germov (2005) agrees with this argument and states that the social model does not deny the requirement for medical intervention, and therefore it coexists with the biomedical model. Thus, the biomedical model focuses on treating

Stop and Think

» What social and cultural factors influence how you perceive health, illness, and well-being?

» How much influence do you think social contexts have on your health status?

illnesses with medical intervention but the social model focuses on social contexts that bring about illnesses in populations (i.e. social exclusion, bullying, and exposure to environmental pollution).

The fifth feature described by Yuill (2010, p. 13) proposes that 'health is not separate from other spheres of society'. In other words, an individual's health is influenced by the provision of health services and resources. This is supported by Perry and colleagues (2010), who conducted a study to examine the use and availability of health services by young people with type 1 diabetes by comparing those living in regional New South Wales with those using city and state capital services. They found that regional services had fewer resources and limited access to specialists compared to city and state capital services. The authors concluded that health service redistribution is required to ensure equity of access to services and resources for young people with type 1 diabetes living in regional Australia.

Last, Yuill (2010) proposes that in understanding perceptions of health and illness, the social model considers viewpoints beyond the medical profession. It can draw on the knowledge and perspectives of lay people, including those experiencing illness. For example, often people with chronic illness are believed to experience social constructions of illness that are considered more relevant and important than healthcare professionals' interpretations (Martin & Peterson 2010; Yuill 2010). By shifting the focus away from a healthcare/biomedical model towards the social model, understandings of health and illness can be viewed within a framework of individuals and society (Habibis 2009).

In summary, the social model allows for a comprehensive understanding of health, illness, and well-being by exploring the range of influential social and cultural contexts within an individual's environment. Some policy and practice responses to the social model of health in the Australian context will now be briefly discussed.

Social model of health: Policy and practice responses

The biomedical model is considered to dominate healthcare practice in many countries, including Australia, but over time it has become more inclusive of the range of social and cultural contexts influencing health and illness (Taylor 2008a). As Taylor writes: 'Public health proponents, for example, have questioned the effectiveness of biomedicine in improving the overall health of the Australian population and socially disadvantaged groups' (p. 28). This has resulted in a move towards adoption of a social model of healthcare, with a range of social and economic determinants being addressed at the level of health policy (Taylor 2008a). For example, the Victorian Department of Health (2010) recently published *Using policy to promote mental health and well-being: An introduction for policy makers*, which is a guide aimed at enabling policymakers in Victoria to consider, when developing or reviewing policy or programs, the range of social and environmental determinants of mental health. Additionally, many local governments within Victoria prepare Integrated Health Promotion Plans that place emphasis on addressing the social, economic, and cultural determinants impacting on the health, illness, and well-being of their communities.

In addition to the social model of health being recognised at a health policy level, it is also acknowledged by many health service providers. For example, Women's Health West (WHW) is the regional women's health service for the western metropolitan region of Victoria. This organisation provides a range of health services including health promotion, community development, research, training, and advocacy around women's health, safety, and well-being (Women's Health West 2008). WHW recognises that women's lives are shaped by political, economic, cultural, and social forces and 'as a result, WHW places great importance on identifying the structural factors that impact on women's health and well-being' (p. 2).

The shift from a biomedical to a social model of health has clearly been adopted by many health policy and healthcare providers within Australia, so it is worth considering how 'health sociology' has evolved to provide a perspective for understanding how health is socially constructed.

Health sociology

> Health sociology...provides a second opinion to the conventional medical view of illness derived from biological and psychological explanations, by exploring the social context of health and illness—the social, economic, cultural and political features of society that influence why some groups of people get sicker and die sooner than others. (Germov 2005, p. 5)

As the above quote suggests, '**health sociology**' encompasses multidimensional ways of thinking about social worlds and recognises that while illnesses are experienced by individuals, they are also influenced by a range of social determinants (Earle & Letherby 2008; Germov 2009). Aligned with the social model of health, health sociology is not necessarily focused on the individual but rather the social group to which they belong (Willis & Elmer 2007; White 2009; Weitz 2010).

Health sociology
A discipline that recognises that health and illness are influenced by a range of social determinants and focuses on the social patterns of health and illness.

Health sociology came to fruition during the 1970s and 1980s when many sociologists working in the area of health and illness began to question the biomedical model of health (Germov 2009; White 2009). They felt that only considering that people become ill because of the incursion of a germ overlooked the fact that living in social groups may also influence why people become ill (White 2009).

White (2009) asserts that when confronted by someone who is ill, sociologists do not think about why that person is ill but rather, what are the characteristics of the group to which they belong that leaves them at risk of becoming ill. Germov (2009, p. 4) agrees with White and states that 'health sociology focuses on the social patterns of health and illness, such as the different health statuses between women and men, the poor and the wealthy, or the Indigenous and non-Indigenous populations, and seeks social, rather than biological or psychological, explanations'. Some relevant examples will now be described to demonstrate how health sociology can inform understandings of health, illness, and well-being.

Life expectancy

Life expectancy is significantly higher in developed and wealthy countries than in developing and poorer countries (Baum 2008; Germov 2009). Baum (2008) suggests that people in poor countries tend to earn lower incomes, are less likely to be educated, and have limited access to safe drinking water and sanitary conditions. Australia has a high life expectancy compared to other countries, with data indicating that a boy born during 2007–09 can expect to live 79.3 years, while a girl can expect to live 83.9 years (ABS 2009a). This long life expectancy could be attributed to the living and working conditions of Australia, such as access to a clean water supply, efficient sewage system, education, and employment. However, not all Australians experience long life expectancy, with data indicating that there is a gap in life expectancy for Indigenous Australians compared to non-Indigenous Australians: 12 years for males and 10 years for females (AIHW 2010a). This gap could be due to a range of social and cultural factors such as lower socio-economic status, unemployment, or lack of access to culturally appropriate health services (Baum 2008; Germov 2009).

Gender

Gender Socially and culturally constructed categories reflecting what it means to be 'masculine' and 'feminine' and associated expectations of roles and behaviours of men and women.

Gender is considered a vital element in the social construction of health, illness, and well-being, as it shapes exposure to health problems, accounts for differences in health-related behaviours, and influences how illness is experienced (Waldron 2005; Broom 2009). White (2009) suggests that women live longer than men (as indicated by the life expectancy example given previously), but they are also diagnosed with illness more than men. Several reasons account for why women experience illness more than men, such as complications related to reproduction, their social roles (working longer hours, being paid less, having a work/life imbalance), and the fact that they are reported to consult health practitioners more often than men (Broom 2009; White 2009). Temple-Smith and colleagues (2007) conducted a study, in Australia, to determine if there are any gender differences in seeking care for hepatitis C. They found that women were more likely than men to consult a general practitioner (GP) specifically for hepatitis C virus (HCV) related symptoms, consistent with previous research. However, they also found that women would seek the advice of a GP even when they had not experienced any HCV symptoms, suggesting that gender influences the health-seeking behaviours of individuals (Temple-Smith et al. 2007). Gender roles have also been found to influence rates of illness and mortality. Waldron (2005) argues that in some South Asian countries, boys receive better healthcare than girls, which contributes to a lower mortality rate for boys. This is largely due to a cultural preference for sons, which results in discrimination against girls in accessing healthcare and health-promoting resources (Reidpath 2004; Waldron 2005).

Income inequality

Social class The position of a person in a system of structured inequality; it is grounded in unequal distribution of income, wealth, status, and power.

Income inequality is reported to be one of the key indicators of **social class** inequality within populations (Germov 2009). Essentially, income inequality is the unequal distribution of income within a society, or in other words, the contrast between 'rich' and 'poor' (or high and low socio-economic status) (Atkinson & Leigh 2006). Societies with more equal income distributions have better health, but the unequal distribution of wealth within countries is believed to be increasing worldwide, and this may result in a range of health inequities (Wilkinson & Pickett 2006; Baum 2008). Cross-national research shows that the greater the degree of socio-economic inequality within a society, the steeper the gradient of health inequalities (Schrader 2004). The fact that class differences in health are smaller in Sweden than the UK and the USA has been attributed to Sweden's more even distribution of income (Schrader 2004). It is important to note that 'income distribution is related to health where it serves as a measure of the scale of social class differences in a society' (Wilkinson & Pickett 2006, p. 14). Wilkinson (1997a) has argued that income inequality in areas that are considered small has been influenced by the degree of residential separation of rich and poor people and that the health of people in disadvantaged neighbourhoods is poorer not because of the level of inequality within their neighbourhoods, but because they are perceived to be disadvantaged in relation to the wider society.

In summary, these examples demonstrate how social patterns of health and illness can be understood from a health sociological perspective. How the Social Skeleton model (Germov 2005) can be applied to understanding health, illness, and well-being will now be discussed.

Social Skeleton: Health, illness and structure-agency

Germov's (2005) **Social Skeleton: health, illness and structure agency model** (see Figure 12.1) represents the social structures individuals are part of and demonstrates how social groups, social institutions, and the wider culture influence perceptions of health, illness, and well-being. Germov (2005) contends that social structures are like the human skeleton; the various body parts (heart, lungs, muscles) need the skeletal frame to function and survive. Social structures include cultural customs and health, government, and education institutions that people experience in their lives and that influence their social interactions (Germov 2005).

Social Skeleton: health, illness and structure agency model Represents the social structures individuals are part of and demonstrates how social groups, social institutions, and the wider culture influence perceptions of health, illness, and well-being.

The model allows us to see how our society is structured and to appreciate that the various components of the social skeleton are interconnected (refer to the two-way arrows). Germov (2005) suggests that a society's economy can influence its political system and culture. He also suggests that religion, via marriage and family, has influenced how personal relationships are structured.

Social institutions such as healthcare services, housing, education, welfare provision, and mass media are defined as 'formal structures within society that are set up to address identified social needs' (Germov 2005, p. 19). These social institutions are said to influence the formation of social groups. For example, different socio-economic classes evolve from the economic institutions in a society, and cultural attitudes and laws influence gender-based social roles (Germov 2005). Additionally, other social relationships can develop, for example, between patients and doctors, students and teachers, and employees and employers.

Another important component of the model is that of the 'structure/agency debate'. Germov (2005, 2009) suggests that this is a key debate in sociology that asks us to determine how much influence we have over our lives and whether we can blame society for some of the actions we take. It also suggests that we perceive structure and agency as interrelated and consider to what extent we shape society and simultaneously are shaped by society. In other words, 'structure and

Figure 12.1 Social Skeleton: Health, illness and structure agency model

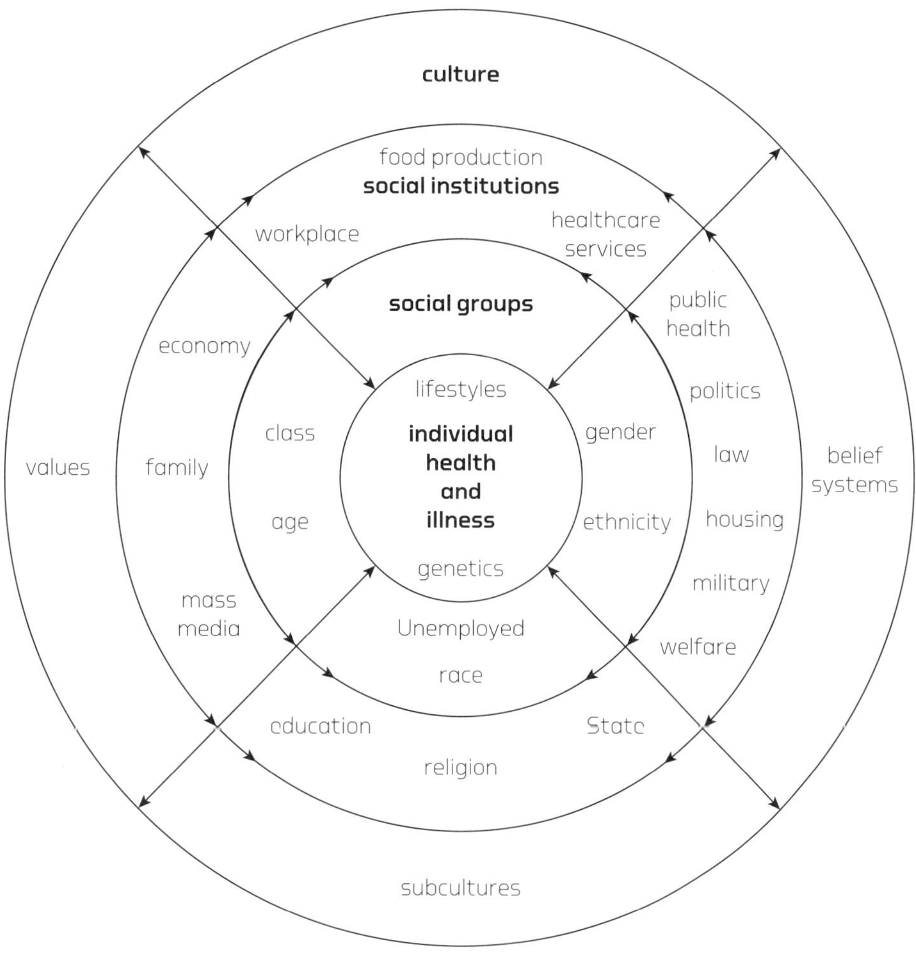

Source: Germov 2005, p. 19

Case Study 12.1 Social Skeleton: Health, illness and structure agency model

The following hypothetical example is provided to briefly demonstrate how key social structures, as represented in the Social Skeleton model, influence an individual's perceptions of health, illness, and well-being.

Katie is an 18-year-old university student living in an outer suburb of Melbourne. She is Anglo-Saxon and of a high socio-economic status. Belonging to these social groups, combined with her lifestyle, influences her perception of health. Katie considers herself to be a very healthy young woman as she consumes a balanced diet, exercises daily, does not smoke cigarettes or drink alcohol, and maintains positive relationships with friends and family members. Although Katie is responsible for controlling her health and lifestyle, a number of social institutions can be said to influence her life. The social relationships Katie shares with her parents would be considered to influence her perceptions of health and illness. For instance, Katie's dad Barry has always been a regular marathon runner and instilled the importance of regular exercise in his daughter from a young age. This no doubt has influenced how Katie perceives health but so too have the mass media. Often, television shows and magazines portray slenderness as equating to healthiness; this could be influencing Katie's perceptions of health. Furthermore, cultural attitudes towards women being seen as healthy if they are slender dominate Katie's society, including via the mass media, and this is another social structure that influences her perceptions of health, illness, and well-being.

Stop and Think

- » If you think about the various parts of the Social Skeleton model, which social structures influence your perceptions of health, illness, and well-being the most?
- » Thinking about the structure/agency debate, how much influence does society have over your health behaviours and actions?

Mythbuster

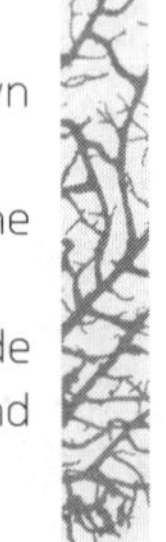

Consider whether you see the following as questionable. What does this tell you about your own values regarding the influence society has over health behaviours and actions?

- There are many who believe that an African male infected with HIV/AIDS can be cured of the infection by having sex with a virgin.
- In Pakistan, decisions about pregnancy and antenatal care are said to be usually made by older women. Often, this is the pregnant woman's mother-in-law, and the mother and father to be are distanced from the process.

These and other examples are reported on <http://en.wikipedia.org/wiki/Sociology_of_health_and_illness>

agency may be in tension, but they are interdependent—that is, one cannot exist without the other' (Germov 2005, p. 21).

In summary, Germov's (2005) Social Skeleton is a useful model for depicting a range of social structures influencing people's perceptions of health, illness, and well-being. However, ecological models are other useful tools for mapping the social, cultural, and other determinants impacting on people's health, illness, and well-being and they will be explored in the next section.

Ecological models

Human ecologists contend that an individual's health is part of a structure of relationships (contexts and determinants) and is altered by changes in that structure (McLaren & Hawe 2005). They are interested in the relationships between humans and the physical, natural, cultural, and social dimensions of their environment (Lawrence 2003). The notion that health is a result of connections between humans and the elements of their broader environments has gained prevalence since the mid-20th century (McMichael 2001). Following the development of the social model of health, a number of ecological models have been developed since the 1970s to show the relationship between humans and elements of their social, cultural, and broader environments that impact on health (Townsend & Mahoney 2004).

For example, Hancock and Perkins (1985) developed the Mandala of Health to demonstrate the links between humans, social and cultural environments, and the broader environment/ecosystem. The model displays human health in a broad context, with four critical factors influencing the health of an individual at the centre (Nicholson & Stephenson 2004). These four factors are human biology, personal behaviour, psychosocial environment, and immediate physical environment (Hancock & Perkins 1985). The Mandala sees health in its holistic sense, so the health of the individual at the centre is shown to have body, mind, and spirit dimensions. Hancock (1993) indicates that the Mandala has been widely used by educators and practitioners to map the determinants of health of individuals and populations.

Following this, Hancock (1993) developed two more ecological models. First, the Health-Environment-Economy model focuses on human development and is based on two key principles of public health first proposed in the 1980s—ecological sanity and social justice. It demonstrates the intersection between health, the environment, and the economy and indicates that 'the economy both underpins human health and the environment and, at the same time...the economy is—or should be—subservient to those broader imperatives. It also ensures that issues of human well-being and social equity are incorporated in the discussion of sustainable development' (Hancock 1993, p. 44). Second, the Community Ecosystem Model demonstrates that community health is found at the intersection of three circles: the community, the environment, and the economy. Hancock suggests that healthy community ecosystems should comprise six qualities within their environmental, economic, and community domains. They should be convivial, liveable, sustainable, viable, and adequately prosperous with equitable wealth distribution.

Social ecological model

Social ecological model
A nested arrangement of interrelated structures comprising the microsystem, mesosystem, exosystem, and macrosystem, which have a trickle-down effect on an individual at the centre of the model.

Urie Bronfenbrenner, a renowned human ecologist, argues that an individual's health and well-being is dependent on their interaction with the environment. He develops an ecological model to depict how various contexts and consequences impact on an individual's health and well-being. This model is now described in detail and a case study will be used to demonstrate the applicability of this model for understanding health as a social construct. Bronfenbrenner's **social ecological model** consists of a nested arrangement of interrelated structures comprising the microsystem, mesosystem, exosystem, and macrosystem, which have a trickle-down effect on an individual at the centre of the model (Bronfenbrenner 1979).

At the centre of the model is an individual and their particular characteristics such as gender, age, and health status (Bowes & Grace 2009). The first layer of the model, the microsystem, is the structure of activities, roles, and personal relationships (family members and peers) experienced by an individual that directly affects health and well-being (Bronfenbrenner 1979; Bowes & Grace 2009). The next layer is the mesosystem, which comprises the relationship between two or more settings (places where people can engage in face-to-face interaction) in the microsystem, such as the level of match between family and work (Bronfenbrenner 1979; Bowes & Grace 2009). A third layer of the model is the exosystem, which refers to one or more settings that do not directly involve the individual, but that affect the individual's health and well-being, such as extended family and community influences (Bronfenbrenner 1979; Bowes & Grace 2009). The macrosystem is the outer layer of the model and consists of cultural norms, values, and attitudes that are passed on through families and social and government institutions to shape an individual's health and well-being (Bowes & Grace 2009).

Traditionally, the social ecological model has been used to determine the range of factors impacting on an individual's development (Bronfenbrenner 1979). But it has also been useful for exploring the influence of family on an individual (Townsend & Mahoney 2004) and can be applied to a number of individuals and contexts. How the model can be used to map the factors affecting the health and well-being of inner-city high-rise residents is illustrated in the following case study.

Case Study 12.2 Adapted social ecological model

For her PhD, the author conducted an exploratory mixed-methods study that investigated the factors, including access to nature (i.e. parks, gardens, and/or bodies of water), impacting on inner-city high-rise residents' health and well-being (see Henderson-Wilson 2009, 2010). The study participants varied in age, gender, socio-economic status, housing tenure (owner-occupiers/private tenants and public housing tenants), city of residence, and degree of proximity to natural environments. Phase 1 of the study involved surveying 221 high-rise residents from inner Melbourne and Sydney to identify and measure relationships between access to nature, high-rise living, and health and well-being. Phase 2 involved interviewing 30 of the surveyed residents to gain a deeper understanding of their experiences with high-rise living, access to nature, sense of community, and sense of place. Analysis of the integrated findings (from Phases 1 and 2) revealed that numerous factors (including accessibility, choice and control, tenure, and community infrastructure) impact on residents' health and well-being, either directly or indirectly. Results of this study indicated that for disadvantaged populations (e.g. public housing tenants), the availability of a park, garden, and/or body of water can enhance residents' quality of life.

The social ecological model was applied to describe the range of factors affecting high-rise residents' access to nature, health, and well-being. The results of the study showed that a range of factors trickle down from the outer, macrosystem level to the high-rise resident at the centre of the model. The following section discusses the range of contexts and consequences at each level of the adapted social ecological model (see Figure 12.2).

Figure 12.2 Adapted social ecological model

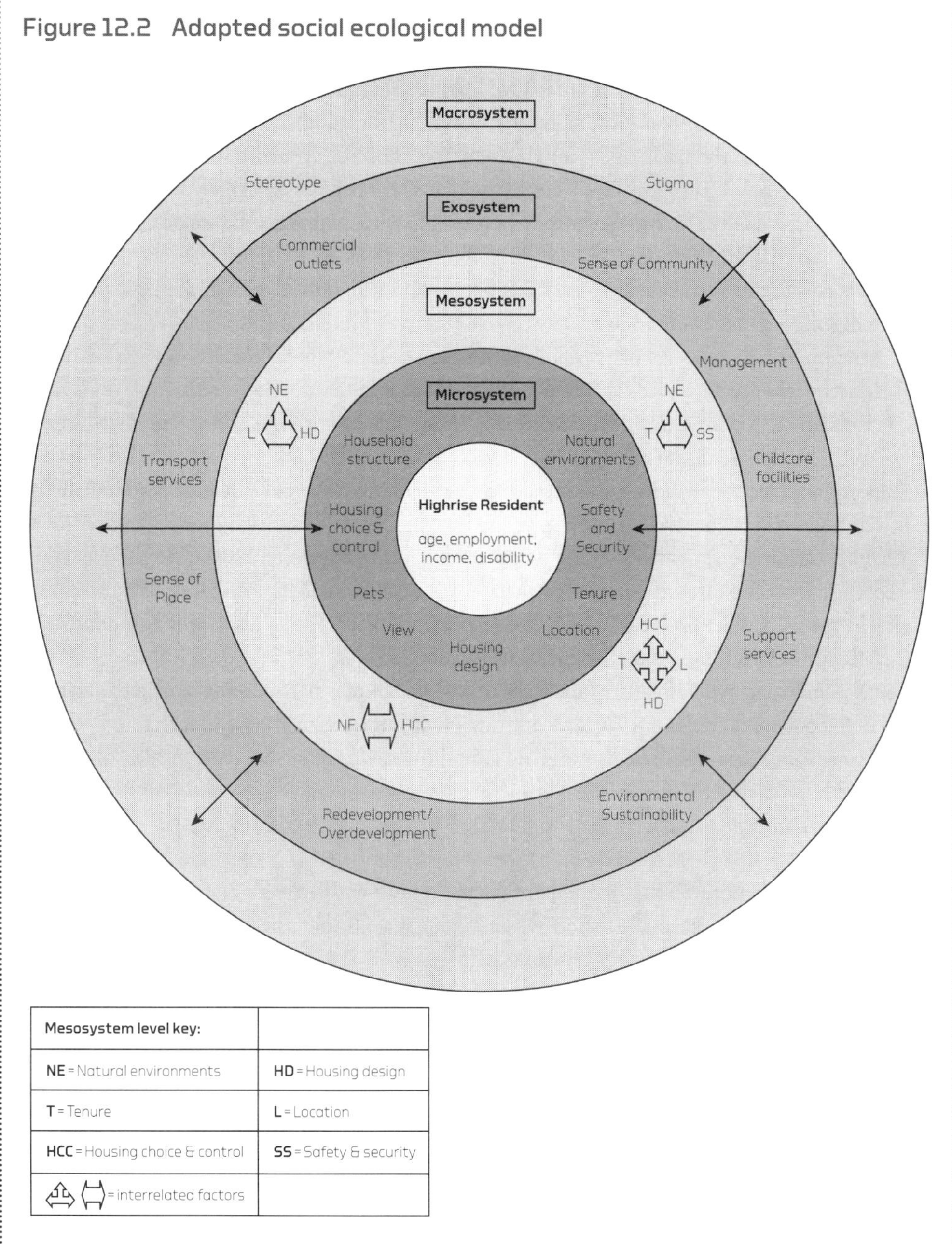

Source: Adapted from Santrock 2004, p. 40

Several demographic factors were found to impact on participants' health and well-being. These are displayed in the adapted model within the individual/high-rise resident level at the centre of the model as including:

- *Age*: being aged 55 years or more resulted in higher well-being. This could be due to the fact that residents at this age are more resilient to changing contexts.

- *Employment*: participating in paid work for 21 hours or more a week resulted in higher well-being. This is not surprising considering that residents who participate in meaningful occupation are likely to have enhanced well-being (Furnass 1996; Trewin 2001).
- *Income*: earning an income of more than $31,000 per annum resulted in higher well-being (linking to the findings on employment). It should be noted that at the time of data collection, 2004, less than half of the participants worked full-time (39.8%); the majority earned more than $15,000 per annum (64.7%), with about a quarter of them earning $90,000 or more (23.5%).
- *Disability*: findings indicated that participants who did not have a disability or medical condition had higher well-being.

At the microsystem level, that which is closest to the high-rise resident, a range of contexts and consequences was found to impact directly on the resident's health and well-being (Bronfenbrenner 1979; Bowes & Grace 2009). These factors are displayed in the first layer of the adapted model (refer to Figure 12.2) and include:

- *Household structure*: Findings indicated that participants who did not have children living with them had higher well-being.
- *Tenure*: Owning or privately renting an apartment resulted in higher well-being.
- *Location*: Satisfaction with housing location resulted in higher well-being. Factors found to influence residents' location satisfaction include access to natural environments, the availability of facilities, and efficient transport services.
- *Safety and security:* Vandalism and security were factors discouraging participants from public housing to access their nearby natural environments. In addition, safety and security within a participant's high-rise and neighbourhood impacted on their health and well-being.
- *Housing choice and control*: Choosing to live in an apartment resulted in higher well-being.
- *Pets:* Findings indicated that participants who do not own pets (majority) had significantly higher well-being. The main reason why residents do not own pets is because they do not feel apartments are suitable for housing them.
- *Natural environments*: Visiting available garden/s and park/s resulted in higher well-being.
- *Housing design*: Being very satisfied with an apartment's size resulted in higher well-being.

The mesosystem layer of the adapted model displays the relationship or congruence between two or more contexts and consequences of the microsystem layer (Bronfenbrenner 1979; Bowes & Grace 2009). A review of the findings indicated that the congruence between the following factors impacts on residents' health and well-being:

- *Natural environments and housing design*: The inclusion of natural elements (i.e. gardens and parks) within residents' development, or nearby, contributes to their accessibility, health, and well-being.
- *Natural environments and housing choice and control*: Good access to natural environments was a motivator for a number of residents to move into an apartment.
- *Natural environments and safety and security*: Residents' access to nature, and satisfaction with available nearby nature, was influenced by its safety and security.

The exosystem layer of the adapted model displays a range of contexts and consequences that, while not directly impacting on the high-rise resident at the centre of the model, affect the resident's health and well-being through a trickle-down effect (Bronfenbrenner 1979; Bowes & Grace 2009). These factors are displayed in the third layer of the model as including:

- *Sense of community*: Residents' sense of community ranged from strong to nonexistent and was influenced by body corporate/management bodies and access to nature.
- *Sense of place*: Residents' sense of place and connection to location varied from strong to nonexistent and, like the sense of community, was influenced by access to nature.
- *Childcare facilities, transport services, commercial outlets, and support services*: Safe and easy access to childcare facilities, transport services, commercial outlets, and support services influenced residents' health and well-being.
- *Management*: Body corporate/management bodies influenced residents' sense of community, sense of control, opportunities for accessing natural environments, and pet ownership.
- *Environmental sustainability*: Developments that were designed to be environmentally sustainable and gave residents the ability to practise environmentally sustainable behaviours enhanced residents' quality of life.
- *Redevelopment/overdevelopment*: The proposed redevelopment of public housing in Sydney was found to have a large impact on the well-being of the public housing tenants. In addition, overdevelopment of apartments was a concern for many residents because they felt it impinged on available open space.

The outer level of the adapted model, the macrosystem, consists of the attitudes and ideologies of the culture which trickle down to impact on the resident's health and well-being (Bronfenbrenner 1979; Santrock 2004; Bowes & Grace 2009). The factor contained within the macrosystem level is displayed as including:

- *Social exclusion*: Many residents experienced stigma and stereotyping, which may be components of social exclusion, i.e. derogatory comments relating to their living in high-rise developments.

As demonstrated, the social ecological model, like the Social Skeleton model, can be used to map the range of social, cultural, and other contexts and determinants impacting on an individual's health and well-being. In this example, the factors impacting on inner-city high-rise residents have been mapped. You may wish to use this model to map determinants impacting on a range of individuals.

Summary

The social model of health has moved beyond the limitations of the biomedical model to allow for an understanding that health is comprised of a dynamic interaction of social structures. Six key features of the social model of health proposed by Yuill (2010) include: 'individual health is enabled or inhibited by social context'; 'the body is simultaneously social, psychological and biological'; 'health is cultural'; 'biomedicine and medical science is something—but not everything'; 'health is political'; and 'other voices matter'.

Health sociology provides a useful perspective for understanding the social and cultural contexts influencing understandings of health, illness, and well-being. It is aligned with the social model of health and focuses on the social group to which people belong and the social patterns of health and illness. Examples of social patterning of health and illness include life expectancy, gender, and income inequality.

The Social Skeleton model can be used to depict a range of social structures influencing people's perceptions of health, illness, and well-being. In addition, ecological models can be useful aids for mapping the range of social and cultural contexts impacting on individuals' health and well-being, particularly the social ecological model.

Tutorial exercises

1 In small teams, debate which is the most effective model for mapping/depicting the range of social and cultural contexts influencing perceptions of health, illness, and well-being: the Social Skeleton: health, illness and structure agency model or the social ecological model? Why?
2 Now use the social ecological model to map/depict the range of social and cultural contexts influencing your health and well-being. How useful was the model in completing this exercise? Why? Discuss your responses with your team mates.
3 Reflecting on your responses to Question 2, which level contained the most contexts? What factors were located at the macrosystem level? What interrelationships were depicted at the mesosystem level? Were your responses similar to your team mates?

Further reading

Bowes, J., & Grace, R. (2009). *Children, families and communities: Contexts and consequences*, 3rd edn. Melbourne: Oxford University Press.

Bronfenbrenner, U. (1979). *The ecology of human development: Experiments by nature and design*. Cambridge, MA: Harvard University Press.

Broom, D. (2009). Gender and health. In J. Germov (ed.), *Second opinion: An introduction to health sociology*, 4th edn. Melbourne: Oxford University Press, 130–55.

Germov, J. (2009). Imagining health problems as social issues. In J. Germov (ed.), *Second opinion: An introduction to health sociology*, 4th edn. Melbourne: Oxford University Press, 3–24.

Habibis, D. (2009). The illness experience: Lay perspectives, disability, and chronic illness. In J. Germov (ed.), *Second opinion: An introduction to health sociology*, 4th edn. Melbourne: Oxford University Press, 288–306.

Taylor, S. (2008a). The concept of health. In S. Taylor, M. Foster, & J. Fleming (eds), *Healthcare practice in Australia*. Melbourne: Oxford University Press, 3–21.

White, K. (2009). *An introduction to the sociology of health and illness*, 2nd edn. London: Sage Publications.

Yuill, C. (2010). The social model of health. In C. Yuill, I. Crinson, & E. Duncan (eds), *Key concepts in health studies*. Thousand Oaks, CA: Sage Publications, 11–14.

Websites

<www.abs.gov.au>

This website provides the latest Australian statistics on everything from health through to housing. It is a useful resource for any health-related studies.

<www.aihw.gov.au>

Visit this website to access the latest 'Australia's Health': a comprehensive profile of the nation's health and welfare status.

<www.health.vic.gov.au>

This is the website for the Victorian Department of Health. Visit this website to obtain the latest health information relevant to Victoria.

<www.chs.unimelb.edu.au>

This is the website for the Centre for Health and Society at the University of Melbourne. Visit this website for links to research investigating the social construction of health.

<www.phac-aspc.gc.ca/ph-sp/determinants/index-eng.php>

This is the website for the Public Health Agency of Canada. Visit this website for information on social factors impacting on health.

Language, culture, and health

Rebecca Fanany

TOPICS COVERED

This chapter covers the following topics:

- what culture is and how it is related to language
- the effects language and culture may have on people's conceptualisation of health
- the nature and importance of cultural competence in health professionals
- the concept of illness behaviour and how it is shaped by culture

KEY TERMS

Cultural competency
Culture
Disease
Health
Illness
Illness behaviour
Sociolinguistics

Introduction

Health There is no definite meaning of health. Its meaning can be different depending on individuals, social groups, and cultures and can differ at different times. In general, it means not just the absence of illness or disease but a total sense of well-being.

The language people speak and the culture they are part of play an important role in shaping their understanding of **health**. The terms and concepts they have available to talk about health and illness and what exactly these terms and concepts mean are determined by the language they speak (Reynaert & Gelman 2007). Similarly, a society's accepted norms about what it means to be healthy or sick, what kinds of symptoms indicate illness, and what is the right thing to do if someone is sick are all determined by culture (Heggenhougan & Shore 1986). These things are not universal. That is, while each person's understanding of health and illness is an integral part of their way of thinking, people from different cultural backgrounds may have a very different idea of what health and illness mean.

It is very important for health professionals to understand that conceptualisations of health in different parts of the world differ as these views underlie many aspects of health behaviour and may be significant in working with patients or clients from a variety of backgrounds. We must be aware of our own culture and language-based conceptualisation of health and recognise that it affects our perceptions just as much as our patients' or clients' affects theirs. This chapter gives an overview of the ways in which the language and cultural background of individuals can affect their understanding of health. The need for cultural competence among health professionals is also discussed along with a consideration of **illness behaviour** and culturally determined expressions of disease.

Illness behaviour The socially acceptable way to act when sick.

Culture

Culture A system of shared ideas, attitudes, and practices that defines the social system of its members.

Culture is a system of shared meaning, representations, and practices that make up our social life. These principles are known and understood in more or less the same way by all members of a given society and are characteristic of that society (Danesi & Perron 1999). Most people never think about the culture they are part of and how it affects their ideas and understanding. We begin to absorb the principles of our culture from birth, and eventually they become the basis for our worldview. We do not need to think about our own culture but we use it as the basis for making decisions about everything we experience.

Culture is reflected in language and is also shaped by it. This is a reciprocal relationship where language acts as the means to express culture, while the demands of culture also contribute to the development of terms to express them (Kramsch 1998). To a great extent language provides a structure for our thoughts and ideas, and culture supplies a set of norms within which we express ourselves such that these two elements make up our cognitive framework. Our cognitive framework gives structure to the way we perceive the world and allows us to interpret and understand our surroundings and experiences. This extends to health; we should not assume that people from different cultures will conceptualise health and illness in the same way.

Any culture has clearly identifiable characteristics that give it a unique identity. We often speak about the national character of various countries or invoke (frequently negative) stereotypes about some group. In many cases, the elements that contribute to these set ideas represent observable but superficial characteristics of the culture in question as seen through the lens of our own culture. Going beyond the superficial, a more objective understanding of other cultures may be useful as a guide to behaviour and perception, although it cannot guarantee any particular reaction from members of the culture. Every society is composed of individuals who may share knowledge and understanding that derive from a shared background but who may also use this common understanding differently according to their particular personalities. It is important to remember that every culture is really composed of subcultures, groups, or individuals whose perceptions may be significantly different from the accepted social norms (Danesi & Perron 1999).

Language and culture cannot really be separated because, as noted, language gives us the means to express the understandings culture gives us. People who are native speakers of the same language, even if they come from different countries, often share understandings of culture. If we think about native speakers of English, who may come from Australia, the USA, or the UK, we realise that the culture of these three countries is quite different but the common language, English, means that these cultures are necessarily more similar than the culture of any one of them would be to people from a non-English-speaking country, simply because the means of expressing culture is the same.

Language

The languages of the world are divided into families that share general characteristics of grammar, lexicon, origin, and so forth. Within linguistic families, individual languages are different, and each has unique aspects. The structures available in a given language are related to how speakers perceive and categorise events and, by extension, how they think about their experience (Crystal 1997).

The Sapir-Whorf hypothesis describes this situation and is taken as an important tenet of the field of **sociolinguistics**, the area of study that relates to the social uses of language. The hypothesis states that differences in languages affect the way speakers think. This is called linguistic relativity (Dirven & Verspoor 2004). Linguistic relativity suggests that while every language can express anything its speakers might wish to say, each language has a unique set of words and structures that are the means by which speakers convey their ideas (Crystal 1997). Because the linguistic material available to discuss a particular issue, health for example, differs, it is likely that speakers of different language will also have different conceptualisations of this issue, and these conceptualisations will be more different for languages that are further apart.

Sociolinguistics The study of language in the social/cultural context.

For instance, the Indonesian language has a single word, *sakit*, that is used to mean both 'sick' and 'in pain'. Indonesian is very dependent on context and position, and speakers have to interpret the meaning of each utterance based on the social situation in which it occurs. In English, by contrast, we distinguish between being sick and being in pain and, in fact, have a number of different terms to further distinguish what exactly is wrong. We might wish to indicate that a pain is an ache or soreness or is stabbing. Indonesian has none of these distinctions. This does not mean that Indonesian speakers do not experience the same physical manifestations of pain that English speakers do, only that their conceptualisation of health does not require that the concept of being in pain be further specified.

The result of these differences in language, which are underpinned by the nature of the culture that uses the language, may be difficulty in understanding or even communication breakdown between healthcare professionals and their clients and patients. We normally expect health issues to be expressed in the way we are familiar with and rely heavily on culturally determined phrases and terms that are part of our cognitive framework (see Reynaert & Gelman 2007). When we work with speakers of other languages (even if they are speaking our language), we often find that they conceptualise their own health problems in ways that are unexpected and unfamiliar because we each tend to use our first language and culture as a template or model for what we say. This is an important issue for healthcare professionals and will be discussed further under the heading 'Cultural competency'.

Another important aspect of sociolinguistics that may affect us as healthcare professionals is the difference between our manner of discussing health and disease and that of the general public (see e.g. Keller & Carroll 1994; Chang & Fortier 1998). Health professionals generally spend many years completing their training, and part of this training is learning the ways of the profession. We can think of each health profession as a subculture that has its own conventions, ways of using language, and means of talking about clients or patients and their conditions. Being able to fit into this subculture is a part of successfully carrying out our duties. The general public who are not trained in our field have a completely different way of talking about health and disease. If we are members of the same culture, we understand what lay people mean when they talk about their health in this way, but it is often imprecise compared to our professional usage. It is easy to forget that lay people may not understand our own way of speaking or may be uncomfortable with it.

The use of medical language is often viewed by patients as a problem for them in understanding what their condition is and what they are supposed to do. Research has shown that patients feel much more comfortable using ordinary language to discuss their health, while doctors, in particular, tend to use the technical language that they use with their colleagues (Castro et al. 2007). It is often nurses who have to mediate by translating medical terminology and phrasing into more ordinary terms patients feel comfortable with (Hadlow & Pitts 1991; Bourhis et al. 2002). It is worth noting that patients and clients often react to non-verbal communicative cues as well as to language. What is considered the usual conversational manner differs considerably from culture to culture, and common hand gestures, making eye contact, smiling, and a whole range of other mannerisms contribute to how comfortable a patient or client feels with a healthcare professional and, indirectly, how much they might gain from the conversation (Larsen & Smith 1981; Harrigan et al. 1985; Griffith et al. 2003).

Language and culture in health

We understand that there are many universal aspects of human experience anywhere in the world and that people everywhere from every culture have the same potential for health and disease. We also understand that the state of health of different populations in different places may vary significantly because of a whole range of factors, including language and culture issues. This extends to what are viewed as signs of health and signs of illness (Kleinman et al. 1978).

The human condition includes a multitude of minor problems and pains that most people have suffered at one time or another. We have all had a headache which we might have treated ourselves with an over-the-counter pain medication. Or we might have done nothing, knowing that the headache would go away itself and did not represent a major problem. Most of us have an idea of what kind of symptoms are more serious and warrant a visit to the doctor for further treatment. The set of symptoms that may be ignored and those that should not are part of our cultural understanding and are often understood quite consistently by members of the same population.

This shared understanding derives from the culture and language shared by the group but also develops from a shared environment with specific characteristics in which the population in question lives. For example, drinking water in many Western countries is fluoridated, and toothpastes and other dental products often contain fluoride as well. Dentistry is highly developed, and awareness of dental hygiene is high among much of the public. For this reason, while still an important public health concern, dental health has improved greatly in Western societies over the course of the 20th century. Tooth loss due to decay or disease, especially among the young, is much less common than it once was, and most people expect to retain all or most of their teeth into adulthood. In other parts of the world, however, there is no treatment of drinking water and fluoride is generally not added to toothpastes and dental products. Dentistry may be less advanced than in the West, and there are generally fewer dentists. More importantly, the public in these areas tend to be much less accepting and trusting of dentistry and may accept much higher levels of pain, disability, and tooth loss than would be tolerated by most people in the West. Tooth loss and dental pain, in many parts of the world, are considered a normal part of life and if people do seek dental treatment it is often too late to save the teeth in question. The idea that there is a great deal the individual can do to prevent dental problems is not well understood, and many people make little effort to protect their own teeth (see WHO 2005c).

This difference in understanding is based on the cultural norms of each population. We often encounter a conflict between expectations when people emigrate from one country to another. In Australia, where oral health is one of the national health priorities, dental health among refugees is a particular concern. Because of the nature of the cultures these individuals come from combined with the effects of the social disruption there that caused them to become refugees, many suffer from serious dental and oral health problems. These can be treated more readily in Australia than in their countries of origin, but in many cases their condition is far advanced, and it is no longer possible to save teeth. This may have the effect of further strengthening the idea among this population that dentists cannot really help, and tooth loss is inevitable. Deeply held cultural understandings are often extremely difficult to change because we are not aware of their subjective (at the societal level) nature and often do not or cannot consider another perspective. For this reason, it may not be possible for the first generation of immigrants to learn the health perspective of their new country, but their children who grow up with them generally absorb the views of the society they live in more readily (Davidson et al. 2006; Finney Lamb et al. 2009).

It is important to understand that people are rarely aware that their actions represent a cultural norm that relates to their background and upbringing. We generally feel that we are behaving in the 'right' way because we are doing something that comes naturally in the social context in which we find ourselves. This subjective perception of appropriateness applies to language use as well. People talk about health in the ways they have observed among family members, friends, and other social groups. For the lay person (someone who is not trained in a health field), as mentioned above, it is more natural to use the imprecise terms common in society to refer to health conditions than to use more technical terms even if they are known. For example, we often read that someone has died 'following a long illness' (often used euphemistically to refer to death from cancer), that someone needs 'an operation' (where the professional might speak of surgery or a procedure or an appendectomy), and so forth.

While it is important to understand the cultural and linguistic factors that may affect perceptions about health, we should also be aware that at best they provide a set of guidelines. It is probably never the case that every member of a given culture or language group shares the exact same attitude and perceptions about health and illness. Similarly, we should not expect that every member of a cultural or language group will use their culture's approach to health as a basis for their own actions, and members of particular groups may act very differently from what we expect. This extends to members of our own culture as well as to individuals from cultural backgrounds we are less familiar with. Overall, then, we should be cautious about making generalisations about expected health behaviour based on cultural and language background but we should be aware of differences in perception due to diverse backgrounds and train ourselves to be sensitive to their existence.

Stop and Think

We all have ideas about health that come from our cultural and language background, including what we learn from the media and from other people.

» What kinds of things does the average Australian believe about health?

» To what extent do lay people's ideas about health correspond to the evidence used by health professionals as the basis for their work?

Indigenous health in Australia and New Zealand

The Aboriginal and Torres Strait Islander populations in Australia and the Maori population in New Zealand provide important examples of how the health of specific population subgroups that possess specific linguistic and cultural characteristics can differ from that of members of the majority culture. In Australia, Indigenous people suffer a greater burden of disease than the general public, tend to have less access to healthcare, and experience higher rates of hospitalisation for a range of diseases and conditions. As a group, they also have more disability and a lower life expectancy than the rest of the population, as well as more emotional and mental illness. Levels of behaviours that tend to be detrimental to health have also been observed to be higher among Indigenous peoples (AIHW 2011). This discrepancy in health outcomes and experience between the Indigenous and non-Indigenous populations is often referred to as a gap that must be addressed through policy, service provision, and change in social attitudes. To address this, the Australian Government has introduced the Closing the Gap Strategy which addresses a range of health concerns affecting the Indigenous population, including basic health, education, and employment as well as social inclusion (Australian Government 2009).

Like Australian Indigenous populations, the indigenous Maori of New Zealand have specific health concerns and issues that differ from those of the non-Maori population. Over the last 50 years, life expectancy for Maori individuals in New Zealand has increased significantly, bringing the discrepancy to 8.6 years for men and 7.9 years for women (Ministry of Maori Development 2009a). Like the Indigenous population in Australia, the Maori population in New Zealand is affected by higher rates of some diseases, especially diabetes, than the general public. Although this group tends to be more physically active than the non-Maori, obesity remains a problem as do rates of smoking, which tend to be higher than for non-Maori despite dropping significantly since the late 1990s (Ministry of Health 2010).

The experience of the indigenous peoples of Australia and New Zealand with respect to health is characteristic of indigenous populations around the world for whom dramatic change in social structures and the living environment has occurred rapidly in the context of colonisation and integration into modern nation states. A range of social inequalities and socio-economic factors associated with globalisation, migration, loss of language and culture, and disconnection from the land have been implicated as the basis for current health discrepancies (King et al. 2009). Another important element of social change that has affected indigenous populations is the shift from the use of traditional languages to the majority language of the nation in which they are located (Gracey & King 2009). As discussed above, our understanding of health is embedded in language which, in turn, develops in such a way as to facilitate cultural conceptualisations, including ideas about health. It has been observed, for example, that indigenous conceptualisations of health, as expressed through traditional languages and cultures, tend to be more holistic and more centred on well-being. Recovering from illness may entail consultation with the wider community and participation in collective practices (King et al. 2009). The importance of the traditional community in indigenous health cannot be underestimated; it has been observed that many indigenous peoples define their personal identity in the context of the group (Durie 2005; Durie et al. 2009). This identity, as a member of a particular culture with its own language, practices, and worldview, is central to the emotional health of the individual and will also contribute to how people perceive illness in themselves as well as in others. It is generally agreed that, in considering the social determinants that affect the health experience of all people, a range of cultural factors in the special case of Indigenous health in Australia—loss of language and connection to the land, environmental deprivation, and spiritual, emotional, and mental disconnectedness—must also be taken into account (Mowbray 2007; Nettleton et al. 2007). The communal aspect of health is significant as well, and recognition of this conceptualisation is part of the rationale for the Australian Government's social inclusion agenda for Indigenous populations (Australian Government 2011). A similar approach has been taken in New Zealand to encourage greater participation by the Maori community in larger social issues and governance with the aim of further closing the gap between indigenous and non-indigenous health and welfare (Ministry of Maori Development 2009b).

Cultural competency

As health professionals, we are required to provide appropriate care to patients and clients that best meets their needs and represents best practice. This means that we have to be aware of the ways in which language and cultural background may affect people's perceptions and understandings about health and take these into account in our work. This is increasingly important as societies around the world become more multicultural; Australia is no exception to this. Our population is made up of people from many different backgrounds, and its diversity is continuing to increase (Department of Foreign Affairs and Trade 2008). For this reason, it is especially important that we are aware of cultural differences and how they may affect health and that we develop cultural competency in working with people from different backgrounds.

Cultural competency
The ability to work effectively with people from different cultural and language backgrounds.

Cultural competency for the healthcare professional means the ability to work appropriately with people from different cultures and who speak different languages. A culturally competent healthcare system is one that acknowledges the importance of cultural practices and the relationship between cultures in achieving health outcomes (Betancourt et al. 2003). Individually, we must be aware of our own cultural outlook and how it colours our understanding of health, but also that the people we work with may have a very different set of perceptions based on different assumptions. In the healthcare system, cultural competency is one way of eliminating some of the inequities in health that are observable in modern society. We know that a number of social factors, such as income (socio-economic status), education, and structural/institutional issues, can have an impact on health, but cultural factors can as well. Cultural competency allows us to address the effects of the social environment that are shaped by culture and language.

It is important to understand why cultural competency has become so important in healthcare and the training of its professionals. There are two main reasons for this. The first is that individuals from different cultural backgrounds may describe their symptoms quite differently according to their own understanding of illness. They may also have limited ability in English (or whatever the language of interaction is in a given situation). Their decisions about when to seek care may vary, and their expectations for treatment and beliefs about their condition may affect their adherence to health advice (Berger 1998; Betancourt et al. 2005). The second is that a great deal of research has shown that communication between health professionals and patients or clients is closely related to patient/client satisfaction, adherence to advice, and health outcomes. In other words, poorer health outcomes may result when sociocultural differences between health professionals and patients/clients are not acknowledged and addressed (Stewart et al. 1999; Williams & Rucker 2000; Institute of Medicine 2001; Smedley et al. 2002).

In Australia, the National Health and Medical Research Council (NHMRC) has produced a set of guidelines about cultural competency for healthcare professionals. Cultural competency is especially important in the Australian context because our population is very diverse, and, like many other countries, we must address a number of health inequities between different population subgroups. The Australian model for cultural competency addresses four dimensions of the healthcare system as a whole: systemic (how the whole national healthcare system is structured); organisational (how the various agencies at different levels of government are structured); professional (relating to the various health professions whose work contributes to the well-being of the population); and individual (how each person in the healthcare system does his or her job). According to the NHMRC (2005, p. 4), a culturally competent healthcare system is one that

> acknowledges the benefits that diversity brings to Australian society; helps health providers and consumers achieve the best, most appropriate care and services; enables self-determination and ensures a commitment to reciprocity for culturally and linguistically diverse consumers and their communities; and holds governments, health organizations, and managers accountable for meeting the needs of all members of the communities they serve.

This emphasis on cultural competency is based on the fact that different Australian population subgroups have a very different experience of health. For example, statistics collected by the Australian Government show that certain communities have higher than average rates of diabetes (immigrant groups from southern Europe, the South Pacific Island states, North Africa, the Middle East, and Asia). The population that emigrated to Australia from the UK and Ireland has higher than average rates of breast cancer and lung cancer, while rates of skin cancer for the population born overseas are less than half those of the population born in Australia (AIHW 2004, 2005).

Stop and Think

It is important that health professionals be aware of cultural differences that might affect the health of the patients or clients.

» Why do you think this is viewed as the responsibility of those who provide healthcare instead of part of the responsibility of the patient/client?

Illness behaviour and culture

The idea that each culture has a 'sick role', a set of behaviours and attitudes that are accepted by members of the culture as the appropriate way for a sick person to behave, is long established in the field of health sociology (see e.g. Parsons 1951). Continuing research in this area has shown that the cultural perspective of health professionals as well as their patients and clients is an important influence on illness behaviour. It is now accepted that the way people behave when they are sick derives from a complex interaction between their particular biological determinants, the nature of their symptoms, the social context in which illness occurs, the characteristics of the healthcare system of which they are part, and learnt responses to illness that are rooted in their language and culture (Mechanic 1995; Kirmayer & Sartorius 2007).

A learnt response to illness comes from all the observations of the behaviour of people around them that an individual absorbs from birth. Young children come to understand what is expected of a sick person, what kind of illness means a person is sick enough not to participate in normal activities, what symptoms require professional assistance, and how various diseases are viewed in the context of their own family, culture, and social group. These culturally determined lay understandings of health often differ dramatically from the evidence-based, best practice approaches of health professionals. For example, evidence indicates that early ambulation is an important factor in recovery after certain kinds of surgery (Oldmeadow et al. 2006; Izumi et al. 2010). However, lay conceptualisations of health in many cultures suggest that a person who has undergone a serious operation should not move around too much, especially if they are in pain. These opposite interpretations may lead to disagreement and conflict between patients and their family members and health professionals.

Illness behaviour has been shown to influence several important dimensions of health, particularly in relation to when and how an individual might seek treatment. First, culturally influenced illness behaviour may affect who is vulnerable to illness (Hartog & Hartog 1983). In this, it is important to distinguish between **illness** and **disease**. *Disease* refers to a clinical condition that is acknowledged to be abnormal and detrimental to a person's health. By contrast, *illness* is the state of being sick or having something wrong as perceived by the individual in question. Many people who have a disease do not feel that they have an illness, but it is also the case that many people who feel that they have an illness do not have a detectable disease. Different cultures

Illness A condition adversely affecting health as perceived by the individual in question.

Disease A condition adversely affecting health that has measurable (clinical) symptoms.

allow, in the sense of deeming it socially acceptable, for certain people to suffer from illness as part of their social role. Second, culturally influenced illness behaviour can determine who decides to become a patient (Hartog & Hartog 1983). That is, some cultures do not recognise certain symptoms or problems as evidence of a health concern, and individuals who experience these symptoms may not be willing to seek treatment. This is often the case in mental illness but may apply to physical symptoms as well (see e.g. Roy et al. 2005; Canino & Alegria 2008). And third, culturally influenced illness behaviour may dictate how a person behaves once they are a patient (Hartog & Hartog 1983), including to what extent they are likely to follow health advice given to them by professionals or what the meaning of illness is in their culture (Bhui & Dinos 2008). For example, for individuals from a low socio-economic background whose earnings allow for few savings, it may be impossible to take on the role of patient and hence deprive the family of necessary income. In socio-cultural contexts like this, there may exist deeply ingrained behaviours and rationales that encourage people to ignore symptoms and continue to work until it is physically impossible to ignore pain or other problems.

Culture-bound syndromes

Culture-bound syndromes are usually said to be locally defined patterns of discrete behaviour (Littlewood & Lipsedge 1985). That is, they are illnesses that occur only in specific communities and are identified by a set of symptoms that derives from the culture of the society that experiences them. For a long time, culture-bound syndromes were seen as exotic, occurring generally in cultures that were viewed by Westerners as less developed, more traditional, and lacking the institutions of modernity (Hughes 1996; Bhugra & Jacob 1997). Culture-bound syndromes depend on the recognition of symptoms reported by the person who is affected that often cannot be confirmed clinically. That is, the symptoms of these conditions typically do not have physiological effects that can be measured by Western tests. For this reason, culture-bound syndromes are usually psychiatric or psychological conditions, as opposed to strictly medical ones.

Case Study 14.1 Being sick in Indonesia

Illness behaviour in Indonesia is very different from Australia or other English-speaking societies. As we have seen, how people act when they are sick and how their condition is perceived are determined by a combination of factors that derive from the language, culture, and shared environment of the people in question. We should also understand that every country has a number of cultures. Indonesia, for example, is very diverse with more than 300 ethnic and language groups. Nonetheless, there are also aspects of culture that are shared by many people in the country. Illness behaviour is one of these.

In Indonesia, illness behaviour is related to how serious a particular health condition is viewed. Some health issues are seen as serious by definition. These include broken bones, fevers, pain of any kind, and recovery from childbirth. Whether a condition is viewed as serious is not always related to how the individual feels but instead is based on how others react to any visible signs and symptoms. It is perhaps for this reason that broken bones or injuries are always considered serious. In Australia, for example, a person with a broken arm would be expected to go about most of their usual activities. The injury would certainly not prevent them from leaving the house or going to work (assuming they were physically able to do their job with one hand).

In Indonesia, when a person is viewed as having a serious health condition, even if this is only a headache, they are expected to lie in bed. Other family members will normally wait on them, bringing them food, helping them walk to the bathroom, and so forth. A sick person is not supposed to watch television, read, or do anything around the house and will not be allowed by family to go outside. If someone is sick, they must rest, and the appropriate illness behaviour will be enforced by others. Needless to say, the sick individual also understands this sick role and tends to adopt the culturally appropriate behaviour. From a Western point of view, Indonesians frequently take to their bed for what we perceive as no reason at all. However, the social need to do so is part of their culture and represents correct behaviour in the context of their shared expectations and experience.

Indonesia does not have a tradition of diagnosis and did not develop techniques for examining and understanding how the body works beyond what is visible to the eye. Traditional medicine relies on what we would call magic, herbal remedies, and basic technical skills such as bone-setting. In the modern era, Western, allopathic medicine forms the basis of the nation's healthcare system, but diagnosis remains much less important than in the West, and many people are more familiar with traditional conceptualisations of health and disease than with the evidence-based understandings of health professionals with modern training. For this reason, the determination of what constitutes a serious illness to the average Indonesian is based on a different set of considerations from those a modern doctor would use. For example, it is common to see people on the street or in the market with coughs so severe it is difficult for them to breathe. A cough is rarely considered enough to require illness behaviour on the part of the sufferer, however, even though to a health professional it might be a sign of serious illness or represent a threat to public health. Similarly, diseases like diabetes, which is very common in Indonesia, that do not have pronounced symptoms very seldom change people's behaviour (including diet), even when they have received a medical diagnosis.

When working with patients or clients from another culture, it is important to recognise that their understandings of disease and what they consider to be appropriate illness behaviour may be very different from what we consider to be usual. It is important to approach these differences without making judgments and without criticism. This is where communication between the healthcare professional and their patient or client becomes central in providing the best care that also meets the needs of all involved.

Although culture-bound syndromes have been viewed largely as occurring in non-Western populations, Western societies do, in fact, experience these illnesses. For example, it has been suggested that the type A behaviour pattern that has received as great deal of attention in the media since the 1970s is a culture-bound condition. People suffering from this condition say that they feel chronically pressed for time, extremely frustrated when they cannot achieve what they expect to, aggressive, overly ambitious, and impatient (Hughes 1996). The type A behaviour pattern has been thought to lead to greater incidence of heart disease, but the evidence supporting this is inconclusive (Matthews & Haynes 1986; Ragland & Brand 1988). Similarly, bulimia nervosa has also been observed to be a Western culture-bound syndrome (Littlewood 1996).

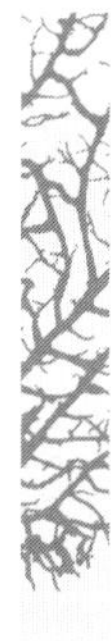

Mythbuster

Emotional response is not universal. While all human beings have the same range of emotions, the events or perceptions that trigger a particular emotion are culturally determined, as is the way in which that emotion is expressed. For this reason, we have to be very careful in interpreting the emotional reaction of people from another culture. Even the experience of war, which might be expected to be universally traumatising regardless of culture, has been observed to produce different reactions in different populations. In fact, post-traumatic stress disorder, the expected response to severe emotional trauma in the West, is increasingly viewed as being culture-bound or determined by the specific cultural understandings of the population affected by it.

There are indications that Western health problems that are culturally defined in terms of their nature and symptoms are spreading around the world. One cause of this may be the dominance of Western health paradigms in health fields and the fact that a large part of research and study in these areas comes from Western societies. Another contributing factor may be the globalisation of healthcare through the activities of multinational companies that may seek to create and maintain global markets for their products (Watters 2010). Examples of Western patterns of illness being transferred to societies where they did not previously occur include depression in Japan (Vickery 2010) and anorexia nervosa (with the Western characteristics of the condition) in Hong Kong (Lee & Lee 1996).

The existence of culture-bound syndromes emphasises the important role that culture plays in people's conceptualisation of health. The fact that a set of subjectively constructed symptoms can be generally understood to indicate the presence of a particular condition that is recognised by members of specific linguistic/cultural groups shows that the nature of health and illness is not necessarily universal but depends to a significant extent on how people think about themselves and their physical and emotional reactions. It is important to understand that perceived health conditions are real to those involved, even when they do not have observable clinical signs, and contribute greatly to how people evaluate their own well-being. As health professionals it is important that we are aware of the degree to which culturally formed conceptualisations of health affect individuals and try to understand how others understand the experience of being ill.

Summary

Language and culture shape our understanding of what it means to be healthy or sick. Language provides the means of expressing perceptions about health and disease, while culture is a shared set of understandings that direct behaviour, attitudes, and views. Language and culture are related, and this relationship is studied in the field of sociolinguistics, which is concerned with the social uses of language.

While knowledge of culture may provide guidelines for how members of that culture may understand their own health, generalisations of this kind are not absolute, and there may be a great deal of variation among members of a group. Nonetheless, it is important to be aware of cultural differences in how people understand health and disease. Cultural competency is the ability to work effectively with people from different language and culture backgrounds. Australia is becoming more diverse, and health professionals have to be increasingly aware of and sensitive to cultural differences. Understanding the specific health needs and experience of Indigenous populations is an important aspect of cultural competency.

Cultural differences are often observed in the context of illness behaviour. These culturally determined behaviours relating to health are often at odds with evidence-based best practice that would be recommended by health professionals, but are often very deeply ingrained. As health professionals, we must be aware of potential differences, be prepared to understand how a patient or client feels, and approach our work with that individual without making judgments or criticisms.

Tutorial exercises

1. Based on your own experience, what aspects of language use or social interaction that are considered usual and appropriate in Australia might be misunderstood by people from a different cultural background?
2. Does the behaviour of health professionals ever contribute to communication problems with patients or clients from another cultural or linguistic background? Explain.
3. What kind of illness behaviour is expected where you come from? Explain and discuss.

Further reading

MacLachlan, M. (2006). *Culture and health: A critical perspective towards global health*. Chicester, UK: John Wiley & Sons.

Ritter, L.A., & Hoffman, N.A. (2010). *Multicultural health*. Sudbury, MA: Jones & Bartlett.

Singer, M., & Baer, H. (2007). *Introducing medical anthropology: A discipline in action*. Lanham, MD: AltaMira Press.

Websites

<www.nhmrc.gov.au/publications/synopses/hp25syn.htm>

The National Health and Medical Research Council offers a set of guidelines as well as other information on cultural competency.

<www.cyf.vic.gov.au/indigenous-initiatives/archive/practice-guides/aboriginal-cultural-competence-framework>

The Department of Human Services of Victoria has developed an Aboriginal cultural competency framework and matrix for working with the Indigenous community.

<www.indigenous.gov.au/About/Pages/closing_gap.aspx>

Close the Gap offers a variety of resources related to narrowing the disparity between Indigenous and non-Indigenous health in Australia.

<www.health.vic.gov.au/cald>

The Department of Health of Victoria offers information and advice on working with individuals from culturally and linguistically diverse (CALD) communities.

READING 5

Health and the media

Linda Portsmouth

TOPICS COVERED

This chapter covers the following topics:

- impact of the mass media on public health
- utilising the mass media to promote public health
- developing media materials to communicate health messages

KEY TERMS

Entertainment-education
Health literacy
Marketing
Mass media
Media advocacy
Public health communication
Semiotics
Social marketing

Introduction

The mass media constitute one of the social determinants of health. They are one of the many features of a society that impacts on people's knowledge, attitudes, and beliefs about health—and thus on their health behaviours. The mass media that people are exposed to, and interact with, have a measurable impact on their health choices and outcomes. Many people gain much of their understanding of health from what they see and hear on television, the internet, radio, and in newspapers and magazines.

The mass media are pervasive and persuasive, reaching population-wide with health information in a way that promotes and normalises the health concepts portrayed. The mass media play a part in the socialisation of children and adolescents—influencing them as to what to expect and what is expected of them in their society.

This chapter will discuss the impact of the mass media on health and how they can be used to promote health. News and current affairs, entertainment, the internet—and the advertising that pays for most of it—often contain messages of significance to public health. Public health professionals seek to explore the impact of the mass media—aiming to describe, quantify, and counter any negative influence on population health. We also study the effective techniques used by media professionals and learn to work in partnership with media professionals. This enables public health professionals to successfully communicate health messages via the mass media in a way that promotes population health. We seek to influence news and current affairs content to increase people's awareness of health issues, often advocating for a change in policy or legislation. We seek to influence existing entertainment and develop entertainment-education media. We have also successfully developed social marketing campaigns that include the use of advertising (among other activities) to promote health.

The chapter will also outline the process by which successful media materials and campaigns can be developed. Working closely with members of population groups at risk allows us to develop concepts, messages, and media materials that will communicate most effectively with that particular group—and thus have a greater impact on their health.

The mass media

Media means 'middle' in Latin and the media lie in the middle of the communication process—between the people who send messages and the people who receive them (O'Shaugnessy & Stadler 2008). The media are the means by which we 'transmit information and entertainment across time and space', with the **mass media** enabling mass communication to a large audience (p. 3). The mass media require technology and electricity to produce—and some mass media also require technology and electricity to consume at the other end. The mass media are one of society's ways of communicating with its members.

Mass media The means by which messages are communicated throughout a society, transmitting the same message to large numbers of people over a large geographical area at the same time, e.g. television, cinema, radio, the internet, newspapers, and magazines.

The mass media can be contrasted with 'limited-reach' media—which communicate with individuals or smaller groups of people within a limited geographical area. Limited-reach media include items such as pamphlets, DVDs, posters, T-shirts, drink bottles, stickers, and fridge magnets. Mass media can also be contrasted with 'folk media' or 'popular media'—the traditional media that humans used to communicate long before we could read and write. People everywhere enjoy music, song, theatre, puppetry, and dance as a form of entertaining communication. Public health professionals use folk media when these are the best way to communicate their health message; they might be the most culturally appropriate form of communication for the health issue and the target group. It may also be that the target group has low literacy levels and/or limited access to those mass media that require technology and electricity. The traditional dividing line between mass media and both limited-reach and folk media has become blurred over the last 15 years as limited-reach media such as pamphlets are now routinely put up on websites and gain frequent hits as people search for health information using their web browsers. Videos of folk media performances can now be seen on YouTube by people all over the world. Some may argue that social network services on the internet are limited-reach media as people need to sign up to access other members—but how many hundreds of millions of members are needed before Facebook can be considered a mass media tool in its own right?

The mass media constitute a powerful, far-reaching social influence—particularly with the impact of globalisation of media and the internet over the past couple of decades. Never before, in the history of the planet, have such a large proportion of the population been exposed to the same messages at the same time. O'Shaughnessy and Stadler (2008, p. 34) argue that the media 'show us what the world is like; they make sense of the world for us' as they represent, interpret, and evaluate the world, noting that many media products 'do not show or present the real world; they construct and re-present reality' (p. 35). The authors also acknowledge that the media are 'not the only social forces to make sense of the world for us, nor do they have total control over how we see and think about the world' (p. 35), noting the influence of, for example, family, religion, and education.

Mass media impact on health

Seeking health information via the mass media

When people look for health information, the media sources they seek out and trust are influenced by their level of health literacy, educational level, age, gender, ability to access the digital media, culture, and religion. **Health literacy** is 'the wide range of skills and competencies that people develop to seek out, comprehend, evaluate and use health information and concepts to make informed choices, reduce health risks, and increase quality of life' (Zarcadoolas et al. 2006, p. 5). Health literacy is related to, but not the same as, the ability to read and write. People can have high educational levels and yet not have highly developed health literacy—and vice versa. In an Australian study, Dart (2008) found that the internet is considered an important source of health information for most people, noting that people from lower socio-economic backgrounds had less access. He also noted well-developed health literacy skills—most people did not fully trust the internet, as they were aware that the credibility of websites varies.

Health literacy The individual's ability to successfully seek out, identify, interpret, and act on health information so as to protect and improve their health.

Mass media representation of health

The knowledge, attitudes, beliefs, and behaviours of many people are influenced by the health messages they are exposed to via the mass media. The health issues reported in the newspaper, explored on a television current affairs program, shared by celebrities on the front cover of a magazine displayed at the supermarket checkout, and experienced by characters on television dramas or in movies enters the public consciousness. People are stimulated to think about the particular health issue and, if they have no firsthand experience of the issue, will tend to think of it in the way it is presented by the media.

It is important to consider how the mass media can impact on the health of some of society's most vulnerable members: children and adolescents. Strasburger and colleagues (2009) discuss, for example, extensive research which concluded that aggression is a behaviour that children can learn from witnessing media violence and that while media violence is not the major cause of violence, it is a 'socially significant...part of a complex web of cultural and environmental factors that teach and reinforce aggression as a way of solving problems' (p. 193). Strasburger and colleagues also review the literature regarding children and adolescents' frequent exposure to sexual material via the mass media. They argue that most of this material is either suggestive or explicit, with few messages about safer sex and sexual responsibility. The authors note that several studies reveal that the media are an important source of information about sex for teenagers. Strasburger and colleagues also discuss several studies which conclude that teenagers who are exposed to a lot of media are more likely to

Stop and Think

Karl is 18. He is planning to go out to a nightclub with a group of his friends. He wants to have fun and would like to meet an attractive young woman and start a relationship. He is a bit shy and worries that he will say the wrong thing and not look or act 'cool'. In movies, he has noticed that the main male characters often seem to be having a drink while romantic things happen to them. A TV ad he has found amusing shows sporty guys having a great time together drinking beer and getting the attention of beautiful women by offering them a drink. Karl decides that he will have a few drinks to relax him and help him have a laugh with his mates.

» What could be the adverse health outcomes of his night out?

» How do you think his attitudes and behaviours are influenced by the media?

Jasmine is 13. She loves to access social networking media and has her own Twitter and Facebook accounts. Her parents have never accessed these media and so do not know how it works or who she is in contact with. She met a new friend in a chat room two months ago. He is a 14-year-old boy who lives a couple of suburbs away. They have been getting closer and closer and he has started to ask her about her body and if she has ever had sex. She has not told her parents about this boy because she thinks they would stop her talking to him if they knew that he had asked her to meet him in the local park next weekend.

» What could be the adverse health outcomes of this social media contact?

» How do you think Jasmine's attitudes and behaviours are influenced by the nature of the media she is using?

overestimate the number of their peers who are engaged in sexual activity, and feel pressure from the media to begin having sex; this increases the likelihood of earlier sexual activity.

The relationship between the mass media and mental health is another important example of mass media impact. In a review of two decades of research, Klin and Lemish (2008) conclude that the mass media have perpetuated misconceptions and stigma about people with mental illness due to 'inaccuracies, exaggeration, or misinformation' (p. 434). They argue that the mass media tend to portray people with mental illness as male, violent, and unpredictable. They note that through news coverage, entertainment, and advertising the mass media have shaped community attitudes towards people with mental illness and this has formed a barrier to such people seeking assistance. There is also a clear link between the mass media and suicide. Stack (2003) discusses the 'copycat effect'—that suicides reported in the media trigger people to emulate what they have seen reported. News reporting of real suicides (4.03 times) and suicides of celebrities (14.3 times) are more likely to trigger suicides than fictional suicides in the entertainment media (Stack 2003). Sudak and Sudak (2005) point to more suicides resulting from media reports that 'romanticize or dramatise the description of suicidal deaths' (p. 495). An Australian study supports these findings, reporting that 39% of media items resulted in increased male suicide and 31% resulted in increased female suicide (Pirkis et al. 2006). The effect noted by the researchers was more likely if there were several media reports, it was reported on television, and the suicides were completed rather than just attempted. Recommendations for media reporting were made by all of the above authors and a later study found more positive or neutral reporting of mental illness in the Australian news media (Henson et al. 2009). Media reporting of major disasters and terrorist attacks has also been implicated as a contributor to mental health problems such as post-traumatic stress disorder in children (Pfefferbaum et al. 2002; Saylor et al. 2003).

Marketing was defined by Kotler and colleagues (2009, p. 7) as 'an activity, set of institutions and processes for creating, communicating, delivering and exchanging offerings that have value for customers, clients, partners, and society at

Marketing The strategies used by commercial or non-profit enterprises—including the use of persuasive communications such as advertising—that aim to change attitudes so that the consumer feels positive towards, and decides to buy or use, the advertised product or service.

Stop and Think

Public health professionals are concerned when the product or service being marketed has a negative impact on health. Tobacco advertising is an important example. Tobacco was advertised in Australia—and still is in many places in the world—despite clear evidence that it damages health. How did the tobacco companies advertise their product? Australians only see tobacco advertising when they travel—or if the tobacco product is promoted by being placed into media they access such as movies at the cinema. Exploration of tobacco advertising gives an interesting insight into how advertising is crafted to be so persuasive to people. Link to these two websites to see some tobacco advertising posters—but do not be too influenced by them!

<http://wellmedicated.com/lists/40-gorgeous-vintage-tobacco-advertisements>

<www.tobaccofreekids.org/ad_gallery>

large'. Marketing is often thought of as just selling and advertising, but Kotler and colleagues (p. 5) describe these as 'the tip of the marketing iceberg'. Marketing discovers and meets the customer's needs, building an ongoing relationship that leads to profit. Marketers aim to provide the right product, at the right price, in the right place, at the right time—and advertising is one method used to promote this to customers. Advertising has an enormous impact on purchasing behaviours—or companies would not have advertising budgets worth millions of dollars.

Semiotics The study of the meaning of signs and symbols (e.g. images and colours) within a particular culture and how they communicate specific information and influence the interpretation of messages.

Semiotics is the study of sign systems and the meanings (feelings, beliefs, or ideas) that people within a culture attach to them (O'Shaughnessy & Stadler 2008). Signs and symbols include language, colours, objects, facial expressions, clothing, and hairstyles. Note the images and words that were used in the advertisements in the above two internet links. What were the advertisers promising when they placed the words and images alongside the cigarettes they were trying to sell? Analyse the semiotics. The people in the images are attractive and many of them are having a wonderful time with other attractive people. They are shown enjoying a golden and wealthy, carefree and relaxing, or highly romantic lifestyle. They are having fun or are quietly satisfied by their success. There are celebrities or trusted community members (e.g. doctors) promoting tobacco. The Virginia Slims ads promise a voice and freedom for women. The Marlboro ads connect their tobacco with a rugged outdoors cowboy lifestyle for men. Many of the ads suggest sexual success. Advertising often presents stereotypes of what is generally agreed in society as what we should aspire to be, do, or have in order to be successful. Stereotypes enable customers to quickly see that desirable people are connected to this product—thus the product must be desirable too. Tobacco advertising offers us a wonderful life if we smoke cigarettes.

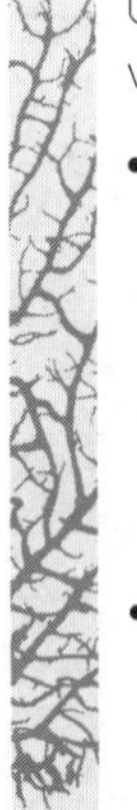

Mythbuster

Consider why you see the following as questionable. What does this tell you about our societal values?

- Tobacco companies, who are unable to advertise their product in Australia, are pouring millions of dollars into advertising in developing countries. Some of the advertising communicates the message–by use of stereotypes and images–that smoking is a thing done by people in rich countries and that if you smoke, you will appear more like them. The companies also use the full range of marketing techniques–such as giving away free cigarettes to young people at music concerts they sponsor. As the number of smokers in richer countries declines, the number in poorer countries is increasing.
- When people search for health information on the internet, some companies pay for advertising so that the link to their product appears at the top of the list of hits. Links to credible health information from reputable health organisations can be lower on the list than information pages put together by community members who do not know much about the health issue they are writing about.
- Some companies use the social media to market their products, particularly to children and young people. Marketers, for example, are able to enter chat rooms, posing as a child or teenager, and start off discussion about the product or service they are employed to promote.

Case Study 16.1 Television food advertising and children

The levels of childhood obesity are increasing globally with overweight and obese children more likely to become overweight adults who are at higher risk of health problems such as cardiovascular disease, diabetes, and some cancers (WHO 2010b). Using BMI measurements, it has been estimated that between 1985 and 1995 the proportion of Australian children who were overweight increased by between 60% and 70% and the proportion of Australian children who were obese more than tripled (Magarey et al. 2001; Booth et al. 2003). The most current Australian statistics, from the 2007 Australian National Children's Nutrition and Physical Activity Survey, indicated that 16.7% of children are overweight with a further 5.7% being obese (Commonwealth of Australia 2008).

Public health professionals have looked for the reason for this rise in childhood obesity. While there is a genetic predisposition to obesity (Wardle et al. 2008), this does not explain the rapid increase over the past two decades. The 2007 Australian National Children's Nutrition and Physical Activity Survey (Commonwealth of Australia 2008) revealed that 26.2% of children did not meet the recommended 60 minutes of moderate to vigorous physical activity per day and 66.6% of children exceeded the recommended two hours of screen time per day. There is a link between the amount of television watched and childhood obesity (Wake et al. 2003; Salmon et al. 2006). Public health professionals wondered if the time spent watching television rather than participating in physical activity has contributed to the development of obesity. The link between physical activity levels and obesity has been explored and it is now thought that the obesity causes the lack of physical activity rather than the other way around (Metcalf et al. 2010).

The Australian National Children's Nutrition and Physical Activity Survey (Commonwealth of Australia 2008) also discovered that Australian children's diets are higher in saturated fat, sugar, and salt—and lower in fruit and vegetables—than recommended by the Australian National Dietary Guidelines. Several Australian and international studies have demonstrated that children's television viewing is associated with a higher consumption of fatty foods, soft drinks, and sweet and salty snacks, and a lower consumption of fruit and vegetables (Woodward et al. 1997; Coon et al. 2001; Coon & Tucker 2002; Lowry et al. 2002; Boynton-Jarrett et al. 2003; Giammattei et al. 2003; Zuppa et al. 2003). Children from families that routinely watch TV during meal-times have been found to consume fewer fruits and vegetables and more fast foods than children whose families do not (Coon et al. 2001).

Australian children have been estimated to watch an average of 23 hours of television per week (just over three hours per day) (Woodward et al. 1997; Story 2003) with an average of eight food ads per hour, and thus are estimated to be exposed to over 10,000 food advertisements every year (Story 2003). Almost 80% of these food ads are for non-core foods and approximately 50% are for fast foods, chocolate, and confectionary (Zuppa et al. 2003; Neville et al. 2005; Chapman et al. 2006). Children of all ages who watch more television have consistently been found to desire more advertised products than children who watch less television (Robinson 2001). Children ask for and eat the foods that they see advertised (Hitchings & Moynihan 1998) and eat more of them after seeing television advertisements—particularly obese children (Halford et al. 2007). Giveaways (such as toys) and messages promoting taste or fun were the most used marketing strategies to Australian children, with the most frequently used features being cartoons and scenes of people eating the food within a social setting (Hill & Radimer 1997). Goris et al. (2010) attribute 10–28% of Australia's childhood obesity to television food advertising.

There has been an international call for the banning of television food advertising to children (WHO 2010b)—and this has already occurred in several countries. The Australian Television Communications and Media Authority has produced the Children's Television Standards 2009 which list standards that advertising to children is required to adhere to: <www.acma.gov.au/webwr/aba/contentreg/codes/television/documents/childrens_tv_standards_2009.pdf>. These standards stipulate that such advertising requirements as popular characters cannot be used to promote foods during children's viewing times, pressure cannot be put on children to ask parents to purchase, children who have the food cannot be shown as superior, and those who buy the food cannot be implied to be more generous. Chapman and others (2006) and Kelly and Chau (2007) have, however, reported frequent breaches of these standards.

Australian parents are concerned about the amount of advertising their children are exposed to and support tighter restrictions on television food advertising (Morley et al. 2008). Advocacy groups (see the media advocacy section below) are lobbying for the Australian Government to ban advertising of unhealthy food to children but this has not yet occurred. Some influential advocacy and information-sharing groups include the Public Health Association of Australia, who have written a policy document, <www.phaa.net.au>; the Australian Council on Children and the Media, <www.youngmedia.org.au>; Coalition on Food Advertising to Children, <www.cancercouncil.com.au/cfac>; and The Parent's Jury, <www.parentsjury.org.au>.

Utilising the mass media for health promotion

Public health communication
Uses a variety of carefully developed communication strategies to improve or maintain the health of a population.

Health communication is the 'study and use of communication strategies to inform and influence individual and community decisions that enhance health' (National Cancer Institute 2002, p. 2). **Public health communication** can be seen as a subset of health communication and 'focuses more on the health of communities and populations', being 'inherently interventionist, seeking to promote and protect health through change at all levels of influence' (Bernhardt 2004, p. 2052). The major mass media communication strategies used in public health communication are discussed in the sections below: social marketing, media advocacy, and entertainment-education. Public health communication aims to change knowledge, attitudes, beliefs, and, ultimately, behaviours. The term 'behaviour change communication' is often used, particularly in developing countries, to refer to those communication programs aiming for behaviour change. In developed countries, 'social marketing' is more commonly used to refer to such programs.

Social marketing
The application of commercial marketing communication techniques to the promotion of health and other socially desirable outcomes.

Social marketing

The most commonly cited definition for **social marketing** is that of Andreasen (1995, p. 7), who explains it as 'the application of commercial marketing technologies to the analysis, planning, execution, and evaluation of programmes designed to influence the voluntary behaviour of target audiences in order to improve their personal welfare and that of society'. Social marketers can be seen as 'selling' health and social development. The advertising on television, radio, and in newspapers—urging the community to quit smoking, drive within the speed limit, watch their waistline or increase their physical activity levels—are very visible examples of this conceptualisation of social marketing.

Social marketing campaigns have successfully influenced population-wide changes in knowledge, attitudes, beliefs, and behaviours of relevance to public health. Campaigns have targeted a range of public health issues; see the list of websites at the end of this chapter to explore some current Australian campaign messages, materials, and evaluations. Social marketing is suitable for communicating simple messages about public health issues that affect a large proportion of the general population. There is a mass media campaign aiming to increase people's physical activity levels to 30 minutes a day, for example, but readers would not see a mass media campaign that promoted safer injecting techniques by injecting drug users (that very important public health message is best communicated in a trusted face-to-face setting). Messages and images that may offend sections of the community are usually avoided. While there are occasional safe sex campaigns in the mass media, for example, the messages and materials are not as explicit as the limited-reach media developed for specific target groups. Most of the links at the end of the chapter relate to physical health, but note the last link to the innovative Western Australian 'Act, Belong, Commit', which is the first population-wide attempt to promote mental health.

Social marketing campaigns are most effective if the mass media campaign is coordinated with limited-reach media and activities within the community that support and extend the reach of the 'brand' and the message (Donovan & Henley 2010). A current, successful, and comprehensive Australian social marketing strategy is the 'Go for 2 & 5®' campaign promoting increased consumption of fruit and vegetables (see Case Study 16.2).

Donovan and Henley (2010, p. 1) take a wider view of social marketing, arguing that it is 'the one discipline to embody, within one framework, most of the principles, concepts and tools necessary for the development and implementation of effective social change campaigns'. They believe that Andreasen's definition needs to be extended to include involuntary behaviours because we now know that behaviours are influenced by environment and are thus not entirely under an individual's control. Social marketing, they state, also needs to target policymakers in order to create supportive environments. They also propose that social marketing needs to enable individuals to reach their potential by seeking to change social structures and influence the social determinants of health. Donovan and Henley would thus argue that both media advocacy and entertainment-education—discussed in the following sections—are actually social marketing activities.

Case Study 16.2 The 'Go for 2 & 5®' Campaign

<www.gofor2and5.com.au>

<www.crunchandsip.com.au>

The 'Go for 2 & 5®' Campaign is a national multi-media campaign successfully using the mass media (television, radio, newspaper, magazines, and the internet). This campaign developed paid advertising, gained publicity via public relations events, and launched excellent websites.

There has also been the development of many limited-reach media (e.g. cookbooks, pamphlets, posters, billboards, signs on taxis), point-of-sale marketing (e.g. signs on supermarket trolleys, cooking demonstrations) and school-based activities (such as 'Crunch & Sip®', a program in which schools take a formal break every day for children to drink water and eat fruit or vegetables).

Australians do not eat the recommended amount of fruit and vegetables for good health and the prevention of many chronic diseases such as cardiovascular disease and some cancers. The 'Go for 2 & 5®' campaign, as summarised by Pollard et al. (2008a, 2009a), was first run by the Department of Health in Western Australia for the three years from March 2002 to June 2005. Research revealed that people knew fruit and vegetables were 'good for them' but they did not know the recommended level of intake and thought that they were already eating enough. Research also uncovered that people did not believe they had enough time or the skills to prepare vegetables. The campaign aimed to increase Western Australian adults' knowledge about the required number of serves, inform them as to what constitutes a serve, increase their perceived need to eat more (especially vegetables), and persuade them that vegetables were easy to prepare and eat. The main target group was the family meal preparer and grocery shopper. All of the campaign materials were strongly branded with the registered, colourful, memorable logo and attention-grabbing vegetable characters based on the celebrities who provided their voices. Explore the 'Go for 2 & 5®' website above to see many current campaign materials. The first message was: 'It is easy to get an extra serving of vegies into your day.' In 2003, a question was added to encourage honest self-assessment: 'How many servings of vegies did you really eat today?'

Pollard and colleagues (2008a, 2009a) also detailed how telephone surveys tracked the responses of thousands of Western Australian adults over time—before, during, and after the campaign. These surveys discovered that 90% of adults in the Perth metropolitan area were aware of the campaign—mainly via the television advertising. The surveys revealed that the campaign successfully increased awareness of the recommended servings and improved attitudes towards eating more fruit and vegetables, and that consumption rose as a result. From 2002 to 2005 there was an increase from 1.6 to 1.8 serves of fruit, and vegetable intake rose from 2.6 to 3.2. The proportion of the adult population who reported eating the recommended two or more serves of fruit a day and five or more serves of veg rose from 7% in 2001 to 13.4% in 2005. Pollard and colleagues (2009b) noted the direct link between increasing knowledge and behaviour change—people who knew what a correct serving size was were more likely to eat more fruit and vegetables. Other Australian states without the campaign did not show this increase and had consumption levels similar to Western Australia before the campaign (Pollard et al. 2008a). These increases were so impressive that the campaign has been implemented by all other Australian states and territories.

This success was not just due to the visible campaign. 'Go for 2 & 5®' also demonstrated the successful impact of taking the wider view of social marketing discussed by Donovan and Henley (2010). Partnerships were developed between government organisations, non-government organisations, and industry in order to increase the availability of affordable, high-quality fruit and vegetables and to increase opportunities for the consumption of fruit and vegetables within different community settings (Pollard et al. 2008b). The authors listed some achievements that targeted the environmental and social determinants of fruit and vegetable consumption.

Examples included the development of nutrition policies for schools and childcare centres; award schemes that rewarded the food industry; promotion of the correct storage, handling, and preparation of fruit and vegetables; and supporting welfare agencies in the provision of fruit and vegetables.

Media advocacy

'Advocate' comes from the Latin word meaning 'to be called to stand beside' (Stafford et al. 2009) and advocacy is 'the pursuit of influencing outcomes—including public policy and resource allocation decisions within political, economic, and social systems and institutions—that directly affect people's lives' (Cohen 2001, p. 7). Chapman (2004a, p. 361) states that **media advocacy** aims to 'develop and shape...news stories in ways that build support for public policies and ultimately influence those who have the power to change or preserve laws, enact policies, and fund interventions that can influence whole populations'. While some advocacy is more behind-the-scenes, such as meetings with politicians or policymakers, media advocacy involves public health professionals carefully planning and telling their 'story' so that it is reported in the mass media in a way that can bring about the changes in society that they desire.

Media advocacy Aims to stimulate public support—and obtain the attention and sympathy of policymakers and legislators—to gain changes in law and policy which impact on public health.

Gaining this kind of publicity for a health issue can be cost-free—as compared to the high cost of a large social marketing campaign, for example—but it is less within the control of public health professionals. Journalists and news editors decide what will be reported—as well as how, when, and where it will be reported. News is also a 'perishable commodity'—it will only be reported for a short time before it is 'yesterday's news' (Howard & Mathews 2006, p. 27).

Public health professionals working in media advocacy need to develop good working relationships with journalists. They need to know what journalists consider 'newsworthy' as this will affect how health messages need to be 'framed' so as to gain maximum media interest. Newsworthy issues, according to Howard and Mathews (2006), are those that are considered important; interesting (e.g. unusual, entertaining, human interest, emotional); timely (e.g. current, new); close to people (e.g. local issues); or prominent (i.e. famous). Public health professionals are more likely to have their message communicated if they can provide memorable stories that will connect with people's emotions. They need, for example, to give local statistics; introduce local members of the target group who are willing to be photographed or filmed and tell their story; give a new angle to the issue such as recent and compelling evidence; suggest powerful images that can be photographed or filmed; and involve celebrities or high-profile spokespeople.

Public health professionals working for large organisations will usually have a public relations or media department to assist them—while those who work for small community-based organisations will need to develop some media relations skills. After careful planning, the issue in question needs to be brought to the attention of journalists. Large organisations have the skills and resources to hold press conferences; this works well when the issue is of interest to journalists and you can be sure they will attend. Many health organisations fax or email media releases (short written pieces summing up the main points about the issue) in order to interest the journalist, to contact them or attend an event. Journalists are often also open to clear, concise emails or clear telephone messages, particularly if they have worked with the public health professionals before. The events can be initiated in order to show that many and/or prominent people feel strongly about the issues. A media release, for example, can invite journalists to a protest, a public meeting, the presentation of a petition to a politician, or the launch of an intervention that is being attended by a politician or a concerned celebrity. Another effective, no-cost strategy is to write a letter to the editor of the newspaper. This way—should the letter be well written and topical enough to be chosen—a public health viewpoint can be put onto the public agenda quickly using a few words in an email. Once media interest is shown in their issue, public health professionals need to plan for newspaper, television, or radio interviews. They need to find and train articulate and credible spokespeople—while being aware that some interviews about urgent issues can happen with little warning!

Stafford and colleagues (2009), in the reading list at the end of this chapter, is an excellent and easily accessible 'how to' guide for public health professionals. This manual describes how public health professionals can plan and implement media advocacy strategies—including how to write media releases and letters to the editor, how to prepare for interviews, and how to influence journalists and politicians.

Case Study 16.3 Anti-tobacco media advocacy

Australia has implemented a highly successful social marketing campaign encouraging people to quit smoking: <www.quitnow.info.au>. It supports cessation activities and is an international leader in the use of media advocacy to create supportive environments that encourage people not to start smoking and assist smokers to quit.

Chapman and Wakefield (2001, p. 274), in their exploration of 30 years of tobacco control in Australia, cited tobacco company documents that stated that 'Australia has one of the best organised, best financed, most politically savvy and well-connected anti-smoking movements in the world. They are aggressive and have been able to use the levers of power very effectively to propose and pass draconian legislation...Australia is a seed-bed for anti-smoking programs around the world'. Chapman and Wakefield went on to chronicle the achievements gained by tobacco control advocacy since 1970: harm reduction via reduction in the tar and nicotine levels in cigarettes; 'civil disobedience' as activists 'graffitied' tobacco advertising billboards with anti-tobacco messages; banning of tobacco advertising and sponsorship; tobacco taxes; replacement of tobacco sponsorship of sport and arts by using some of the tobacco tax income; warnings printed on cigarette packs; banning of the small packs popular with children; banning of smokeless tobacco; and the banning of smoking in transport, workplaces, and domestic environments.

Smoking rates in Australia have fallen from their peak levels of 72% for adult males in 1945 and 31% for females in 1983 (Chapman & Wakefield 2001) to some of the lowest in the world: 18% for males and 15.2% in females aged 14 years or over—as estimated from the 2007 National Drug Strategy Survey (AIHW 2010a). This survey also revealed that more than half the Australian population have never smoked and approximately a quarter of people are ex-smokers. Statistical projections released in 2006 estimated that if current trends continue, smoking will disappear in Australia by 2028 (Daube & Walker 2008).

Chapman and Wakefield (2001, p. 278) noted that media advocacy 'challenges radio and television audiences and newspaper readerships—including the politicians at whom it is often ultimately directed—to locate themselves in a moral debate'. They argued that casting the tobacco industry as 'pariahs' who require heavy regulation has been an essential part of this process—giving the examples of how advocates 'framed' tobacco as a series of 'newsworthy' issues such as advertising seducing vulnerable children, and the hidden and dangerous chemical additives in tobacco which should be revealed. Advocacy's role was to successfully frame the public health issue so it gained the support of the public and politicians—and to communicate problems which require solutions that politicians are usually responsible for finding (Chapman & Wakefield 2001).

The media advocacy in Australia was first undertaken by the advocacy group Australian Council on Smoking and Health (ACOSH), which was formed in 1967 out of frustration with the government response to calls for tobacco control (Daube & Walker 2008). ACOSH worked in partnership with government health departments and non-government organisations such as the Heart Foundation, Cancer Council, and the Australian Medical Association. Daube and Walker described ACOSH's attention-getting media strategies which reduced the credibility of the tobacco industry, increased the sympathy of the media, and eventually gained the required legislation. These strategies included buying shares in tobacco companies so they could attend AGMs and ask questions; holding a press conference releasing a report on the number of body parts removed each year due to smoking; a 'death cards' campaign where doctors sent postcards to politicians when their patients' deaths were smoking-related; a report for each MP showing the impact of smoking in their electorate; and presenting statistics in forms that could be easily understood and reported on—such as bookies' odds.

It is interesting to note that, after exploring the concepts of deviance and stigma in Chapter 15, 'smoking, smokers and the tobacco industry are today routinely depicted in everyday discourse and media representations in a variety of overwhelmingly negative ways' (Chapman & Freeman 2008, p. 25). Mass media advocacy and social marketing, according to Chapman and Freeman, have been so successful in 'denormalising' smoking behaviour that this national 'culture change' may be impacting on the mental and social health of people who smoke. Smoking is now seen as dirty and smelly and smokers are now publically framed as selfish, undesirable, undereducated, lower class, or addicts, who are a drain on health services and should not be employed (Chapman & Freeman 2008). A 2007 Western Australian survey revealed that smokers now feel like 'social pariahs' and reported that they receive 'disdainful looks' and 'social verbal bashing' when they smoke in public—with many stating that they would consider quitting so that they could 'rejoin society' (Carter 2008, p. 28). This situation presents an ethical dilemma. Public health professionals used effective media strategies that aimed to reduce the population level of smoking—placing the overall population health 'good' above the mental and social health of the minority of people who smoke. Public health would normally seek to promote the health of all population groups—so this is a rare case where public health is culpable of a negative impact on the mental and social health of a particular group in society.

Entertainment-education

The terms **entertainment-education** and *edu-tainment* have been used interchangeably in the past. De Fossard (2008) notes that a clear difference between the two is becoming widely accepted and described the key difference. Edu-tainment is education made entertaining, by the use of a story for example, so that learners are emotionally engaged in the educational experience.

Entertainment-education
A mass media 'vehicle' which is designed to entertain a wide general audience while changing societal attitudes and norms. It models and normalises behaviour change that promotes health and social development.

Entertainment-education is an entertainment experience that is sought out and appreciated by a general audience who are emotionally involved with characters they identify with. Within this entertainment experience, the 'behavior change messages are woven and modeled gradually, naturally and subtly' (De Fossard 2008, p. 19). Entertainment-education connects with people in a unique way, becomes a part of the social fabric of their lives, and thus a social influence on their health.

Most interestingly, Singhal and Rogers (2004) point out that the first recognisable entertainment-education intervention was in Australia with a radio series called 'The Lawsons' in 1944—which encouraged farmers to adopt new agricultural innovations. However, they also note that for a long period the most common form of entertainment-education was donor-supported television and radio soap opera in developing countries which communicated health messages to audiences without much mass media exposure. According to Barker (2005), one soap opera was based on the successful formula pioneered by Miguel Sabido in the late 1970s and early 1980s, who made an enormous impact on family planning in Mexico using serial television dramas (telenovelas). The 'Sabido Methodology' results in a serial drama that captures people's attention and emotions over several months or years. This allows the audience to increasingly identify with the main characters as they change their behaviour slowly, in a realistic way, in a realistic social context—with various subplots enabling the introduction of different issues in a believable way through different characters (Barker 2005). Techniques used to keep the audiences thinking and wondering about the storylines include mystery, suspense, dilemmas, and 'cliffhangers' at the end of episodes (Singhal & Rogers 2004). Piotrow and De Fossard (2004) point out that when communicating health risks that are routine or longer-term, well-written drama scripts can make the health issue appear more important, urgent, or dangerous. They mention examples such as contraceptive pills being thrown into the fire, highlighting that they need to be taken daily, and a fruit seller who contaminates his fruit due to poor personal hygiene, resulting in a stampede of people to the latrine. Singhal and Rogers (2004) note that evaluation of this type of entertainment-education reveals that it is memorable—people can recall health messages years later—and it has resulted in millions of people changing their health behaviours.

Entertainment-education is now widely applied and many forms of entertainment media are utilised. Some entertainment-education reaches a local audience—particularly when folk media such as theatre is used. Other media, such as comics and fotonovelas (stories told by the use of photos with brief dialogue in 'bubble text'), are reaching an increasingly wider audience due to dissemination via the internet. The scope of mass media entertainment-education ranges from the placement of a few lines of dialogue into an existing mass media program (e.g. the Harvard Alcohol Project; see Case Study 16.4) to an ongoing multi-media TV, radio, internet, and print program spanning several countries over several years (e.g. Soul City; see Case Study 16.5).

Case Study 16.4 The Harvard Alcohol Project, USA

The Harvard Alcohol Project (Winsten 1994; Winsten & DeJong 2001) is the first, biggest, and most famous example of public health working with the existing commercial mass media to successfully promote a health message to an entire population. This project was launched across the USA in 1988 and ran until 1992. It demonstrated how a new concept and new behaviour could be introduced and disseminated via entertainment programming to a whole society—and actually shift social norms (i.e. what is considered normal behaviour).

All of the major Hollywood studios and the ABC, CBS, and NBC television networks worked with the Center for Health Communication at Harvard School of Public Health to promote the idea of the 'designated driver'. The designated driver is the one in the group who does not drink alcohol because they are driving—and getting everyone else home safely. It was intended, according to Winsten (1994), to give the non-drinker's role 'social legitimacy' and to encourage people to plan for their transport if they intended to drink. The author outlined how he met with more than 250 television producers and writers who agreed to insert drink-driving prevention messages, including mention of designated drivers, into scripts of top-rated television programs, such as 'Cheers', 'L.A. Law', and 'The Cosby Show'. The characters of the shows acted as role models for safer behaviours. Over four years, more than 160 prime-time television programs, with audiences of up to 45 million, incorporated the health message. At the same time, the networks also agreed to air frequent Public Service Announcements promoting the designated driver concept; a number of prominent individuals and organisations endorsed the message and the campaign was widely reported in the news media (Winsten 1994; Winsten & DeJong 2001).

The term 'designated driver' became a household phrase in the USA, appearing in the 1991 edition of Webster's College Dictionary (Winsten 1994). Research revealed that, by 1998, 62% of adults who were frequent drinkers had been designated drivers or had been driven home by one (Center for Health Communication 2011). The Center for Health Communication reported that a 30% reduction in alcohol related traffic fatalities was gained over the six years following the launch of the campaign—compared with a reduction of 0% in the three years preceding the campaign. This was equated to 50,000 lives saved by the end of 1998.

Case Study 16.5 Soul City, South Africa

<www.soulcity.org.za>

'Soul City: Institute for Health and Development Communication' is a highly successful mass media entertainment-education program. It is a highly recognised and trusted source of health information in South Africa and was the first to address national health priorities with an ongoing nationwide multi-media strategy.

Soul City was established in 1992 by two medical doctors, Garth Japhet and Shereen Usdin, who wanted to prevent the serious health and social issues they saw impacting on the lives of their patients. Dr Japhet had been writing a newspaper column but realised that he was only reaching people who were literate (UNAIDS 2005). He then discovered that educational programs on South African television might reach an audience of 500,000 while 'prime-time' television drama would reach an audience of more than 7 million (UNAIDS 2005). Drs Japhet and Usdin brought together government, donors, and business to develop prime-time, health-promoting mass media that is entertaining and well made (Singhal & Rogers 2003; UNAIDS 2005).

Singhal and Rogers (2003), UNAIDS (2005), and Usdin and colleagues (2004) describe the media materials produced by Soul City and how success is ensured by undertaking extensive research with audience groups to develop realistic scripts that resonate powerfully with their audience. Each year Soul City produces a 13-part one-hour television drama on the most popular television channel; 60 episodes of 15-minute prime-time radio drama (with different characters and storylines to the television series) in nine languages covering all regional stations on a daily basis; and three nationally distributed 36-page booklets which are designed around the television characters and serialised in 11 major newspapers. Soul City also has relationships with newspaper journalists who regularly publish features based in Soul City activities. In 2000, for children aged 8 to 10, they began 'Soul Buddyz', which also includes a television series, radio series, and print materials.

Soul City reaches millions of people in South Africa and in the neighbouring countries of Botswana, Zimbabwe, Lesotho, Swaziland, Namibia, and Zambia. The most recent evaluation available from Soul City (Health and Development Africa 2007) is of Series 7, which broadcast in 2005 and 2006. Research revealed that 87% of the total adult population of South Africa was exposed to at least one Soul City program component in 2006—with wide reach across rural and urban areas and all educational levels—particularly among black Africans; 76% of women and 69% of men watched Soul City on television in 2006—with 60% of those watching nine or more episodes. This series had a measurable impact on the HIV issues it raised including increased HIV testing, increased condom use, and an increased willingness to accept and assist people living with HIV/AIDS. Soul City has been identified by the World Health Organization as an example of best practice in the use of mass media to communicate about HIV/AIDS (UNAIDS 2005).

Soul City has also had an influence on knowledge, attitudes, and behaviours relating to many other health and social issues. Usdin and colleagues (2004) detail the famous example of the impact that 1999's Series 4 had on community practices relating to domestic violence. In one episode, people in a neighbourhood gather around a house where a husband was beating his wife, loudly banging cooking pots and pans to show their disapproval. This newly suggested practice of pot beating—or making other loud banging noises—was reported to occur in response to domestic violence in several locations after this episode was broadcast. This series also resulted in communities organising several protest marches to highlight violence against women. An evaluation of this series reported that it stimulated public discussion of domestic violence; increased recognition of the abuse of women; increased knowledge and use of a telephone hotline; and many viewers subsequently did something to stop domestic violence in their lives or in the lives of others. Interviews with viewers revealed that some women had invited their husbands to watch episodes so that they could recognise their perpetration of domestic violence—and that some men who saw it recognised for the first time that their violence against their wives was wrong.

Developing media materials to communicate health messages

The National Cancer Institute (2002) in the USA has developed a useful way of conceptualising the process of developing health communication media materials. Media materials are most successfully developed when public health and media professionals follow the four stages described below. This process can be used for the development of mass media, limited-reach media, and folk media materials. The process is a cycle because, after evaluating the health communication program they have undertaken, public health professionals are better informed as they plan for future communications.

Figure 16.1 The stages in the health communication process

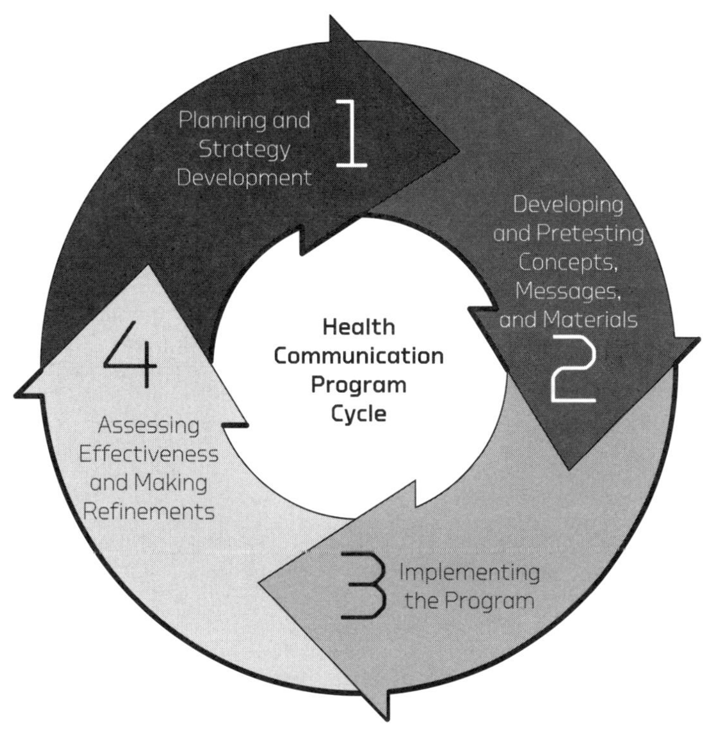

Source: NCI 2002, p. 11

Stage 1: Planning and strategy development

Adequate time spent at this vital stage will ensure a greater chance of success at later stages, and for the health communication program's overall objectives. Some people want to rush into developing their media materials as the first stage of their intervention; these people need to be held back and made to wait.

Public health professionals first need to assess the health issue and identify all parts of a possible solution. It could be that communication to the community via media materials is not the best plan of action—or that it is an excellent idea but needs to happen concurrently with communication with policymakers about changes in policy or with healthcare providers about changes in health services. It could be that the communication needs to be accompanied by changes to physical infrastructure or the social environment. It can be impossible for individuals to decide to change their behaviours if the things they need to do this are not available. We cannot, for example, produce a social marketing campaign encouraging women to go for breast screening if they are unable to access affordable, acceptable screening services close to where they live. It is difficult for people living in remote and rural areas of Australia to 'Go for 2 & 5' when the local shops do not stock affordable, high-quality fresh fruit and vegetables.

Public health professionals need to find out as much as possible about their intended audience. The target group may be of a different culture, language, religion, gender, age, and educational level than the public health professionals. Research will often reveal that the target group is made up of different audiences that require different media and messages. Surveys, interviews, or focus groups can be used to ask members of the target group such questions as: What do you know about this issue? What are you doing now? What have you tried before? What happened then? What do you think about it? What do you believe has caused it or is making it worse? What would help you to change? What is stopping you from changing? What would be the benefit—or the cost—of change to you? Do you think it is worth changing? What media do you pay attention to? What media do you believe? What media would you trust communicating about this health issue? Where are you and what are you doing when you access this media? The answers to these sorts of questions are invaluable in developing communication objectives and planning for the communication program. If these questions were not asked, public health professionals would develop media materials that made sense to them—not to a target group with a different understanding and lived experience of the particular health issue.

Stage 2: Developing and pretesting concepts, messages, and materials

The first thing public health professionals need to do in this stage is to review existing media materials and discover if there are any that meet their needs. If the decision is made that new materials need to be developed, it is useful to work with experienced media professionals who have expertise in research to ensure the concepts, messages, and materials are going to be the most effective for that particular target group. The concepts and messages need to be put together (in terms of words, images, colours, and sounds) in a way that is understandable, believable, convincing, and culturally appropriate. All of the information discovered in Stage 1 needs to be considered as this will shape the concept and the message. It is good practice to involve members of the target group in developing the concepts, messages, and materials. It is essential to then test the materials with different members of the target group to check that they are having the intended effects.

Stage 3: Implementing the program

The concepts, messages, and materials implemented are as varied as the health issue and the target group. Mass media approaches can be expensive and may not be the correct approach for the issue and target group. Mass media campaigns have been found to work best when an appropriate range of limited-reach media and person-to-person approaches also form part of the plan of action. Public health professionals can discover the kinds of messages and media that have worked for other people in similar projects—but must always be most influenced by what their target group tells them. Members of the target group are the experts on what will work for them, and it might not be what the public health professionals expect to be doing. Public health professionals may find that directly involving the target group in the program implementation (e.g. peer outreach and support) may enhance the impact of the media materials produced.

Stage 4: Assessing effectiveness and making refinements

Public health professionals need to ask such questions as: How appropriate was the message for the target audience? How effective were the media channels? How well did the message reach the target audience? What changes resulted? To what extent were the goals achieved? Were the benefits worth the cost? Evaluating the health communication program is not something that can be left until the end. Stage 1 activities include putting plans in place for evaluation. The program, methods, and media materials need to be evaluated while they are being developed and used. Surveys, interviews, and focus groups can assist in gaining the required information, but information can also be collected while the program is running. The people delivering the program can record useful information while they work (e.g. number of calls to the telephone information and support line or hits on the website after advertising appears in print, television, or radio).

Summary

The mass media constitute a powerful social determinant of health. Many people gain much of their understanding of health from messages in the mass media. This influences their health knowledge, attitudes, beliefs, and behaviours.

The mass media can have a negative impact on health. Media representation and reporting of violence, sexuality, body image, mental health, and suicide, for example, have been implicated in poor health outcomes. The marketing of products and services detrimental to health (such as tobacco) are of public health concern. Public health professionals need to recognise and study these negative impacts—and then act to counter them.

Once the mass media impacts on health are understood, the public health professional can use this knowledge to work in partnership with media professionals to utilise the mass media to promote health. Social marketing, media advocacy, and entertainment-education are the forms this activity usually takes—and all have demonstrated a strong, positive impact on public health.

Public health professionals need to carefully plan, implement, and evaluate health communication programs. It is vital, at all stages of the health communication process, to work closely with members of the media audience (target group) in order to successfully develop media materials to communicate appropriate health messages.

Tutorial exercises

1 Watch the American documentary *Super Size Me*, which won the Academy Award for best documentary in 2004. It is accessible in most university libraries and video shops. This film documents one man's decision to consume McDonald's food and drink for every meal for 30 days—with the resulting negative impact on his physical and mental health. What role do you think fast food marketing plays in the 'obesity epidemic'? Note how the documentary was made. What choices did the filmmakers make (in terms of words, vision, sound, music, and graphics) in order to make the film more persuasive?
2 Watch a commercial television station during a timeslot for children's programs. Note the advertisements for food and drink. Choose one of them and record it if possible to bring to

class. What messages are being communicated by the advertisement? What stereotypes, images, sounds, music, and colours were brought together to make the advertisement more persuasive to children? Do you think the advertisement adheres to the Australian Children's Television Standards?

3 Find an internet site that is potentially harmful to health. It may contain incorrect information, have information presented with bias (e.g. a commercial site selling 'cures'), or openly promote poor health choices (e.g. anorexia, suicide). Note the URL. What are the main messages being communicated? How were they communicated? What words, images, colours, and sound were used—and what do those choices communicate? Is the site presented as being more credible than it really is? Does it contain references for scientific information given? Does it contain advertising? What other sites does it link to? Is it clear who wrote it and how you can contact them? How might it harm health?

4 Link to the examples of the Australian social marketing campaign websites listed below. Watch their television advertisements. For each advertisement, answer the following questions: Who do you think the target group is? What is the key message? Note the way the advertisement has been constructed. What do you think the initial research revealed about the target group?

Further reading

Cancer Council Western Australia (2008). *The progress of tobacco control in Western Australia: Achievements, challenges and hopes for the future*. Perth: Cancer Council Western Australia. <www.cancerwa.asn.au/resources/2010-07-07-Tobacco-Control-Monograph.pdf>.

Donovan, R., & Henley, N. (2010). *Principles and practice of social marketing: An international perspective*, 2nd edn. Melbourne: IP Communications.

Howard, C.M., & Mathews, W.K. (2006). *On deadline: Managing media relations*, 4th edn. Long Grove, IL: Waveland Press.

National Cancer Institute (2002). *Making health communication programs work*. Bethesda, MD: National Institutes of Health, US Department of Health and Human Services. <www.cancer.gov/pinkbook>.

O'Shaughnessy, M., & Stadler, J.M. (2008). *Media and society*, 4th edn. Melbourne: Oxford University Press.

Stafford, J., Mitchell, H., Stoneham, M., & Daube, M. (2009). *Advocacy in action: A toolkit for public health professionals*, 2nd edn. Perth: Public Health Advocacy Institute of Western Australia. <www.phaiwa.org.au/index.php/component/attachments/download/35>.

Websites

<www.comminit.com>

The Communication Initiative Network connects people from all over the world so they can share their work in media communication to promote health, peace, and social development.

<www.cdc.gov/healthcommunication>

The Centers for Disease Control and Prevention's 'gateway' to many health communication and social marketing resources.

<www.jhuccp.org>

Center for Communication Programs, Johns Hopkins Bloomberg School of Public Health promotes international public health through partnering organisations to assist them in health communication. This website links to many resources such as downloadable publications/reports and examples of health communication materials.

<www.populationmedia.org>

The Population Media Center works to improve global health through the use of entertainment-education strategies. This website shares their current projects and links to many resources.

<www.communicationforsocialchange.org>

The Communication for Social Change Consortium is a non-profit organisation working globally to help people living in poor communities to communicate in such a way as to influence the change they need in their societies and in their lives.

<www.drinkingnightmare.gov.au>

<www.alcoholthinkagain.com.au>

<www.rta.nsw.gov.au/roadsafety/speedandspeedcameras/campaigns>

<www.ors.wa.gov.au/Campaigns/Pages/campaign.aspx>

<www.drugs.health.gov.au>

<www.quitnow.info.au>

<www.safesexnoregrets.com.au>

<www.findthirtyeveryday.com.au>

<www.drawthelinewa.com.au>

<www.actbelongcommit.org.au>

Interesting examples of Australian social marketing interventions and their media materials.

<http://social-marketing.org>

<www.hc-sc.gc.ca/ahc-asc/activit/marketsoc/index-eng.php>

Useful social marketing sites in the US and Canada.

<www.phaiwa.org.au>

The Public Health Advocacy Institute of WA.

READING 6

Employment, Working Conditions, and Health

Objectives

By the end of your study of this chapter, you should be able to

- understand how employment, unemployment, and health interrelate;
- appreciate the health implications of recent changes in the labour market;
- see how on-the-job experiences affect health and well-being;
- assess how policy responses to employment and working conditions impact on population health.

Synopsis

Chapter 8 reviews the research relating to the health effects of employment, unemployment, and working conditions. It examines the changes that have taken place in the labour market and the workplace over the past few decades as globalization and neo-liberalism have changed the employment landscape. The chapter ends with a discussion of positive changes that can be made to working conditions and employment benefits.

The Centrality of Employment to Adult Health

Pause and Reflect • Employment, Health, and Well Being

What features and consequences of employment influence the health and well being of the individual?

Employment in the Americas, western Europe, and Australia is the principal source of personal income and, as we have seen, income is the single most important determinant of health. But employment is more than a source of income. Individuals, especially men, define who they are and their social position through their employment. One's working life is a key source of personal identity. Moreover, the workplace accords many opportunities to build social networks, garner social support, learn new skills, and exercise a sense of mastery and control. Employment shapes our non-work responses and behaviours. Whether you go to the opera after work or home to watch sports on television, or whether you go to a coffee bar or a cocktail lounge at the end of the day, depend largely on what work you do and with whom you do it. Paid work determines where and how and with whom you spend most of your waking time and significantly conditions where you live.

Sometimes, the workplace may not be positive and supportive. Superiors or fellow workers may subject an employee to coercion or harassment. The conditions under which the work is performed may be unsafe, impose restrictions on movement, require physically repetitive actions, or the work environment may be too hot, too cold, or poorly ventilated. Task allocation, shift assignment, or pay and benefits may be unfairly decided. There may be a lack of opportunity to exercise meaningful control over work timing, pace, and process. The workplace might be characterized by poor communications, a lack of respect, or other conditions that undermine dignity. Some job types—unskilled labour and many positions in the service industry—combine unhealthy working conditions with low levels of control over the work, the potential for poor treatment, even abuse, by supervisors or customers, and job insecurity—creating an atmosphere of perpetual fear that the job and associated income will disappear.

Box 8.1

Case Study ○ Low Wages, Abuse, and Job Insecurity: The American Waitress

Chelsea Welch was a server in an Applebee's restaurant in Saint Louis. She was paid $3.25 per hour, plus tips. Ms Welch was expected to work up until 1:30 a.m. and then return at 10:30 a.m. to open the restaurant, unless it was quiet, in which case she would be sent home and not be paid. Late in 2012, a customer wrote on the bill "I give God 10 per cent. Why do you get 18?"—presumably referring to (a) tithing to his/her religion (common among Mormons and Catholics, and tax deductible in the US) and (b) Applebee's suggested tip of 18 per cent. He or she left nothing by way of a tip. Ms Welch took a picture of the bill and posted it online (with the customer's name blanked out). The ensuing publicity caught the attention of the customer, and he or she demanded that Applebee's fire all the employees in the Saint Louis restaurant. Applebee's investigated and promptly fired Ms Welch, an employee about whom no complaints had been made and whose work record and reputation were solid. (Ms Welch was not the server of the customer who left the nasty note and no tip; that was a fellow employee.)

In the US, starvation wages plus tips are accepted because it is widely believed employees will work harder and provide better customer service. In reality, employees are harassed, abused, and fired on whim, in addition to living below the poverty line, even though they are working full time. Moreover, it is difficult to contend that the work ethic and service is better in the United Kingdom (low wages plus tips) than Australia (high wages, no tips); the opposite would be closer to the truth. If service is better in America, something many would contest, it likely arises from employees' terror at being fired for annoying a customer. Only the US affords almost no job protection to its service workers, and therefore employees must continuously strive to please their supervisors and customers if they want to keep the job. No wonder service industry workers, especially in the US, have such poor health.

Health and Jobs

In general, people in stable, well-paying jobs are healthier than people in unstable or poorly paying work. Being employed promotes health (Lavis et al., 2003). And as the Whitehall Studies show, the higher the quality of the job, whether measured by job status, income, or degree of control the employee has over his or her work, the better the person's mental and physical health.

Marmot remarked that patterns of employment both reflect and reinforce the social gradient (Marmot, 2010). He was pointing out that people higher up on the socio-economic scale are those with the education and other resources to secure the highest-quality jobs. These high-quality jobs, in turn, reinforce—through high income, capacity to build social networks, and control over the work—the good health associated with education and other benefits accrued over the life course. There is a virtuous circle, a positive cumulative effect. Conversely, people lower down on the socio-economic ladder compete for lower-quality

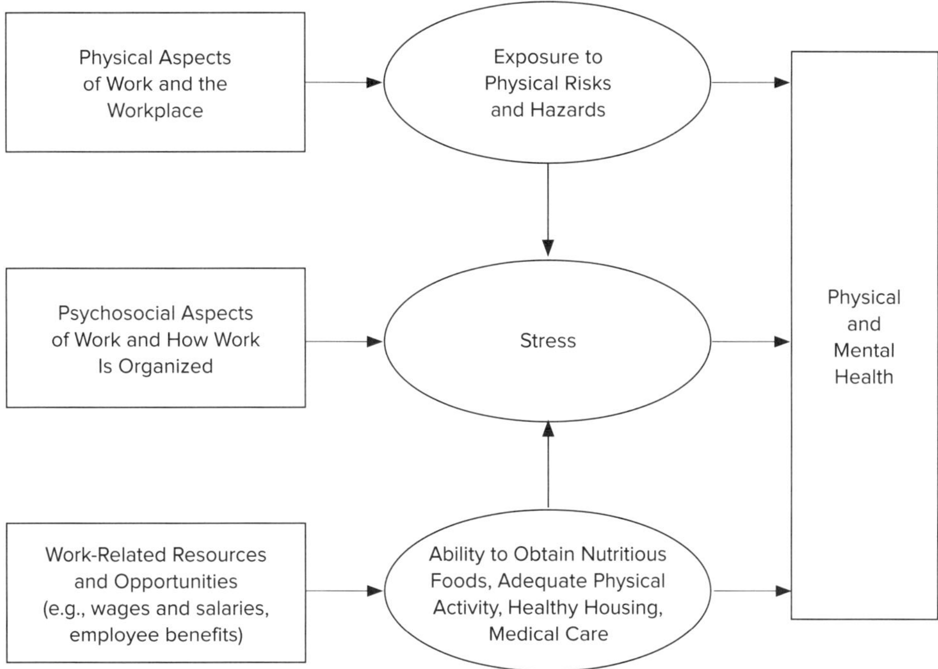

Figure 8.1 How Work Affects Health

Source: From Robert Wood Johnson, *Foundation Exploring the Social Determinants of Health: Work, Workplaces and Health*, May 2011. Reproduced with permission of the Robert Wood Johnson Foundation, Princeton, NJ.

jobs. These jobs, in turn, reinforce existing and generate new health problems through low income, monotonous work, limited social interaction, adverse working conditions, and limited control over the work. There is a vicious circle, a cumulative negative effect. In short, good jobs are health enhancing; bad jobs are health destroying. Hence the gradient in health is reflected, reinforced, and magnified by employment patterns.

We can readily see the health effects of higher- or lower-quality jobs. Figure 8.2 shows the odds of developing **metabolic syndrome**. Employees in the lowest-government jobs, clerical staff, are 2.7 times as likely to develop the syndrome, a precursor to heart disease and diabetes, than employees in the highest ranking government jobs (Marmot, 2010).

Unemployment and Health

In the capitalist West, North America, Europe, and Australia, people in the lowest quality, worst-paid jobs are at the greatest risk of unemployment, whereas people in the best quality, highest-paid jobs are at the least risk of unemployment. The quality of the job is largely a function of education, which in turn is largely a function of social class at birth. In recent years, pockets of highly paid jobs for workers with limited education, for example

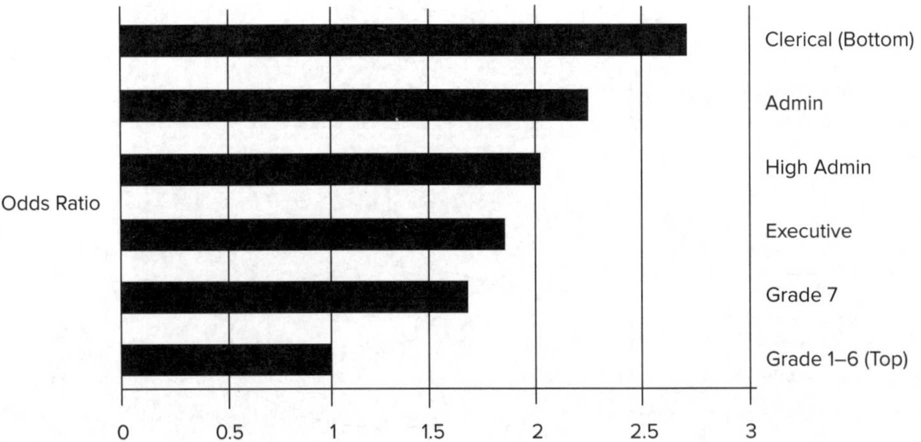

Figure 8.2 Odds of Developing Metabolic Syndrome by Occupational Position (Whitehall II)

Source: Based on Marmot, 2010.

factory-manufacturing work, have almost entirely disappeared in North America and Britain. Today, the relationship between socio-economic position of origin and quality of work obtained in adulthood is stronger than ever. Thus, too, is the relationship between risk of unemployment and social class. The lower a person's socio-economic status, the higher their risk of unemployment.

Unemployment affects health in several ways. The most obvious is the loss of employment income. From this we would deduce that negative health effects are greatest where unemployment insurance and welfare schemes for the unemployed are weakest. And that, in fact, is true. Unemployed Swedes suffer fewer health effects than unemployed Americans because Swedish citizens receive more generous unemployment assistance in the forms of guaranteed income and publicly funded job retraining (Kim et al., 2012). But loss of employment also means loss of socialization outlets, truncation of social networks, loss of self-actualization possibilities, and potential loss of sense of personal identity and self-worth. The extent to which these are important could at least in part, hinge on the qualities of the job lost. If the job was bad, exposed the worker to poor working conditions, and provided few positive outlets, its loss may have no more than the income effects, which may be partly offset by no longer being exposed to the poor conditions.

Unemployment may run through three levels of causality: (1) there may be individual effects, such as loss of personal resources and increased personal stress (the proximal or individual level); (2) there may be effects at the level of the family, such as family breakdown or the effects on the family of a forced re-location (the intermediate or household level); (3) there may be contextual effects of living in a community where unemployment is rising, such as perceiving one's own unemployment differently, reductions in public service levels, and deterioration of the neighbourhood (distal or population level). All three levels, proximate, intermediate, and distal may impact on the health of an unemployed person. Areas adversely affected by economic change such as the "rust belt" (mid-western and northeastern US) have large numbers of residents who are chronically unemployed, who belong to families who have lost their homes, and live in neighbourhoods that have degraded schools, parks, libraries, and other public services. De-industrialization has robbed many areas in central Canada, the mid-western US, and northern England of jobs. Consequently, life expectancies, general health, and well being have declined.

Box 8.2

Case Study ○ Unemployment

Many companies in fields as diverse as textiles, shoe manufacturing, machine parts, and electronics have moved their assembly operations "off shore," mostly to China and south Asia. Plants involved in large-scale assembly have, consequently, closed and the many well-paying jobs in historic manufacturing centres in Canada (mostly Quebec and Ontario), the US, and Britain have vanished. How might job-loss affect individuals? How might extensive job-loss affect communities? What health consequences ensue?

Sophisticated modelling and multi-level analyses are required to untangle the individual and contextual effects of unemployment on health. Moreover, there are direct, indirect, and buffering effects to consider. Direct effects, such as income effects, must be separated from other individual-level direct effects of unemployment. Some effects might be buffered by other factors. For example, "supportive social contexts will buffer the effect of an individual's unemployment" (Beland et al., 2002). Being a member of tightly knit, loving family situated in a safe neighbourhood can reduce the negative effects of job loss on an unemployed person.

Empirically, it has been shown that unemployment increases the risk of cardiovascular disease (Gallo et al., 2004), suicide (Voss et al., 2004), and use of prescription medication (Jin et al., 1997). Unemployment is associated with increased smoking and alcohol consumption (Marmot, 2010) and worse recovery following illness or surgery (Leslie et al., 2007). The negative effects of unemployment increase with the frequency of periods of unemployment and the duration of each period of unemployment, demonstrating a clear cumulative impact (Marmot, 2010). And, as Marmot points out, "the longer a person is unemployed, the risk of subsequent illness increases greatly, and therefore further reduces the likelihood of returning to employment" (Marmot, 2010).

Changes in the Nature of Employment

Globalization and the transition to the "knowledge economy" have had dramatic effects on work. "Globalization" refers to the complex interaction of contemporary factors that include rapid and inexpensive communications and transportation (mostly due to technological change) and the systematic removal of barriers to travel, communication, transporting goods and services, and moving money and other resources from one geographic place to another (mostly due to changes in government policies). "Knowledge economies" refers to the belief in, and pursuit by, governments and companies of economic growth by seeking to capitalize on technical innovation and providing cutting-edge goods and services (which, in theory, ought to have greater value and fetch higher prices than old-fashioned production of basic goods and services).

Commitment to economic growth, globalization, and the emphasis on building a knowledge economy create steadily growing pressure for increased productivity—doing more with less, greater work intensity, increased hours of work, and decreased wages and benefits. The push for greater product innovation at lower cost spawned just-in-time and flexible production modalities which in turn have dramatically increased the use of part-time, temporary, casual, and contract employees. They have also increased reliance on shift-work.

A good example of the revolution that has taken place in the past 20 years is the automobile industry, which used to introduce new models every five to seven years, making only modest and largely cosmetic changes between changeovers. Parts were ordered, manufactured, and inventoried for years; assembly lines using the same equipment and workers ran virtually unchanged. Now no manufacturer who hopes to stay in business can avoid continuous innovation, ordering only the components needed in the next few days or weeks, and switching suppliers and assembly modalities to keep costs down and quality up. Today's production techniques are incompatible with large, stable workforces, and the numbers of full-time and continuing jobs have been slashed. Perhaps an even better example is consumer electronics, where even large and successful companies like Sony and Panasonic are teetering on insolvency as they shuffle their product lines, open and close new manufacturing facilities, and shed jobs.

The emerging knowledge economy functions through projects, not ongoing routine work. Less continuous production means more contract work and less regular employment. Not surprisingly, globalization and the shift to a knowledge economy have been linked to degraded health (Blouin et al., 2009).

Traditionally, both unions and companies pursued the goal of a stable workforce, albeit for different reasons. Now, in the Anglo-American world, the only large-scale labour-intensive work conducted in stable environments is found in government offices, universities, schools, institutional health care, and the few remaining assembly plants, mills, and large-scale mining operations. Traditional production jobs have been replaced by service jobs, mostly low-end jobs, such as sales clerks and restaurant workers. The less skilled are increasingly competing for low-paid, unstable jobs with few or no fringe benefits.

We are currently experiencing the collective effects of four related trends: de-industrialization, de-unionization, de-skilling, and privatization. We already referred to de-industrialization and its impact on jobs in the old manufacturing heartlands of Canada, the US, and Britain. The so-called post-industrial or service-economy countries of the Anglo-American world now import rather than manufacture the vast majority of finished goods, from shoes and socks to mobile phones. This is because corporations have sought out lower-wage and lower-taxation places to site their manufacturing activities, a process made possible by the innovations in the communications and transportation sectors, the abundance of cheap energy for global shipping, and changes in international trade rules and tariffs. Relatively well-paid jobs for relatively low-skilled workers have vanished along with the assembly plants, forcing large numbers of people to seek work in the lower-paying service sector (e.g., retail sales, restaurants, maintenance, and cleaning).

De-unionization, employers' successful efforts to exclude unions from workplaces, is connected to manufacturing's move off-shore because remaining industrial employers have demanded wage and contract concessions and new employers have pursued low-wage/no union labour practices to bring wages and benefits closer to those of the developing world. Governments in Canada, the US, and Britain have contributed to the trend by making it more difficult for unions to organize workers and easier to get unions de-certified.

De-skilling is multi-dimensional and includes increased use of automated processes and routines, importation of prefabricated materials, rather than skilled construction on site, and modular construction of consumer items such as automobiles so that component assemblies are swapped rather than the vehicle repaired by a skilled mechanic. In labour-intensive areas like health care, less expensive, lower-trained nursing assistants and aides have replaced qualified nurses. The effect of de-skilling is depression of wages and replacement of higher-quality jobs with higher-job satisfaction by lower-quality, more routinized work.

Finally, governments at all levels and quasi-governmental bodies like health authorities and universities have aggressively privatized. Privatization includes contracting out and changing ownership of assets. Rather than employing people directly to undertake tasks like cleaning, maintenance, grounds work, garbage removal, and the like, governmental and quasi governmental bodies in the Anglo-American world now typically contract with private companies (almost always low-bid, non-union companies) to take over the service. The reason is to achieve (short-term) cost reduction. Wages, benefits, skill levels, opportunities for training and advancement, and quality of work are all driven downward. In the case of changing ownership of assets, governments turn over a public asset (such as a publicly owned nursing home) to a private operator. The usual effect of the transfer of ownership is to have higher-paid (usually unionized), skilled workers replaced by lower-paid (usually non-unionized) employees who experience less job security, less control over the work, and lower wages and benefits. Again, the motive is reduced cost.

Apart from the damage to health done by low wages and physically challenging working conditions, diminished job security is itself a serious threat to health. Job insecurity is linked to both physical and mental health problems (Ferrie, 2001). Higher use of medical services, increased sick days, obesity, psychological problems, and elevated-blood pressure and blood glucose have all been linked to job insecurity.

Working Conditions and Health

Chronic stresses and excessive demands at work that are not compensated by adequate social support constitute **isostrain**—isolated high-strain work. Many routine jobs over which the worker has little control—a server in a busy restaurant, a bus driver, a sales clerk, a junior office worker—involve high strain, limited control by the employee, and little or no support from others.

Isostrain is linked to **metabolic syndrome**—extra fat around the mid-section, insulin resistance, elevated blood pressure—a constellation of risk factors, which together increase the risk of diabetes and heart disease. Bus drivers, for example, have been shown to have a more elevated risk of diabetes and heart disease associated with factors such as traffic congestion, time pressures, social isolation, poor passenger behaviour, lack of control over features of the work and so on (Evans and Carrere, 1991). In addition to isostrain, the physical features of the work, immobility, and the quality of seating and ergonomics, contribute to elevated levels of musculoskeletal disease, making bus drivers amongst the least healthy people in the affluent world.

While stress at work, and the associated psychosocial impact on health, are clearly important, we must be a bit cautious about pushing work-related stress explanations of ill health too far. A recent Canadian study found that only 27 per cent of Canadian workers reported moderate or high levels of stress and 40 per cent of those identified the major sources of their stress to be non-work related. The researchers found no correlation between reported stress and gender nor between reported stress and education (Crompton, 2011). As one would expect, less-educated people reported more stress associated with financial matters, but this was compensated for by more-educated people expressing stress over family matters.

Box 8.3 Case Study ○ Work and Pregnancy

Working throughout pregnancy in a job that is physically demanding or involves a substantial amount of standing is associated with impaired fetal growth and reduction in head circumference of the child (Snijder et al., 2012). Women who have low incomes and limited-educational attainment are much more likely to be engaged in physically demanding work or hold jobs, such as sale associates in shops where they have to stand for sustained periods of time. They are also more likely to work throughout their pregnancies because they cannot afford to take time off. As we saw earlier, children of low socio-economic mothers are pre-disposed to impaired fetal growth for reasons such as maternal nutritional status. Maternal-working conditions may compound the risk (cumulative risk or "pile up" of risk factors). What are the long-term implications for the health and well-being for the mother and child? What workplace and social policy measures might mitigate risks of less-than-optimal health outcomes?

Explanatory Models of Workplace Impacts on Health

Two models have been developed to explain how work can make you sick. Those are the "demand–control" model and the "effort–reward" model. While they feature different elements, they are not mutually exclusive and both may be applied to a work situation. The **demand–control model** attempts to measure the relationship between the demands made of an employee and the capacity to meet those demands. A junior clerk in an office who works for several managers likely has an overflowing in-basket of work and superiors who all think their work is the top priority. She faces heavy, in fact impossible demands, yet has no control over how much work comes her way. A significant discrepancy between what is demanded of the employee and what can be accomplished is associated with fatigue, headache, body aches and pains, sleep disturbances, anxiety, elevated blood pressure, and stroke (Van der Doef, 1999). The **effort–reward model** attempts to measure the relationship between the work effort of the employee and various rewards received including pay, bonuses, recognition, and workplace social support. Many low-end jobs such as labourers in the construction industry must make maximal effort to maintain their jobs but they receive little or no recognition or support from their employers. Again, a significant discrepancy between the effort the employee makes and the rewards received is predictive of emotional, psychosomatic, and chronic disease outcomes (de Jonge et al., 2000). Because the demand–control and effort–reward models are independently predictive of health outcomes, various efforts have been made to combine them.

Forced Inactivity in the Workplace

Many jobs today, as the bus driver example illustrates, combine high isotrain derived from demand-control and effort-reward imbalances with environmental factors inimical to good health. Commonplace is sedentary work involving long periods of sitting—office workers, drivers in the transport sector, check-out cashiers. Not only does prolonged sitting contribute to musculoskeletal problems, but lack of physical activity compounds the isostrain effects on metabolic syndrome, notably by promoting central obesity and hence the risks of heart disease and diabetes. Thus, pathways to chronic diseases such as arthritis, coronary heart disease, and diabetes can be found in the workplace.

Research has recently demonstrated links between sedentary work and many negative health outcomes, including shortened life expectancy (Thorpe et al., 2011). Sedentary lifestyle, even if the individual engages in episodic vigorous exercise, can shorten life expectancy by more than two years.

Box 8.4

Case Study ○ Different Employment Situations, Different Health Risks

Sonya is a 34-year-old woman with a 3-year-old daughter, whose neighbour babysits at a rate of $25 per day while Sonya works. Sonya only has her grade 12 and a certificate from a secretarial school. She holds two jobs currently: she works part-time for a private long-term care home as a clerk/receptionist and picks up as many shifts as she can as a server in a local restaurant. Sonya gets paid $10.25 an hour at the care home and $8.75 plus tips at the restaurant. She has no benefits on top of her pay. Rent in her one-bedroom apartment is $600 per month, plus utilities.

What health challenges confront Sonya?

continued

Sara is a 34-year-old woman with a 3-year-old daughter. Her daughter goes to a neighbourhood play school every weekday. Sara is in a stable relationship with John, her partner, who has a law practice. Sara has a degree in business administration and runs her own small advertising company. Sara and John own their house, making mortgage payments of $1,200 per month. They both own cars.

What health challenges confront Sara?

The Workplace and Health Behaviour

The modern, high-pressure workplace also structures some of our behaviour. In addition to forcing us to be more sedentary, the workplace encourages bad eating habits—grabbing something and eating it at our workstation or behind the wheel—and bad food choices—something quick and easy that we can eat out of hand. Muffins, burgers, wraps, and snack foods are amongst the worst things we can eat but are the mainstays in today's work world.

Policies Affecting Employment, Earnings, Job Benefits, and Working Conditions

We already noted how central employment is to our adult lives. Most adults receive virtually all of their income through paid employment, and most adults spend roughly half of their waking time at work. Securing reasonably paid work with safe and healthy working conditions and benefits, such as paid leave, are among the strongest determinants of our overall health and well-being. Public policies affect employment levels, earnings, job benefits and working conditions. Government spending determines the number of jobs in areas as diverse as construction, education, and health care. Government regulations determine maximum working hours and minimum wages. Thus government policies that might at first glance appear "economic" are, in fact, important from a population-health standpoint. In this section, we will begin by discussing the near-universal policy commitment to full employment and why governments, at least those in Canada, the US, and Britain, abandoned that commitment. We will then look at policies regarding unemployment insurance, wages, benefits, and working conditions.

Keynesianism and Its Demise

Until the end of the 1970s, governments throughout the developed world held a common understanding of macro-level economic principles derived from the work of the great economist John Maynard Keynes (1883–1946). Keynesian economics holds that modern governments need to intervene in order to ensure that employment remains at the highest-sustainable level, as close to full employment as possible, because only under those conditions is economic growth sustainable.

Keynes pointed out that companies can expand their production, spurring economic growth, only if there is enough demand in the economy for their products. Consumer demand is highly sensitive to income and as most people's income is derived from work, employment levels and wages determine overall (aggregate) demand. Thus boosting employment (and wages) is the chief prerequisite for steady economic growth. That growth is also the prerequisite for governments to be able to pay down public debt and, hopefully, build up budget surpluses for a rainy day. High-stable incomes maintain consumer demand for products, and provide high-stable tax revenue, while simultaneously reducing the need for government spending on social programs. Moreover, as the economy grows and government revenues and expenditures stabilize, governments can reduce taxes. Maximizing employment is thus the key to everything we are striving to achieve.

According to Keynes, near full employment can be achieved by increasing the money supply through reducing interest rates and increasing government spending. But once near full employment is achieved, low-interest rates and a tightening of the labour market together tend to drive up prices and wages, which sparks inflation. Governments should respond to accelerating inflation, according to Keynes, by gentle braking, a slow, step-wise increase in interest rates, a slow cutting back on public expenditures, accompanied by a slow, step-wise increase in taxes. Once the economy starts to "cool," taxes should be lowered, interest rates dropped, and public spending picked up, even if that requires heavy government borrowing, until the economy starts to overheat and so on into the next cycle. The aim of it all is to keep as many of those able to work working full-time, thus effectively ending the "boom and bust cycle" typical of capitalist market societies. Keynes, after all, was most interested in providing the economic theory and practical advice that would prevent another great depression such as the collapse of the Anglo-American economies in 1929.

From the end of the Second World War until the mid-1970s, Keynesianism seemed to work. All the affluent countries of the west enjoyed a fairly sustained period of economic growth and near full employment. But by 1975, the massive debts piled up by the United States in pursuing the Vietnam and Cold Wars put huge upward pressure on interest rates worldwide. The sudden rise in oil prices following the 1973 Israeli-Arab war put huge downward pressure on industrial production due to the sharp increase in the cost of producing and transporting goods. Suddenly rich countries had the twin problems of economic recession and rising unemployment, coupled with inflation and rising prices. That was not supposed to be possible. According to the usual reading of Keynes, an economy either grows too fast, causing inflation or contracts causing recession. In theory, at least in Keynesian theory, inflation and recession cannot occur together because the former, inflation, is caused by rapid economic growth whereas the latter, by definition, is a shrinking, failing economy.

Starting with the United States, countries abandoned Keynesianism and resorted to manipulation of the money supply as a means to control inflation ("monetarism"), a strategy that at once drove interest rates even higher and the economic downturn even deeper. Again, starting with the United States, governments then resorted to cutting government programs and services while lowering taxes. Typically, they had more success with the latter—cutting taxes—than the former—cutting spending—because so much of the spending was bound up politically, especially in the United States, with the military, pensions, and big, powerful lobbies like the food and agriculture industries. That meant in practice cherry-picking programs serving minorities, the poor, and other politically insignificant social groups. Out of this was born **neo-liberalism** and a new-found tolerance for high levels of unemployment. Seven to 10 per cent, numbers considered disastrous in the 1940s, 50s, and 60s, became not only thinkable, but increasingly commonplace.

High Chronic Unemployment in Britain, the US, and Canada

At the time of writing, the United States faces chronic unemployment in the order of 8 per cent and a Congress firmly opposed to Keynesian economics—i.e., politicians who refuse to spend in order to create more jobs. The situation in the UK is worse and that in Canada is not much better. In spite of all the evidence that it does not work, the political consensus has hardened around low taxes and limited government spending as the route to economic growth and, eventually, more jobs. The employment situation is marginally better in Australia (mostly because of Chinese demand for raw materials). In Canada, the unemployment situation would be worse but has stabilized in the seven per cent zone mostly due to high oil prices and the resultant construction boom in the Alberta oil sands. Recognition that a slowdown in the oil sands would drive Canada deep into recession recently led the Canadian government to gut environmental protection regulations and sponsor new pipeline construction.

It is important to understand that official unemployment figures do not really reflect how many people are unemployed. To count as unemployed, you must be (a) recently out of work, (b) actively seeking work, and (c) available to take a job if one should be offered to you. The long-term unemployed and those who currently have some commitment like looking after a child or an aging parent that limits their availability, drop out of the numbers. Thus paradoxically, the worse the employment situation, the longer it remains bad, the poorer the pay, the less secure the work, and the higher the hardships a jobseeker must face, proportionately fewer people will count as unemployed. Or to put the point differently, many more people in Canada, the US, and Britain than those currently labelled "unemployed" would seek and obtain work if the jobs were available. That is why unemployment figures tend to spike when economic conditions improve—the "hidden unemployed" flood into the job market hoping for work.

Table 8.1 Unemployment (December 2012)

Jurisdiction	Unemployment Rate
United States	8.1
United Kingdom	8.0
Canada	7.3
Germany	5.5
Australia	5.2
Japan	4.4
Norway	3.2

Source: US Central Intelligence Agency World Fact Book, www.cia.gov/library/publications/the-world-factbook/rankorder/2129rank-html.

From a population-health perspective, the important points are (1) governments can heavily influence levels of employment and (2) those levels of employment heavily influence health outcomes. Unemployment, insecure employment, and poorly paid employment are major determinants of poor health outcomes in affluent countries. The current hands-off attitude of Canada, the United States, and the United Kingdom (less so Australia whose government continues to follow full-employment policies) directly consigns many of their citizens to low income, job insecurity, and unemployment. A recent study (Kim et al., 2012) shows that governments' policies regarding full-time, stable employment have profound effects on the health of their populations. Anglo-American countries with high unemployment and precarious work have poorer self-rated health, more musculoskeletal disorders, and higher incidence of mental illness than countries that have stuck with Keynesian economics, full employment, and progressive income tax (Northern Europe and Australia).

The Anglo-American countries of the world, except Australia, have abandoned full-employment policies and now tolerate very high levels of unemployment. This is justified according to their governments because it reduces inflationary pressure (employees have little bargaining power to increase their pay) and increases economic productivity (by lowering labour costs and by forcing existing workers to work longer and harder). But the hidden cost, of course, is significant hardship, reduced personal income, and diminished health.

Unemployment Insurance

Along with allowing rates of unemployment to rise, Anglo-American governments also acted to tighten eligibility for unemployment insurance, turning what were once essentially social welfare mechanisms, designed to provide income support to part-time, seasonal, and casual labour, into contributory schemes. Canada is currently "reforming" unemployment insurance, making it harder to collect and incentivizing low-paid work rather than benefits. In Canada and the United Kingdom, worker eligibility now depends on the length of employment service and the amount contributed to the insurance plan. No longer are the unemployment insurance plans backed by tax dollars, but instead rely on contributions from the currently employed to provide minimal benefits to those who lose their jobs. Most affected by these changes are women who work part-time, seasonal workers such as loggers, fishermen, and construction workers, and people in "sunset industries," failing enterprises such as the Canadian pulp and paper industry where work is sporadic. Communities where much of the work is seasonal or where whole sectors of the local economy are in difficulty, suffer alongside the individual workers from the loss of spending power derived from unemployment-insurance sources.

As in so many matters relating to income support and employment, Australia is an exception to the Anglo-American pattern. In Australia, unemployment benefits are part of the income-tax system. There is no insurance fund and no compulsory premiums to be paid by workers. For single, unemployed people aged 21 to 65, a maximum of $228 AUD ($250 CAD) is paid per week in support plus up to $58.90 AUD ($65 CAD) per week for accommodation. Amounts payable depend on income, assets, and actual cost of accommodation. Payments are statutory rights and there is no cut-off; benefits run indefinitely. However, people on benefits are required to enter into Activity Agreements which specify a set of obligations the person must meet to maintain eligibility for support, including training and an acceptable level of job seeking.

The high level of income security and the relative generosity of the benefits are contributory factors to the superior health of Australians compared to Canadians, Americans, and residents of the United Kingdom. However, the guaranteed income program is also controversial. Australian conservative politicians have argued against the scheme and claim it contributes to a "welfare mentality." As with conservatives in the UK, the US, and Canada, they believe very low or no benefits are a better approach because then the unemployed would be forced to seek work.

Education and Training for the Workforce

In most of Europe and in Japan, employers are required to provide much of the education and training needed by their employees. Often this is formal in nature, such as apprenticeships, internships, and the like. The government provides general education, numeracy, literacy, and foundational science, with the employer providing specialized knowledge and skills. In Anglo-American countries, the arrangements are quite different. Employers expect their workers to be pretty much "job ready" and it is the joint responsibility of the individual and the government to ensure that the requisite training (much of it at the individual's expense in technical schools or college) has been completed. What is an employer's responsibility and cost in much of the world is a taxpayer's and individual-worker's responsibility and cost in Canada, the United States, and the United Kingdom.

Commitment between worker and employer is obviously much stronger in non-Anglo American systems because each party has a great deal invested in the other. In consequence, job security, full-time work (as opposed to casual and part-time work), and more robust rights and benefits typify the European- and Asian-labour markets. This is reinforced by much deeper penetration by labour unions, which collaborate with employers on training, job security, and other matters in ways that are unfamiliar to the Anglo-American world where relations between unions—where they still exist—and employers are often adversarial. In Germany or Japan, for example, automobile manufacturers hire employees more or less for life, providing them with the training and re-training they need as the companies' needs change. The unions and the employers work together to ensure layoffs do not occur, and that the fit between existing employees and the companies' production requirements remains tight. In Canada and US, automobile-industry unions and employers are adversaries with the former trying to protect as many jobs as possible and the latter trying to lay off as many workers as possible. In the UK, those adversarial dynamics completely destroyed the British automobile industry, a loss of tens of thousands of highly paid jobs.

Because of an employer's responsibility for developing skills in their own workers, the common problem in the Anglo-American world of disconnects between the training workers have and what employers are seeking is avoided in many other countries. Not so in Canada: it is common to have health-care facilities desperate for health-care technicians with training slots in colleges for those self-same technicians going unfilled or students flooding into some hot new field only to discover when they graduate that there are no jobs.

Similarly, governments in Canada and the United States mount (or fund colleges and other agencies to mount) training programs to make welfare recipients and the recently unemployed more competitive in the labour market. But again, those training efforts are often misaligned with the job market or, alternatively, are aimed at low-end entry-level work where there are already more qualified applicants than positions. In Canada, at the time of writing, the Canada Economic Action Plan and the BC Job Plan both target marginalized populations and low-skill jobs. Why does Canada repeatedly offer ad hoc, ineffectual job training? Training efforts of this type are cheap, easy to mount, politically popular, create the impression governments are doing something, and require nothing of the business community.

Solutions for the Anglo-American problems of education and training of the workforce are not easy to come by. Employers are not at all keen to assume new costs such as a more robust role in educating and developing their workforces. The amount of coordination required amongst government, employers, and unions is alien to the more free-market oriented countries, especially the United States, but also Canada and Britain. (Something akin to European coordinated labour-market approaches exists in Australia.) Unfortunately, the misalignments and lack of commitment by employers to their employees in Canada, the United States, and Britain mean wastage of human resources, underemployment, and job insecurity. This is not only inefficient, but it is also harmful to the health of the population.

Some countries have pioneered alternative approaches to education and training. Over the past 50 years, Denmark developed Continuous Vocational Training. Skill-development services geared directly for workplace opportunities are provided to both employed and unemployed people. The program is a joint government/industry venture with funding provided from government sources (CSDH, 2008).

The Danish Ministry of Education is legally responsible for Continuous Vocational Training (CVT), but CVT is managed at the community level by employers, unions, and local government. For the last 20 years, Danish policy has required that collective agreements between employees and employers include educational provisions and at least two-weeks' annual leave for training purposes (funded by government).

Wages and Benefits

As one might expect, the minimum wage a government permits employers to pay is lowest in the United States, roughly similar in the United Kingdom and Canada, and significantly higher than other Anglo-American countries in Australia. In 2011, rates were $7.25 USD per hour in the United States (federal), 6£ ($9.85 CAD) per hour in the United Kingdom, and a range between $8.75 (British Columbia) and $10.25 (Ontario) per hour in Canada. The United States, Canada, and the United Kingdom allow for lower-minimum wages for youth and trainees and differential (lower) wages for people who may receive tips (primarily food and beverage workers). In all cases, working full time would leave the employee on minimum wage well below the poverty line and incapable of acquiring the resources required for healthy living. Without some other special income supports, single parents working at or near the minimum wage would remain unable to provide the means for a healthy life for themselves and their children.

Table 8.2 Minimum Wage

Jurisdiction	Minimum Wage
United States (federally mandated)*	$7.25
Alberta, Canada	$9.75
United Kingdom	$9.85
Saskatchewan and New Brunswick, Canada	$10.00
Ontario and British Columbia, Canada	$10.25
Netherlands	$12.50
France	$12.80
Australia	$17.50
Denmark**	$18.65

*Applies to federal government and federal government contractors; employees of private companies such as servers in restaurants may be paid as little as $3.00 per hour plus tips.
**lowest government-permitted wage for private and public sector collective agreements

Poverty and low income are, of course, closely linked to the labour market. "In 2000, more than 11 per cent of the US population resided in poor households with at least one employed person, while only 4.1 per cent resided in poor single-mother households and 2.6 per cent resided in poor households with no one employed" (Brady, Fullerton, and Cross, 2010). Contrary to common prejudices, most poor people in the Anglo-American world are employed, albeit in low-paid jobs.

The exception to the Anglo-American pattern is, once again, Australia. Fair Work Australia is the national workplace relations tribunal that, amongst other things, sets minimum wages across employment sectors. The current minimum-wage order is $589.30 AUD per week ($17.50 CAD per hour). Of all the Anglo-American countries, Australia alone guarantees a "living wage." The approach not only solves the working-poor problem, but also eliminates the reliance of food- and beverage-sector workers on tips.

Guaranteed benefits such as stable, steady hours of employment, mandated rest breaks, vacation time, sick leave, and health-care benefits are minimal in the Anglo-American world. With the exception of gender equity in Canada, governments in the United States and Canada have deregulated employment standards, shifting policy in employers' favour over the past 25 years. Minimum-wage workers are now least likely to enjoy the security of hours, consistent shifts, regular paid breaks, or any other significant employment benefits. Again, the exception is Australia where the Fair Work Australia tribunal establishes industry-wide standards that must be followed by employers, providing greater levels of employee benefits and more consistent (and fair) treatment of workers than is typical of Canada and the United States.

Life at the bottom, then, except in Australia, has generally gotten worse over the past 25 years. The number of working poor has risen and lower-income people are working longer and harder in less and less secure employment settings. But life at the top is quite otherwise. In the United States, in 2009, workers at the twenty-fifth percentile of the income distribution earned close to $8 per hour, about the same or slightly less than they did 30 years ago.

Employees at the ninety-fifth percentile earned $48 per hour, a substantial increase. Chief executive officers in American companies soared from an average pay of $2 million per annum to $6 million over the same period. CEOs, earning on average about 150 times their factory floor workers in 1980, now earn about 400 times as much (Hallock, 2011).

Improving Working Conditions and Employee Benefits

In general, fewer Anglo-American workers today than in the past are exposed to the dangerous working conditions associated with mines, forestry, the fishing industry, and heavy manufacturing, mostly because these activities have been outsourced to poorer countries. But sizeable pockets of dangerous work remain, such as the construction trades and vehicular transport. More common are the risks associated with sedentary work in shops and offices, repetitive strain injuries associated with keyboards, back injuries (also associated with extensive sitting), and hearing loss arising from noisy worksites and driving trucks and other heavy vehicles. Overall, regulation of worksites has greatly improved workplace safety throughout the Anglo-American world, but the sedentary and repetitive nature of modern work remains a serious health threat for many. Few workplaces, unlike their Japanese counterparts, require group exercises. *Rajio taiso*, an institutionalized feature in Japanese life, involves stretches, knee bends and arm windmills.

More problematic than lack of exercise is a lack of worker control over the work, how it is to be done, and scheduling. Few Canadian, American, and British workplaces accord meaningful input by workers into the work process, thus fail to close the gap between worker control and job demand that is known to foster mental and physical disease. Other countries such as Germany and Japan do much better, involving workers and their unions in workplace decisions. Volkswagen, for example, enables its employees to shape company plans and work processes through workplace participation in formal joint committees.

Box 8.5 Case Study ○ Health Circles

Some workplace interventions such as Health Circles, implemented in German industrial enterprises, have been shown to be effective in reducing stress and in improving worker satisfaction (Aust and Ducki, 2004). Health Circles are structured discussion groups convened at work and charged with exploring health-related problems and solutions. The goals are to improve working conditions and enhance employee health.

Do you see potential for instituting something along these lines in British or North American workplaces? What resistance might there be? How might it best be overcome?

Fairness in the allocation of tasks and even-handed payment of bonuses and perks remain important, unresolved issues. Consequently, the gap between effort and reward remains large in Canada, the United States, and the United Kingdom. But fairness extends well beyond processes used for decision-making about the work. Many workplaces tolerate health-harming power imbalances ranging from gender inequity to discrimination, to worker harassment by supervisors, fellow workers, or clients.

However, considerable progress has been made on a number of fronts. Canada, in particular, moved aggressively to improve gender equity in the workplace. Canada also, through provincial and federal human rights codes, imposed clear employment standards with respect to race, religion, and ethnicity. Some employers, such as universities, have attempted voluntarily to become exemplars of best practices, forbidding harassment and bullying of employees, establishing internal human rights offices and protocols, enforcing hiring guidelines intended to better represent women and minorities within the workforce, and regularizing promotion through transparent, democratic workplace processes. Other employers, notably in the information technology sector, have, in order to retain their valued employees, established health and wellness programs, provided access to recreation, and created more flexible work processes that align better with their employees' wishes.

Overall, however, there has not been a stampede toward healthier workplaces and much of the progress in the late 1990s and early 2000s is at risk of being lost with the current economic slowdown, the political tide toward conservatism, and persistent high levels of unemployment. The Anglo-American world remains well behind leading countries such as the Netherlands and the Nordic countries in creating fairer, healthier workplaces.

Family-Friendly Policy

Other key issues in the Anglo-American context are child-care and maternity/paternity benefits. None of the Anglo-American countries provide universally available, licensed, subsidized child care, although many European countries do. In the absence of quality, affordable child care, many women are faced with paying for child care of uneven or unknown quality, the cost of which can challenge or even exceed their total earnings. Child-care tax credits come nowhere near offsetting those costs, amounting typically to well under 10 per cent of the cost of care. Canada came close to an agreement amongst provincial and federal governments over a universal child-care plan in 2004 but the subsequent election of a Conservative federal government put plans for such a scheme on indefinite hold. The current situation embeds a serious gender bias against women, precludes many women with younger children from working, and impacts significantly on the disposable income of women with families, especially sole-support mothers. The lack of support for women and families is unlikely to change in Canada, the United States, or the United Kingdom in the foreseeable future.

Anglo-American countries, in comparison with other wealthy ones, are also unwilling to provide significant maternal/paternal benefits, whether in terms of mandated employment leave or government-funded payments to new parents. In the United Kingdom, a woman may apply for up to 26 weeks of "ordinary maternal leave" and 26 weeks of "additional leave." In order to qualify, she must have worked 26 weeks with the same employer. In order to qualify for the maximum 39 weeks of paid leave, she must have earned at least £102 ($165 CAD) per week. If eligible for paid leave, she may receive up to 90 per cent of her earnings for the first 6 weeks and up to £128.73 ($211 CAD) per week for the next 33 weeks. In Canada, the leave provisions are governed by employment insurance rules. A woman must have worked enough hours to qualify for employment insurance, at which point either she or her spouse may apply for "parental leave" upon the birth of their child. Employment insurance pays 55 per cent of the woman's salary up to a maximum of $468 per week for 52 weeks. In contrast, Sweden entitles all parents to 16 months of 100 per cent paid leave for each child, whereas the US does not mandate any form of paid parental leave (even poverty-ridden Cuba provides 18 weeks at 100 per cent of salary).

Shift Work and Commuting

Also of concern, especially in the Anglo-American world, is the growth in both shift work and lengthy commuting to the workplace. Shift work is strongly associated with coronary heart disease, sleep disorders, anxiety and depression, substance abuse, and family breakdown (Scott, 2000). It has implications not only for the health of the worker, but also, especially in the case of women, negative ramifications for the emotional and intellectual development of her children. Shift work can impair emotional bonding and attachment, as well as degrade the quality and quantity of interaction between mother and young child.

Distances travelled by private vehicle to work, the time required, and the density of traffic encountered have all increased dramatically in Canada, the United States, Britain, and Australia. Commuting by car is a major contributor to sedentary lifestyles and hence obesity and its negative health correlate. It is also a major source of stress in many working people's lives. The average commuting time in Canada is 26 minutes—appreciably longer in larger urban centres (Turcotte, 2011b). In Toronto 29 per cent of commuters are caught in traffic jams daily. Thirty-six per cent of commuters with longer commutes (>45 minutes) report being "quite" or "extremely" stressed (Turcotte, 2011b).

Processes of assigning shift work and longer-term urban planning, coupled with affordable housing and public transit designed to reduce the burdens of commuting, are matters amenable to public policy. Many countries, notably in northern Europe, have already made significant strides in addressing both sets of issues. Norway and the Netherlands, for example, have focused on coordinating urban planning with patterns of work and commuting, encouraging more use of bicycles, public transit, pedestrian only zones, and staggered opening times of businesses to reduce congestion.

Theoretical Considerations

Employment is the confluence of a range of material and psychosocial factors. Income, personal safety, training opportunities, and the informational and emotional support of others all derive from employment. So do dangerous exposures and physical risks. On the psychosocial side, how we feel about ourselves and others is deeply influenced by workplace conditions, especially the fit between the demands made of us and the control we feel we have over the nature and pace of the work and the congruence between how hard we feel we are working and how well we feel we are rewarded for that work. Employment and workplace studies are thus a kind of vehicle for test driving hypotheses from both the material and psychosocial traditions. The review we conducted in Chapter 8 shows us clearly that both material and psychosocial factors are important, and complete analyses must incorporate both theoretical traditions. Moreover, employment studies neatly show how we must also attend to levels of analysis. Many factors are properly treated as individual, such as my experience of workplace realities, but others such as area-level unemployment are clearly population-level variables. As the chapter pointed out, it is important to consider individual-level, household-level (family), and community-level variables associated with paid work.

Summary

Paid employment is one of the central features of adult life in capitalist societies such as the Anglo-American countries. Work experiences and the level of income derived from employment shape beliefs, values, and health behaviour; provide or undermine social support; and substantially determine the conditions under which we live. Paid employment is especially important in Anglo-American countries because there is little income support outside of the labour market, little social housing, and limited unemployment insurance.

Some policy conclusions that emerge from the discussion in Chapter 8 are as follows:

- A policy that aims for adequate income for the population but does not promote full employment at fair wages cannot succeed. Rather than focusing on safety nets to support those who are excluded from work (or who cannot earn enough money through paid employment to support themselves and their families), governments must do more to ensure jobs are available, people are appropriately prepared in terms of skills and knowledge to assume those jobs, and that the jobs pay wages and provide benefits that are adequate to support healthy living. Of the Anglo-American countries, only Australia comes close to recognizing these realities.
- Closer collaboration between governments at all levels and employers is required to improve the fit between education and training and available work.
- For health of the majority of the population to improve, minimum wages and minimum benefits must be raised in Canada, the United States, and the United Kingdom. Evidence does not support the right-wing contention that higher minimum wages and improved benefits "kill jobs," making the less well-off even worse. In fact, economic recessions are so intractable in the Anglo-American world precisely because lower-income people cannot afford to buy the things they need, even when they go deeply into debt.
- Governments should structure tax and employment policy to discourage insecure forms of employment and incentivize long-term employer commitment to employees. Many non-Anglo-American countries already do this (e.g., Netherlands, Germany, Finland).
- Adequate child care and maternity/paternity leave should be mandated everywhere. Without such policies, we cannot achieve the healthy start for every child that is the cornerstone for improved population health.
- Healthy workplaces and healthy communities go hand-in-glove and policy and planning must be coordinated to ensure both move ahead together.

Critical Thinking Questions

1. In Chapter 4 we discussed some of the determinants of health associated with infancy and in Case Study 8.3 we looked at one aspect of work's impact on fetal development. More broadly, how might employment and workplace policies support early childhood development? Alternatively, how might employment policies and workplace practices harm children and young families?
2. The effort–reward model depends on our sense of fairness. In particular, it assumes that a sense of unfairness will cause considerable distress which in turn will affect our emotional, mental, and physical health. The demand–control model depends on our sense of self-efficacy. In particular, it assumes that we will experience our work life as "out of control" if other people or mechanical processes determine the amount and pace of work. A sense of lack of control over what we must respond to, in turn, will generate stress-causing emotional difficulties and illness. How adequate are these psychosocial models? What other assumptions about health-relevant mechanisms do they incorporate?
3. How do gender and employment interact? Which employment conditions typically affect mostly women? Men? How might working conditions be experienced differently by women than men?

Annotated Suggested Readings

The best resource on employment and health is the publication *Work, Stress, Health: The Whitehall II Study*. Written for an educated lay audience, the short report covers the background to and findings of this seminal prospective cohort study. The document may be acquired at www.ucl.ac.uk/whitehallII/pdf/Whitehallbooklet_1_.pdf.

An excellent book on the health effects of stress in the workplace is Jennie Grimshaws *Employment and Health: Psychosocial Stress in the Workplace* (London: British Library, 1999). While somewhat dated and focused on Europe, the book does a good job of exploring the relationships among the changing nature of work, government policies, and employee health.

For a more current and comprehensive overview of employment conditions and health, consult *Employment Conditions and Health Inequalities* (Geneva: World Health Organization Commission on the Social Determinants of Health) available at www.who.int/social_determinants/resources/articles/emconet_who_report.pdf.

Annotated Websites

Robert Wood Johnson Foundation produced Issue Brief 4: Work and Health in 2008. While relying on US experience and data, the brief is highly relevant to Canada, as well as the US and Britain. It provides a comprehensive overview of the relationships among work, unemployment, working conditions, and health, as well as provides policy recommendations and a blueprint for creating a healthier workplace. The brief is available at www.commissiononhealth.org/

PDF/0e8ca13d-6fb8-451d-bac8-7d15343aacff/Issue%20Brief%204%20Dec%2008%20-%20Work%20and%20Health.pdf

While covering a number of topics related to the social determinants of health, Sir Michael Marmot also speaks about his work on employment. Along the way, he draws out a large number of policy recommendations flowing from his analysis. This video is an excellent review of the subjects covered up to this point. It can be accessed at www.youtube.com/watch?v=FF2SV-VfaC0.

For specifically Canadian content (although the site provides articles of an international and scientific nature as well), the Institute for Work and Health (www.iwh.on.ca/) is an especially rich resource. Articles range from workplace safety to issues of gender in the workplace to fair compensation.

READING 7

The social determinants and the healthcare system

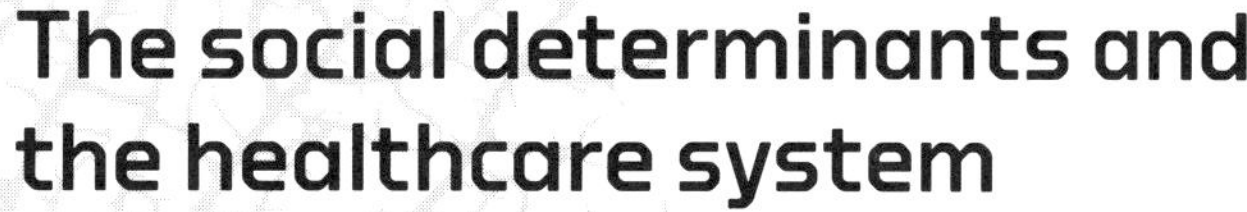

Yvonne Parry and Eileen Willis

TOPICS COVERED

This chapter covers the following topics:

- the healthcare system as a structural determinant of health
- models of healthcare and the social determinants of health
- access to healthcare as an intermediary determinant of health
- the Australian healthcare system and the social determinants of health
- policy initiatives for promoting the social determinants of health

KEY TERMS

Bulk billing
Health access
Intermediary determinants of health
Interest groups
Market-based model
Public policy
Quintile
Role substitution
Separation rates
Structural determinants of health
Welfare state

Introduction

Many of the chapters in this book have stressed that social factors, rather than biological or genetic ones, determine people's health. In this chapter, one specific social factor is examined and analysed for how it impacts on the health of individuals and population groups. This socio-political factor is the type of healthcare system available to a nation's citizens. In previous chapters, the authors have identified a range of social, cultural (including media), environmental, economic, and discriminatory practices that impact on the health of individuals and populations, including the way people may be stigmatised and suffer discrimination. In this chapter, the focus is on how the provision of health services and access to these services can be seen as a social determinant of health. The chapter will argue that access to consistent, timely, and appropriate health services is necessary to maintain and promote effective health outcomes for individuals and populations, especially disadvantaged groups.

In order to demonstrate how a nation's healthcare system can be understood as a social determinant of health, the chapter will draw on the World Health Organization's CSDH framework (2007), particularly the work of Solar and Irwin (2007). The first section of the chapter will summarise the CSDH argument that the healthcare system is a structural determinant of health and access to health services is an intermediary determinant of health. Second, it will describe the Australian healthcare system, specifically Medicare. It will then identify those features of the Australian healthcare system that are positive social determinants of health, and those features that contribute to and maintain inequalities in health. In the final section, examples of public policy that might contribute to good health outcomes and overcome some of the structural and intermediary determinants of health are provided.

The social determinants of health

The Commission on Social Determinants of Health (WHO 2007) has divided the social determinants of health into two broad categories: the structurally determined or 'upstream' factors, and the intermediary or 'downstream' factors. The **structural determinants of health** refer to those factors that impact on people's socio-economic position. These include such factors as an individual's income, occupation, and education. Other factors include welfare and taxation policies, or policies that allow equal opportunity for all groups regardless of gender, race, disability, or class. These social factors impact on life chances, which in turn impact on the health status of individuals. The evidence is that an individual's socio-economic position, in interaction with the overall socio-political climate of a country, determines health outcomes such as life expectancy (mortality) or rates of illness (morbidity) (Wilkinson & Pickett 2009). Individuals cannot control the socio-political context of a country, although groups such as political parties or **interest groups** or social movements might be able to bring about policy changes to improve health status.

The **intermediary determinants of health** are shaped by the structural determinants. They can best be understood as the way the structural determinants impact on individuals and the way they react to these determinants. They include

Structural determinants of health Those aspects of a society that influence an individual's health. These include the provision and availability of welfare services such as free healthcare, redistributive taxation practices, and policies to ensure that groups are not discriminated against.

Interest groups Groups of citizens that organise to influence government or public policy.

Intermediary determinants of health Those factors such as social position, access to healthcare, type of housing, or psychosocial risks in the environment or workplace that impact on health status.

factors such as access to healthcare, transport, adequate and safe housing, and safe working conditions (Solar & Irwin 2007). For example, populations in outer, lower socio-economic suburbs of large cities may not have access to the same efficient transport as people in inner suburbs. These people may react to this by not seeking specialist healthcare when it is needed. The intermediary determinants create a causal chain of influence over a person's life span and include factors such as their material circumstances, social position, environmental risks, and housing stress (Solar & Irwin 2007). For example, many social democratic countries have **public policies** around employment that protect workers who are made redundant from sinking into poverty by providing unemployment benefits to tide the worker over until they get a new job. Such welfare polices are part of the structural determinant of health and a key component of the **welfare state**. At the intermediary level, occupational health and safety policies ensure that individuals do not get injured on the job and are able to work in healthy environments. However, the intermediary determinant requires the individual worker to engage in a two-way process of adhering to work safety policies through appropriate workplace behaviour. Because the intermediary determinants of health include individual behaviours they also provide the means of direct delivery of interventions. In the above example, this might include health promotion campaigns directed at safety at work. Figure 19.1 illustrates the two social determinants.

Public policy Policies brought in by governments to administer education, healthcare, water, sanitation, etc.

Welfare state Provision by government of social services such as education, healthcare, old-age pensions. Usually free and funded through taxation.

Figure 19.1 The structural and intermediary social determinants of health

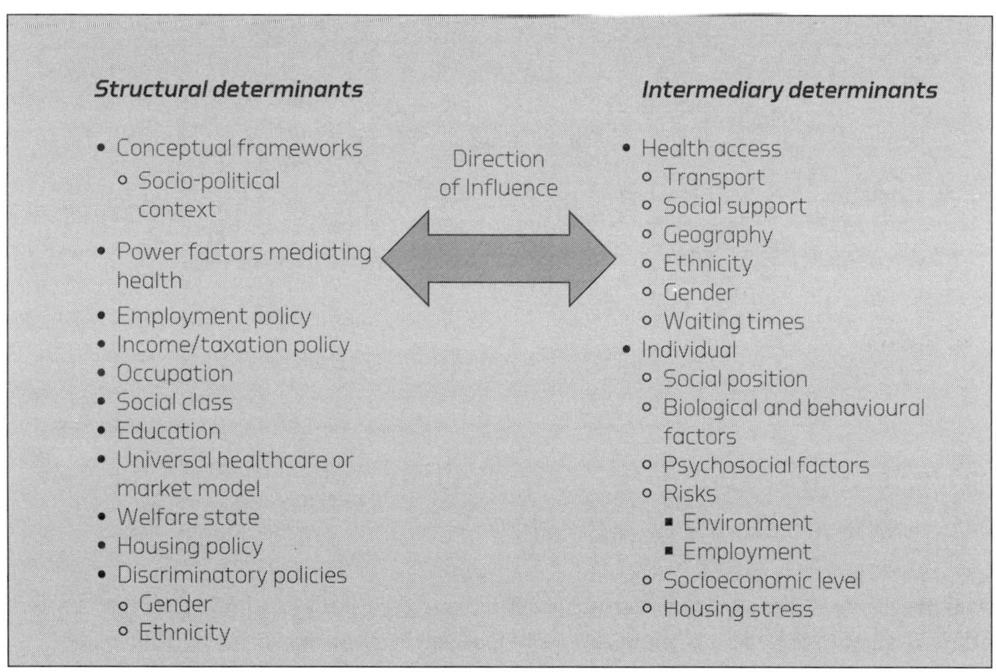

Source: Parry 2009

Stop and Think

Wilkinson and Pickett (2009) in their book *The Spirit Level* provide an evidence-based comparison of the richest 23 countries globally (with populations of over 3 million). They establish that it is more than income, both individually and nationally, that determines the health and social well-being of a population.

Health and social problems are linked to the size of the inequality within a nation, or the gap between rich and poor. Those countries that have smaller gaps between the haves and the have nots and provide support for their people, are more equal, and have fewer health and social problems overall. Conversely, those countries with large gaps have many more social and health problems to tackle. For example, the USA, one of the world's richest nations, has poorer outcomes across a range of health and social issues than many less wealthy countries.

The ability of a country to provide health and social services to its populace in an equitable manner also has a profound influence on population outcomes and the problems faced by the society as a whole. This is captured by the quote below:

> First, the differences between more and less equal societies are large—problems are anything from three to ten times as common in the more unequal societies. Second, these differences are not differences between high- and low-risk groups within populations which might apply only to a small proportion of the population, or just to the poor. Rather, they are differences between the prevalence of different problems which apply to the whole population. (Wilkinson & Pickett 2009, p. 173)

» How can this be? This seems counter-intuitive as surely those countries with more income and with affluent populations have fewer health problems.

» Do you have a view on why this is so?

The healthcare system as a structural determinant of health

As illustrated in Figure 19.1, the structural determinants of health go beyond income, occupation, and education to include the values and social policies in place in a country. This includes the kind of healthcare system. For example, if the government sees health as a human right, rather than an individual responsibility, it is likely to have some form of universal and free healthcare. If the prevailing value is individual rights, the healthcare system may be a user pays or private one.

The type of healthcare system a country has is a structural determinant of health, but as you can see, so too are our values.

Health policies, including the healthcare system, are maintained because they serve the interests of particular powerful interest groups who have sets of values about what they see as important. Besides the government in power, other powerful interest groups might include employer associations, private health insurers, unions, and health professional associations who all have ideas on how healthcare should be organised. Depending on their power, these groups are able to promote and maintain their interests because of their access to powerful decision-makers in government. These groups prevail upon the government to change or alter health policy in their interest or in the interest of members. This can be either positive or negative for particular populations. For example, a public free healthcare system is positive for low socio-economic groups, but a private user pays system may suit the needs of wealthier population groups who can afford private health insurance.

Types of healthcare systems and impact on access

One way of examining how the healthcare system is a structural determinant of health is to examine how the service is financed and whether this system allows for universal and relatively free coverage for all citizens. According to Docteur and Oxley (2003), there are three basic models of health delivery and financing. These healthcare systems differ in several ways: whether the funding is public or private, whether the care is provided by private practitioners or publicly paid providers, and who accepts responsibility for the provision and management of public or private healthcare.

The first is the *public-integrated model*. In countries that have this model, public hospitals and services are funded by the government as part of the welfare state. This makes it a *welfare-based model*. They do not separate insurance and provision functions. Doctors and other health professionals can be either public employees paid on a salary, or if in private practice contracting their services to the government. There is universal population coverage, regardless of income, and this coverage is simple to provide. Thus, **health access** is not dependent on the person's ability to buy health, but on the government's responsibility to provide healthcare as a right for all citizens. Healthcare is paid for through taxation. Those earning more income pay higher taxes and levies towards the healthcare system. Costs and the delivery of the system are directly covered by the government (Docteur & Oxley 2003; Davis et al. 2010). In this system, growth of overall health costs is easier to contain as the government provides both the universal coverage and the provision of services free from competition. The model is used in Australia (in the public hospital sector), Greece, Ireland, Italy, New Zealand, and Spain. Public hospitals are central to the provision of care in this model (Docteur & Oxley 2003).

Health access The opportunity or right to receive affordable, timely, and appropriate healthcare in a manner that promotes optimum health.

The limitations of this model include the lack of incentives to increase productivity or efficiency or to be responsive to patient's needs since the health professionals are waged. There is also a limit on the degree of consumer choice for the provider of services (Docteur & Oxley 2003).

The second approach is the *public-contract service delivery* model. This approach to healthcare funding uses public funds to contract private companies to provide healthcare (Docteur & Oxley 2003). An example of this in Australia is the primary healthcare services provided by general practitioners.

GPs are private providers paid on a fee-for-service basis by the Commonwealth through Medicare (NHHRC 2009a). The public contract model does provide incentives to prevent ill health and can be very responsive to patient needs. For example, in Australia the Commonwealth is able to provide incentives for GPs to become more efficient, increase their productivity, and offer new services. As there is only one funding body, this model is efficient, with low administration costs (Docteur & Oxley 2003). This model is also used in Germany, France, Netherlands, the UK (GP Trusts), and Japan. It requires high levels of government regulation and control to protect public funds and consumer health outcomes (Docteur & Oxley 2003), but despite this has the limitation of not being able to completely control service provider fees. As a consequence, access can be limited by the fact that the patient may have to make a co-payment or pay a gap fee.

The third and final model, the *private insurance model*, is an insurance-based system where delivery relies on the private sector, with the insurance and services delivered by private companies. In some countries, such as Switzerland, it is compulsory to take out private health insurance, while in others it is voluntary, as in the USA (Docteur & Oxley 2003).

There is a high degree of choice in this system and responsiveness to the patient's needs such as very short waiting lists or none. However, there is little or no cost control by government, insurance companies, providers, or individuals. Private insurance companies charge what the market will pay and in some instances limit access to care depending on the type of insurance cover. Affordability for the consumer is an issue with this model. In the 1990s, in an effort to manage increasing costs, the USA introduced managed care plans (Docteur & Oxley 2003). This change allowed insurers to select clients and providers and restrict patient treatments and service access (Docteur & Oxley 2003; Davis et al. 2010). More recent reforms by President Obama have attempted to ensure people are fully insured by private insurers, although how successful this will be is yet to be determined. Where private health insurance is the major form of health cover, unless the government provides some members of the society with healthcare, such as the poor and elderly, large segments of the population may not be covered by any form of health insurance and therefore have limited access to health. Examples of countries using this system include Switzerland (compulsory insurance), USA (voluntary insurance, although health insurance is a standard benefit of employment including in many minimum wages jobs), and Australia, where 50% of Australians have some form of private health insurance (Medicare Australia 2011). Table 19.1 summarises some of the differences in the three models around issues of access such as funding source, the extent of coverage, choice of practitioner, and waiting times.

Table 19.1 Models of healthcare access

Model	Funding Source	Health Access	Cost	Coverage	Choice	Waiting Lists
Public-integrated	General taxation	Universal primary and acute	Relatively free	Universal	No	Yes
Public-contract	General taxation or levy	Universal primary and acute	Relatively free, but may have gap fees	Restricted	Some	Yes

(continues)

Table 19.1 Models of healthcare access (*continued*)

Model	Funding Source	Health Access	Cost	Coverage	Choice	Waiting Lists
Private insurance	Consumer pays	Can be universal where legislated	Based on insurance premium costs and type of cover	Limited	Yes but restricted	No

Source: Adapted from Docteur & Oxley 2003; Davis et al. 2010

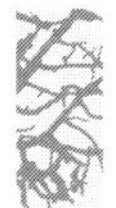

Mythbuster

Consider the claim that the USA has the best healthcare system in the world.

» *From the data presented so far why might this be an accurate statement? Why might this be an inaccurate statement?*

Health access as an intermediary determinant of health

Health access is defined as the opportunity or right to receive affordable, consistent, timely, and appropriate healthcare in a manner that promotes optimum health (Mahnken 2001). The particular model of healthcare impacts on access, but there are also intermediary factors such as waiting times for services, the number and amount of co-payments, barriers to particular services such as dental care, geographical isolation, or obstacles linked to gender, ethnicity, or age.

When people do not have access to good healthcare there are a number of negative consequences. These are not just limited to individuals, but include the entire population. They go beyond health to include negative outcomes for an individual's education, employment, and engagement in the social life of a community. For example, limited access to healthcare services is associated with a significant increase in infant mortality and morbidity (Frankenberg 1995; Sandiford et al. 1995; INDEPTH Network 2007), poorer economic outcomes and poverty (Wadsworth & Butterworth 2006; McCally et al. 2008), lower levels of social and community support (Hendryx et al. 2002), and lower education attainment (Solar & Irwin 2007; Doley et al. 2008). Further, limited access to healthcare in childhood is thought to cause disengagement from schooling (Doley et al. 2008), deleterious adult physical and psychological health outcomes (Wadsworth & Butterworth 2006), an increased incidence of poverty (Wadsworth & Butterworth 2006; McCally et al. 2008), and decreased participation in society, including the capacity to produce and consume goods (Hendryx et al. 2002; Shaw et al. 2006; Solar & Irwin 2007).

Limited health access can also lead to further health problems or deterioration in an existing condition (Bartley et al. 2005, 2006). This in turn may impact on a child's education, or an adult's income, or their capacity to care for their children. It may prevent them from returning to work, or increase the number of sick days they take. Accessing healthcare services is presumed to be an individual responsibility and behaviour; this is why the CDSH defines it as an intermediary determinant. However, as the case study below notes, while deciding to go to the doctor is an individual one, the factors that influence this decision may be out of the person's control. The case study illustrates one way in which health access, the cost of paying for medical care, impacts on a family's health.

Stop and Think

Research in Australia of patients admitted to hospital for a pre-existing condition found that 16.6% of the admissions were 'preventable but not prevented' (Hart 2006, p. 85). These patients had illness conditions that could have been prevented had they sought earlier medical care. If these patients had accessed appropriate primary healthcare services in a consistent, timely manner almost a fifth of the admissions would not have been necessary. Accessing healthcare and services in a manner that enables the cycle of illness to be interrupted or prevented is not only cost-effective, it is also less physically and psychologically tiring for those suffering illness episodes (Hart 2006).

Case Study 19.1 Access to healthcare by different social groups in Australia

In research conducted on access to primary care services, Parry (2011) interviewed a number of parents who took their children to the Emergency Department of a large public hospital for illnesses that were not life-threatening, instead of seeking more appropriate care from their local GP. Parry found that cost was a major factor in parents' decisions on seeking care for their children and themselves.

In the quote below, Gail, a single mother of two children, explains why she takes her child to a hospital Emergency Department rather than the more appropriate local GP clinic, and in her own case puts off consulting a medical specialist for several years.

> I just really wish the doctors wouldn't charge that big a gap, because that's the problem I have with the whole thing and that's why I wait years to get anything done. If I had the money I could see a specialist. My GP knows I'm a single parent and have a Healthcare Card and he still charges a gap fee to see the kids if I arrive at the surgery after 4 p.m. Sometimes you can't get an appointment before then, then there's a gap fee...They charge the gap they want, it's not fair.

In this case, the GP charges low-income patients a fee for a medical consultation. The clinic does **bulk-bill** if parents make an appointment before 4 p.m., but as Gail notes this is not always possible, particularly as she works. These high gap charges (intermediary determinant of health) are outside Gail's control. The Medicare model of service provision limits Gail's access to care because costs cannot be controlled by the government. In this case study Gail does not delay accessing healthcare when her children are sick; she either takes them after 4 p.m. to the clinic and has to pay a gap fee, or travels to the

Bulk billing The practice whereby the doctor accepts the Medicare scheduled fee rebate from the Commonwealth Government as the sole payment for a service rather than the additional cost of a gap fee.

Emergency Department of a public hospital where it is free. However, she does delay accessing healthcare for herself because of the high gap fees for medical specialist care. Delaying care can exacerbate an illness.

Adapted from Parry 2011

The Australian healthcare system

Market-based model A system where access to education, health, and housing must be paid for by the individual, or those who are sick or incapacitated must provide for their own income protection.

As we noted above, healthcare systems around the world can be divided into three broad categories, the first two welfare-based models and the third a **market-based model**. A welfare-based model assumes that health is a basic human right and that all citizens should have equal and timely access to healthcare. As a consequence, governments usually take some responsibility for organising and funding the healthcare system. A market model argues that in a democracy citizens should be able to choose how much and what kind of healthcare they wish to purchase. Under the market model, citizens pay for healthcare; under the welfare model, the government provides and manages the care through a state-run system or the funding of an insurance scheme. Pure market or pure welfare models do not exist. Most countries have a mix of both.

The Australian healthcare system is a mixture of market (private insurance model) and welfare provision (public-integrated and public-contract models). The foundation of the current Australian healthcare system is Medicare. It was established in 1984 by the Hawke Federal Labor Government at a time when up to 35% of Australians had no health cover (Willis 2009a). In recent years, funding has extended to some allied health and nursing services for people with chronic illness (Willis 2009a). The first point to note about Medicare is that it is a compulsory (everyone must be in the scheme), universal (everyone is covered by the scheme regardless of income), health insurance scheme based on the principle of equal access for all Australians. It is funded through taxation and a progressive levy on all taxpayers. This levy is set at 1.5% of each person's income or 2.5% for people on higher incomes who do not have private health insurance. The Medicare levy does not cover the full cost of healthcare, so in reality most Medicare-related health costs are funded through taxation (Leeder 1999; AIHW 2009).

Medicare is divided into two distinct parts: funding for hospitals and funding for primary care and other medical, allied health, and nursing services. Funding for hospitals can be viewed under the public integration model. The Commonwealth funds all public hospitals to around 50% of costs through tied grants to the state and territory governments, who must provide free and timely access to healthcare for all Australians and other eligible persons (Commonwealth of Australia 1993). While not a national health service, this component of Medicare effectively provides free hospital care to all Australians and as a healthcare policy is illustrative of a positive structural determinant of health. For example, if you were involved in a motor vehicle accident, had a heart attack, or a mental health event a state-funded ambulance would convey you free of charge immediately to a public hospital where you would receive free hospital, medical, nursing, and allied healthcare, including free pharmaceuticals during your hospital stay. Follow-up care in rehabilitation or part of the hospital's outpatient clinics would also be free, although you might have to pay a small charge for ongoing pharmaceuticals and wait several weeks or months for an outpatient appointment.

Similarly, if you required elective surgery such as a hip replacement this could be provided in a public hospital free of charge.

The second part of Medicare, also funded by the Commonwealth, provides funding for the patient to cover primary care from a medical practitioner, and some allied health and nursing services. This aspect of Medicare conforms to the public contract model. When the Hawke Labor Government introduced Medicare in 1984 they hoped funding for these medical services would be free through bulk billing. The Commonwealth sets the scheduled fee for all medical services and pays the doctors 85% of this fee. If the doctor bulk-bills the patient is not charged the gap fee, so the service is effectively free, but the doctor only receives 85% of the estimated cost of the service. If the doctor charges the scheduled fee the patient pays the additional 15%. This is called a gap payment. In its original design Medicare provided relatively free access to primary medical care with a low gap fee. Underlying both features of Medicare is an acknowledgment that health and access to affordable care is a basic human right that should be managed and provided by government and paid for through taxation or some form of universal insurance. These aspects of Medicare make it a positive structural determinant of health and in theory should ensure health access.

The limits of access to hospital care

The original 1984 Medicare agreements between the state and territory governments and the Commonwealth noted that hospital care must be timely. Timely care is defined as care that is offered within a clinically appropriate period. For example, as noted above, if you had a heart attack you would receive immediate care. But since not all medical conditions need to be treated straight away, some patients are assigned to elective surgery or outpatient waiting lists. While waiting lists must be made public, and the patient must not wait beyond what is considered safe, this is an area where health access becomes problematic. There are three problems associated with timely access to hospital care that illustrate the complexity of access to healthcare as a social determinant of health even in systems that take as a premise that health is a human right. The first problem is the increase in the population requiring care either as an emergency admission or for elective surgery. The increased pressure on public hospitals is partly explained as a result of population growth, the increase in the percentage of people living into their seventies and beyond requiring care for chronic conditions, the increase in education which leads people to demand quality healthcare, the drop in the number of people with private health insurance, and the high cost of medical care. As a result, elective surgery in public hospitals may not always be as timely as needed for the patient's comfort or convenience. This can impact on people's general well-being, but also on their capacity to earn their living and function in everyday life. The high demand for healthcare services may lead governments with publicly funded hospital systems to use a quota system to restrict the number of procedures as a cost containment strategy, since price is not a deterrent to patients (Hurst & Siciliani 2003). While there is logic to this strategy, it assumes that considerable numbers of patients demand, and their doctors perform, unnecessary surgery.

A second factor is geography. Not all Australians have equal access to public hospitals providing emergency or elective care. Examples include those living in rural and remote areas, particularly Indigenous Australians, and even those living in outer suburbs. Travelling to the city for hospital care brings with it added expenses, although the Patient Admission Transport Scheme, a welfare scheme that reimburses patients from rural and remote areas for their travel and accommodation costs while in a city hospital, provides some additional financial assistance. A major problem for these populations is that it is difficult to entice health professionals to work in isolated communities, or the population may be so low that it is not economically efficient for governments to provide the service. The model of healthcare is a factor here in influencing governments to provide the service.

A third factor relates to socio-economic status, including cultural and ethnic disparities in health access. Over 26% of those admitted to a public hospital for elective surgery come from the *Most Disadvantaged* quintile, while only 13% come from the *Most Advantaged quintile* (AIHW 2010d, p. 131). However, the disadvantage does not stop here. People in higher income brackets have higher rates of elective surgery. Sixty-nine per 1000 persons accessed elective surgery from the highest **quintile**, while only 38 per 1000 did in the lowest quintile (AIHW 2009, p. xv). This points to an underlying problem with the mixed nature of the Australian healthcare system. Those with private health insurance are able to seek timely and usually quick elective surgery or medical care in a private hospital with the doctor of their choice. Waiting lists are not as long in private hospital. People without private health insurance must wait until their name comes to the top of a public hospital waiting list. The problem is that in many cases emergency admissions take precedence over elective surgery, the lists of people needing surgery are long, and the number of procedures a hospital may perform in any one year may be capped.

Quintile A quintile represents 20% (a fifth) of the population. The lowest quintile is the poorest group; the highest group is the wealthiest.

Being poor, and therefore likely to be sicker, is not the only difficulty for low socio-economic populations. Their access to healthcare is also stratified. For example, data from the Australian Institute of Health (AIHW 2010d, p. 131) shows that the median waiting time for patients on public hospital waiting lists was 34 days. However, those in the second lowest quintile (or *Second Most Disadvantaged*) waited 37 days, while those in the highest quintile (*Most Advantaged*) only waited 24 days (AIHW 2010d, p. 261).

Figure 19.2 Separations per 1000 population for public and private elective surgery, by remoteness of area of usual residence

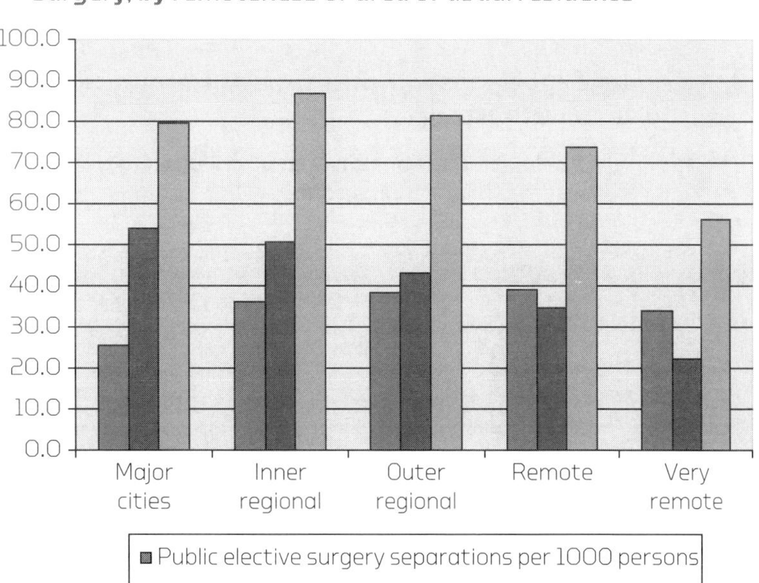

Source: AIHW 2010d

The impact of disadvantage can be examined through **separation rates** for elective surgery, this time looking at the issue of remoteness. Data from the 2008–09 report on Australian hospital statistics 2008–09 (AIHW 2010d) illustrates the impact of remoteness on access to elective surgery for people in the cities, outer suburbs, rural, and remote regions (Figure 19.2).

Separation rates The percentage of people who leave hospital before midnight on any one day either discharged, transferred to another facility, or who die.

Stop and Think

We know that geography makes a difference to rates of illness. People in rural areas in Australia have higher rates of illness, yet the graph above indicates that they are disadvantaged in access to elective surgery. This is partly because they do not have access to private hospitals as there are few in regional, rural, or remote areas.

» If you were Minister for Health how might you go about remedying this disadvantage?

Presumably, access to timely acute care should simply be a matter of increasing resources to the public system. However, how funds are allocated is a political issue that reflects the values of a society and the power of particular interest groups. For example, in order to encourage people to take out private health insurance, the Howard Federal Coalition Government introduced a 30% rebate for individuals and families with private health insurance. This policy decision diverted resources from the public health system to providing financial incentive to wealthier people. It increased the percentage of people with private health insurance, which in turn increased profits for private insurers, private hospitals, and doctors in private practice (Laris et al. 2008), but of course it may

Figure 19.3 Percentage of persons with private health insurance by quintile for Adelaide, South Australia

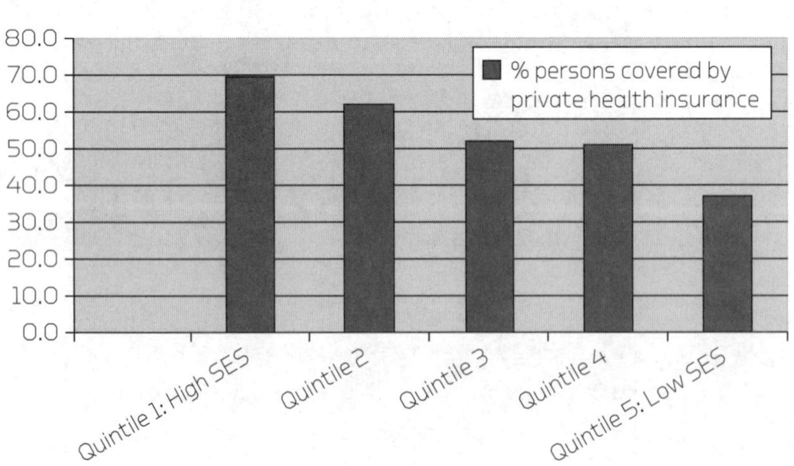

Source: PHIDU 2010

also have increased timely access to care for this population. Data on private health insurance shows that those in the *Most Disadvantaged* quintile have lower rates of private health insurance. Figure 19.3 provides the figures for Adelaide in South Australia by quintile. Readers can readily see that people in the *Most Disadvantaged* quintile have lower rates of health insurance. This means that elective, surgical, acute short-term health access is funded in the private sector, in favour of chronic, emergency, and costly health services provided in the public sector (Laris et al. 2008), given that 75% of the doctor's fee is covered through Medicare. Attempts by the Federal Labor Government to reduce this rebate have been politically difficult, indicating the power of interest groups to maintain health policy that supports the rich over the poor.

The limits of access to primary care

Just as access to hospitals can be problematic, so too is access to primary medical care. Costs, distance, and the problem of supply are major barriers to accessing primary care such as GP services. When Medicare was first introduced it was hoped that the majority of doctors would bulk-bill. However, as the story of Gail (Case Study 19.1) notes, doctors are free to charge any fee they like and many charge above the scheduled fee, leaving patients with an additional gap fee. To assist low-income individuals and families to manage the costs of primary care various Commonwealth governments have introduced safety nets to assist individuals and families manage the rising cost of co-payments. The first is the Family Safety Net. In 2010 the gap fee was $388.80 for an individual or family, after which point Medicare reimburses the individual or family the full scheduled fee. However, since many doctors charge above the schedule fee (Willis 2009b) the patient may still have a high gap fee to pay. To counter this a second safety gap, called the Extended Medicare Safety Net, was introduced by the Howard Government (1996–2007) to cover this gap. In early 2010, the safety net was $562.90 for disadvantaged individuals and families and $1126 for other families and individuals. Thus, disadvantaged families on low incomes or Commonwealth Benefits need to spend $562.90 in Extended gap fees before the rebate is provided. This rebate then provides for 80% of out-of-pocket expenses (Medicare Australia 2011).

The issue of fees for primary medical care is further complicated by the corporatisation of medicine (White 2001). Many small GP clinics have amalgamated to form large multi-purpose clinics either controlled by the doctors themselves or multinational firms. These clinics provide access to care without an appointment, so attract patients who cannot access a family doctor. However, access to the same doctor is not guaranteed. While the positive side of this development means patients can access the diagnostic tests they may need on-site, and get immediate medical care, the profit motive for owners has led to increased charges and a lack of continuity of care. For example, some large multi-purpose medical clinics that previously bulk-billed patients now require a co-payment or charge a significantly high gap fee that may mean that people on low incomes may put off seeking medical care that could prevent further illness (Vaughan & Harvy 2009). The issue of continuity of care goes to the heart of primary medical care. Wong and Regan (2009, p. 6) conducted research into client's experiences of access including the quality and consistency of healthcare they received. Patients in their research identified three types of continuity:

> i) relational—the ongoing therapeutic relationship between a consumer and provider; ii) informational—the use of information on past events and personal

characteristics to make care appropriate; and iii) management—a consistent and coherent approach to the management of a health condition. Participants believed that the inability to maintain a continuous relationship with a provider contributed to challenges in maintaining people's health.

Their data provides the basis for improvements to be incorporated into any future policy and health provision changes, and increasing compliance with treatment.

Distance, supply, and access

In addition to costs, distance and the shortages of GPs and medical specialists in rural and outer suburbs in Australia creates access problems. The problem manifests in two ways. First, there are fewer health professionals per population working in rural and remote regions, and second, the structure of the primary care component of Medicare (public contract model) means that health services in rural and remote regions are anti-competitive. For example, in rural and remote areas the number of GPs per population is considerably less than the higher-income densely populated urban areas of the capital cities. The low populations in rural areas create regional monopolies as the rural GPs are self-employed practitioners with no or restricted competition. This gives these medical practitioners the significant advantage of charging gap fees strengthened by medical shortages, professional dominance, and limited alternatives for services (Kenny 2004). The result is significant disparity in health access between rural and urban populations (Kenny 2004).

This inequity in access also extends to some urban populations. For example, many outer suburban areas have limited health access. This limits after-hours access and places a strain on other services (PHCIS 2006). Areas of socio-economic disadvantage also have higher numbers of patients per GP. Table 19.2 gives examples for five suburbs or towns in South Australia. Since Salisbury has a fertility rate of 2–3 children per women, while the Adelaide metropolitan area average is 1.61 (PHCIS 2006), there is a higher percentage of families with children in these areas with limited or no access to GPs. This table also shows that people living in Burnside have greater access to GP services than those living in outer suburbs or in rural and remote areas. The likely outcome for people in the Flinders Ranges or Salisbury is that they will have to wait for an appointment, whereas people in Burnside may be able to get a same-day appointment.

Table 19.2 Ratio of GP to population; selected SLA, South Australia

Statistical Local Area	1 Gp Per Head of Population	Designation
Burnside	659	Urban-inner
Playford	2,883	Urban-outer
Salisbury	2,883	Urban-outer
Mallala	4,172	Rural
Flinders Ranges	6,340	Remote
SA Average	**1,126**	

Source: Adapted from PHIDU 2006

Cost, access, distance, undersupply, and long waits for an appointment can deter people from accessing primary care, or they may seek inappropriate care such as attending a public hospital emergency department. For example, in 2009–10, 44% of presentations to public hospital emergency departments were for what is referred to as GP-type presentations. These are for illnesses that could be dealt with more effectively by the patient's family doctor. For large public hospitals this rate rose to 51% of all presentations (AIHW 2010d, p. 13). What this data indicates is that between 40% and 50% of people who present at a public hospital emergency department for primary care should really have seen their local GP. While it is not clear exactly why these people do not seek primary care from their GP, the research does show that low socio-economic groups the world over cannot afford appropriate primary medical care or do not have access to it. From this, we can assume that the key to health access is cost; this might be the cost to the consumer or the impact on profits made by the provider (Bell et al. 2007; Kelaher et al. 2008).

Health access reform

Most Western countries have attempted to deal with the problems of health access over the last 20 years through a series of reforms. In the early 1990s, these reforms focused on increasing productivity and efficiency of existing services by setting targets that attempted to ensure better access. Examples included providing hospitals with incentive funding if patients on elective surgery waiting lists did not have long waits. In Australia, public hospitals have to publish waiting times so that the public can see how efficient they are (Willis 2009b). More recent reforms to increase patient access have included increasing the number of health professionals educated and trained, and extending the skills and practice of health professionals other than doctors through a process of **role substitution**. Nurse practitioners are one example of this. Nurse practitioners can prescribe a limited number of drugs and order diagnostic tests. Another strategy has been to design new models of care. Case Study 19.2 provides information on GP Plus and Super Clinics—two policy initiatives aimed at reducing costs and ensuring speedy access to care.

Role substitution The process whereby one profession takes up the role and skills of another.

This discussion on health access has assumed that all sick people need is access to a GP and a hospital. This is not always the case. Comprehensive healthcare also means access to pharmaceuticals, dental care, and ongoing services for those with a mental illness or a chronic condition and for the elderly. Where these services are not provided in a free and timely manner, because they are outside the remit of the welfare state, some populations will have reduced life chances. Of course even where there is excellent health access, if populations do not have access to employment, education, or housing their health status will deteriorate.

Case Study 19.2 GP Plus and GP Super Clinics: Policy futures

In an attempt to improve access to health in areas where there is high need and limited services, the South Australian Government has introduced GP Plus Centres in low socio-economic suburbs and the Commonwealth will fund a number of GP Super Clinics around the country. These clinics were developed in conjunction with service providers to improve access and decrease the inappropriate use of services such as emergency departments for primary healthcare conditions. These services are located in areas of high need and low GP coverage.

The GP Plus clinics provide allied health and community support services such as parenting and counselling sessions. They may also provide access to speech pathologists, community paediatricians, mental health services providers, and kindy gym classes. The clinics are also able to provide after-hours access to GP services provided there is no alternative GP practice in that area. Where after-hours GPs are provided by the GP Plus Clinic all patients are bulk-billed if they have a Medicare card ensuring free access.

In addition, the GP Plus Centre also provides x-ray, blood screening, and other pathology services in order to decrease the need for patients to access acute care services for diagnostic purposes. However, GP after-hours services are not provided if the community has alternative access to a GP. For example, one GP Plus Centre in Adelaide is co-located with a daytime and after-hours private GP service. As a consequence, no GP services are provided by the GP Plus Centre until the private service closes each day at 5.30 p.m. The GP private service only bulk-bills healthcare card holders. Other patients need to pay an upfront gap fee of between $30 and $60 before seeing a GP. This has the potential to limit access and divert patients to emergency departments where the services are free.

Stop and Think

The establishment of GP Plus and GP Super Clinics is an attempt by state and Commonwealth governments to increase patient access to free primary care. However, the way in which Medicare is organised means that the profits of doctors must be safeguarded. Aspects of the Australian Constitution do not allow governments to insist that doctors become salaried employees.

» If you were Minister of Health, how might you go about remedying this disadvantage?

Summary

The social determinants of health are divided into the structural and intermediary. Health access is an intermediary determinant of health. An examination of health access as a social determinant of health requires understanding what kind of healthcare a particular country has in place. Most countries in the developed world have one of three types of healthcare systems. The first is the public-integrated model, which is usually funded by government. The second is the public-contract service delivery model, which uses public funds to contract private companies to provide healthcare. Both models have the capacity to provide universal and relatively free access to healthcare. The third model is the private fee-for-service approach. This model limits health access to those who can afford the care. The type of healthcare system a nation has is influenced by the values of that society, the kind of government, and its social policies. Health access as a social determinant is also underpinned by an understanding of health as a social right, rather than health as an individual responsibility.

In order to examine the health access of a particular system it is necessary to investigate the policies governing the provision of healthcare. In Australia, for example, Medicare both facilitates and limits access to healthcare. Access to GPs is based on the public-contract service delivery model whereby GPs are paid to deliver the service as private providers. As a consequence, they may not offer after-hours services or services to people in remote or rural areas. An example of recent policy initiatives to overcome this is the establishment of Medicare Locals across Australia. These will have a brief to ensure there are after-hours services in their region.

Tutorial exercises

1 Go to <www.equalitytrust.org.uk/why>.
   Read the front page. Watch the video report. On the right-hand corner at the bottom is a PowerPoint show. Watch this. Select a social determinant of health and see the results. The places will be either countries, or states in the USA. Bring some observations that you make to the class for discussion.
2 Go to the interactive features/graph on the website below. The biennial report compares healthcare system performance over several OECD countries. Review the results with the class.
3 Read the report *Mirror, Mirror on the Wall: How the Performance of the U.S. Health System Compares Internationally*, <www.commonwealthfund.org/Content/Publications/Fund-Reports/2010/Jun/Mirror-Mirror-Update.aspx?page=all>.
   This website provides a set of interactive graphs that discuss patient satisfaction, health system performance, and quality and safety issues in health systems. The US health system as a private insurance system is the most responsive to patient needs. So, why does it score so poorly on patient satisfaction, etc.? Discuss.
4 Identify those aspects of the social determinants of health that are part of the healthcare system. Identify those factors that are not part of the healthcare system. Discuss what can be done by health professionals to address the social determinants of health. What limitations do health professionals face?
5 What are the strengths and weaknesses of the Australian health system in terms of its approach to the social determinants of health?

Further reading

Davis, K., Schoen, C., & Stemikis, K. (2010). *Mirror, mirror on the wall: How the performance of the U.S. health system compares internationally*. The Commonwealth Fund. Report No 1400. <www.commonwealthfund.org/Content/Publications/Fund-Reports/2010/Jun/Mirror-Mirror-Update.aspx?page=all>.

Docteur, E., & Oxley, H. (2003). *Health-care systems: Lessons from the reform experience. OECD Health Working Paper 9*. Paris: OECD.

Hart, J.T. (2006). *The political economy of healthcare: A clinical perspective*. Bristol, UK: Policy Press.

Hendryx, M., Ahern, A., Lovrich, N., & McCurdy, A. (2002). Access to healthcare and community social capital. *Health Services Research*, 37(1), 85–101.

Marmot, M., & Wilkinson, R.G. (eds) (2006). *Social determinants of health*, 2nd edn. Oxford: Oxford University Press.

Websites

<www.phcris.org.au>

This website is the home of the Primary Healthcare Research and Information Centre. You can use it to keep up to date with policy reforms in general practice in Australia.

<www.publichealth.gov.au>

This web page is the home of the Public Health Information Development Unit. You can use it to access data on socio-economic status and health in Australia.

<www.who.int/social_determinants/thecommission/finalreport/en/index.html>

This is the home page for the WHO Commission on Social Determinants of Health.

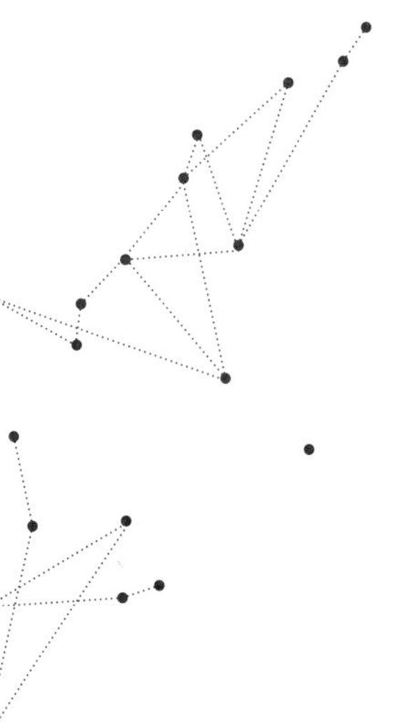

GENDERED HEALTH

Dorothy Broom, Maria Freij, and John Germov

Overview

- What gender differences exist in the experience of health and illness?
- What have been the origins and main activities of the women's health movement and the men's health movement?
- What are intersectionality and gender mainstreaming, and how can they be used to improve our understanding of gendered health?

GENDERED MORTALITY RATES IN THE SOVIET UNION

Contrary to general improvements in global mortality patterns, mortality rates in the Russian Federation (formerly the Soviet Union) worsened in the 1990s and early 2000s, and have only recently begun to recover (UNDP 2013). Researchers have been puzzled by this anomalous trend, but because the rise has occurred chiefly among adult men, part of the explanation must be sought in the gendered lives of the population. The question is: how do Russian women and men differ in the nature of their daily lives, paid and unpaid work, recreation and relaxation, sociability and social networks, family, and other personal relationships? Somehow, these factors apparently expose men and women to very different risks of the serious illnesses and injuries that lead to premature death.

Of course, gender is not operating by itself; there have also been dramatic transformations in the political environment, the economy, and in the opportunity structure that shapes access to the resources necessary to protect and promote health. Deterioration in infrastructure (agricultural and industrial plant and machinery, for example) also appears relevant. The stark sex difference suggests that these significant structural dimensions are expressed and experienced very differently in the lives of Russian women and men—so differently that they can make the literal difference between life and death.

Key terms

chronic illness
class (or social class)
ethnicity
gender/sex
gendered health
health literacy
health promotion
men's health movement
norms
'race'
randomised control trials (RCTs)
risk factors
sexism in medicine
sexual division of labour
women's health movement

Introduction

Because **gender** is such a significant dimension of social difference in contemporary Western societies, we tend to take it for granted. It is hard to imagine that gender could be less socially important or organised very differently from the familiar patterns that we see every day. So it can be surprising to learn that, while gender is socially recognised in all known societies, there is wide historical and cultural variation in the way it is expressed and experienced. In every society, at least some work is allocated on the basis of gender; this allocation is called the **sexual division of labour**. In some societies, females and males undertake sharply differentiated activities, and may be physically segregated for substantial periods, either because of social **norms** or as a consequence of the sexual division of labour. In other societies, children of both sexes are treated in much the same ways, but gender difference becomes important in adolescence or early adulthood. In many cultures, only a few activities are specific to one sex, and the sexual division of labour is minimal. Men dominate overtly in certain cultures; elsewhere, the lives and powers of the two sexes are largely balanced and complementary. In developed economies, the norms and symbols that govern gender tend to vary according to class, subculture, and ethnicity. And everywhere, gender patterns are dynamic: they change over time.

Indeed, the terms themselves are continually contested. In the early 1970s, a distinction was drawn between sex (biological) and gender (psycho-social) (Oakley 1972). Subsequent theoretical discussions have unsettled that clear dichotomy (Gatens 1983; Walsh 2004), and although the contrast is still often invoked, in this chapter the words are often used interchangeably. In the context of such variation and fluidity, making useful generalisations about gender and health is a challenging task. As with both class and ethnicity, the relationship between health and gender is a complex interaction between material circumstances, physical entities, cultural processes, and social organisation. The discussion here concentrates on the interplay between health and gender in Australia and in similar contemporary developed societies.

GENDER/SEX
This pair of terms refers to the socially constructed categories of feminine and masculine (the cultural identities and values that prescribe how men and women should behave), and the social power relations based on those categories, as distinct from the categories of biological sex (female or male).

SEXUAL DIVISION OF LABOUR
The nature of work performed as a result of gender roles. In contemporary English-speaking societies, the stereotype is that of the male breadwinner and the female homemaker, even though this pattern is far from an accurate description of most people's lives.

NORMS
Shared expectations about how people ought to act or behave.

BOX 7.1
DOING HEALTH SOCIOLOGY: GENDERING MEDICAL TRAINING

For decades, many women feared and avoided pelvic examinations and Pap smears because of their male doctors' lack of skill or sensitivity. The women's health movement (discussed later in this chapter) and the health consumers' movement lobbied together for the greater involvement of consumers in medical training.

As a result, in recent years, some medical schools have employed female tutors to act as pseudo-patients and train doctors to perform these procedures respectfully, so as to be able to make female patients as comfortable as possible. Some tutors are actually examined by medical students, and give feedback to the trainees on how to improve, sensitising trainee doctors regarding the impact of their behaviour on their patients, as well as equipping them with improved technical skills. These arrangements challenge the traditional model of medical expertise and professional power by investing authority in patients, particularly female patients, who have previously been the objects (and occasionally the victims) of what was considered to be normal medical practice.

Gender and health

One might think there is little to explain about the link between gender and health. Humans have sexually specific organs and processes, and malfunction in those organs and processes is the relationship between gender and health. Females can get ovarian and cervical cancer; males can get testicular and prostate cancer. According to this view, the rest of health is just human, not **gendered**.

GENDERED HEALTH
A term used to acknowledge the different experiences and exposures to health and illness that result from gender.

A discussion of sexually specific complaints hardly exhausts the topic. Many of the conditions that occur in both sexes appear more often in one sex than the other, or they occur at very different ages. For example, stomach cancer is much more common among males than females, whereas cardiovascular disease is common in both sexes, but tends to occur at later ages among women than among men, and with different symptoms. Because women present with nausea and back pain rather than crushing chest pain, like men, they have often been under-diagnosed and under-treated (Klinge 2010). These kinds of comparisons suggest that the health of women and men is a product of many elements, and not only their reproductive organs. The sexes differ in the types of lives that they typically live, and these differences can influence health; thus, gender is a significant and complex element in the social production of health and illness.

DISEASE AND DEATH: SEX COMPARISONS

Except for a very few nations (mostly in South Asia), there are slightly more females in the population than males because women typically live longer than men, and this is true for contemporary Australia (AIHW 2012). The Australian population is evenly balanced (50.3 per cent female), but because female life expectancy exceeds male life expectancy by nearly five years, there are proportionally more women in the older population (twice as many women as men aged 85 years and over) (Australian Government Office for Women 2009, pp. 3–4). The gender gap in longevity is gradually closing as male life expectancy has been improving more rapidly than female. Life expectancy for the Indigenous population is markedly shorter than for the total Australian population, but sex differences in longevity prevail among Indigenous as well as non-Indigenous people. The main causes of death are largely similar for both sexes, and sexually specific diseases contribute only a small proportion of the overall death rate, as is evident in Table 7.1. Dementia looms larger as a cause of death among women than men (because of the higher proportion of women among the elderly), while lung cancer still causes proportionally more deaths among men than women (although this gap has been narrowing).

THEORYLINK
See Chapter 8 for more about Indigenous health.

Health surveys usually find that the majority of the adult population has some health problem or other at any given time. Many of these health problems are comparatively minor, such as headaches or colds, but substantial proportions of people have a long-term health condition (lasting six months or more). While some of these are minor problems such as visual deficiencies that are readily managed, some are disabling sensory or mobility impairments, or life-threatening diseases such as cancer. In Australia's 2007–08 National Health Survey (NHS), females reported more diagnosed long-term conditions, and were more likely to report psychological distress, more likely to see a GP, and slightly more likely to be hospitalised (ABS 2012).

TABLE 7.1 LEADING CAUSES OF DEATH BY SEX, ALL AGES, 2009

	MALES			FEMALES		
Rank	*Cause of death*	*Number of deaths*	*% of all male deaths*	*Cause of death*	*Number of deaths*	*% of all female deaths*
1	Coronary heart disease	12,047	16.7	Coronary heart disease	10,476	15.3
2	Lung cancer	4761	6.6	Stroke	6706	9.8
3	Stroke	4514	6.2	Dementia and Alzheimer's disease	5491	8.0
4	Chronic lower respiratory diseases	3209	4.4	Lung cancer	3025	4.4
5	Prostate cancer	3111	4.3	Breast cancer	2772	4.1
6	Dementia and Alzheimer's disease	2786	3.9	Chronic lower respiratory diseases	2769	4.0
7	Colon and rectum cancer	2253	3.1	Diabetes	2050	3.0
8	Blood and lymph cancer (including leukaemia)	2175	3.0	Heart failure	1884	2.8
9	Diabetes	2120	2.9	Diseases of the kidney and urinary system	1818	2.7
10	Suicide	1631	2.3	Colon and rectum cancer	1812	2.6
	Total 10 leading	**38,607**	**53.4**	**Total 10 leading**	**38,803**	**56.7**
	Total all causes	**72,320**		**Total all causes**	**68,440**	

Source: Adapted from AIHW 2012, p. 93

Analyses of the gendered experiences of illness have often been summarised by the cliché: 'women get sick; men die'. This apparent paradox is at least partly a consequence of oversimplifications—attempts to make sweeping generalisations about the sexes. On closer inspection, the statistics are not so contradictory. Men tend to experience comparatively higher rates of several life-threatening conditions (such as heart disease and lung cancer), and **risk factors** such as alcohol abuse and dangerous driving. Women, on the other hand, have relatively higher prevalence of painful, unpleasant, but not lethal conditions such as migraines and arthritis. For example, according to most measures, psychological distress appears to be more common among women than among men (ABS 2012), and a particularly gendered experience of illness is the prevalence of disordered eating and eating disorders among young women (Hepworth 2008); but men die from suicide more frequently than women. Furthermore, over the life course, there are variations in certain conditions. Younger men are more likely than younger women to have elevated blood pressure, but by the age of 65, more women are hypertensive. Such variations mean that we must regard simple contrasts between the sexes with caution, since they can conceal as much as they disclose (Macintyre et al. 1996).

RISK FACTORS
Behaviours or circumstances that are known to increase people's likelihood of injury or illness.

An emphasis on sex differences tends to focus our attention on those health conditions for which simple contrasts can be drawn. But in many respects, the sexes are more alike than different, and variations within gender categories (by age or ethnicity, for example) may be more significant. As we have seen in Table 7.1, cancers and cardiovascular disease are the major causes of mortality for all adults. Although there are sex contrasts in the distribution of specific malignancies, cancer is a major threat to the survival and health of adults of both sexes. Furthermore, everyone falls prey to colds and the flu, and long-term health problems such as sensory impairment can affect anyone. The fact that both sexes can get a condition—even that they get it equally frequently—does not necessarily mean that gender is irrelevant to that condition. Instead, we must look to more subtle patterns to detect the interplay between health and gender, as gender can shape both exposures to health problems and the experience of illness.

Gendered exposures

While the main causes of many illnesses remain uncertain, others have clearly identified risk factors. Smoking is a well-known hazard for a range of serious diseases, and smoking behaviour is sexually differentiated. Among Australians over the age of 18, more men than women smoke daily—22 per cent compared to 18 per cent—and in the past this sex difference was very much more marked (ABS 2009). Consequently, it is not surprising that more men than women die from lung cancer. Smoking also contributes to the higher male rates of premature morbidity and mortality from cardiovascular and respiratory diseases. Indeed, it has been suggested that a substantial portion (perhaps half) of the sex difference in longevity may be attributable to smoking (Waldron 1995). These comparisons illustrate a dynamic interaction between gender and exposure to a major illness risk factor. Most of the illness effects of current exposure will appear many years in the future, when the relationship between smoking (the 'exposure') and gender may have changed yet again. If young women continue to take up smoking, the sex difference in lung cancer will probably diminish further or even disappear. Already, deaths from lung cancer among women are nearly as common as deaths from breast cancer, although not yet as common as lung cancer deaths among males, which are still significantly more numerous than deaths from prostate cancer (AIHW 2012; ABS 2009).

Certain occupations are significant sources of injury and disease, and the sexual division of labour has tended to concentrate men in the occupations in which such hazards are greatest. Construction, mining, waterside work, and farming are examples of comparatively hazardous occupations mainly done by men. Few female-dominated occupations are as dangerous, although the health hazards of work done mainly by women (such as office jobs, nursing, and unpaid household and care giving work) are often harder to detect and may be underestimated (Broom 1986; Doyal 1995; Strazdins & Broom 2004). The nature of the hazards may also differ. For example, the low levels of autonomy, pay, and other rewards in many female-dominated jobs may contribute to women's poor mental health. Such work conditions are also known to be related to comparatively poor physical health (Bosma et al. 1997).

Exercise is a health-beneficial behaviour that helps prevent a wide range of significant illnesses, and most young children engage in regular vigorous activity. While for many years it was reported that there was a difference between men and women as regards physical activity, participation in exercise is now 'similar across all age groups except for adolescence (15–17 years), where males were more active' (AIHW 2012, p. 204). While physical activity generally improves health, some forms of exercise, particularly contact sports, also expose participants to injury.

Males, especially young men and adolescents, are more likely to engage in a range of dangerous activities such as contact sports, risky driving, and physical aggression. Consequently, males suffer higher rates of accidental and non-accidental injury.

There is considerable debate about gender differences in exposure to violence and its health consequences (Hurst 1996). Males are the main perpetrators of physically violent acts, but they are not the main victims of all kinds of violence (Fletcher 1995). The most visible kinds of violence—such as mugging, street assault, and fights in public places—usually involve males as both aggressor and victim. But sexual assault and domestic violence are overwhelmingly crimes against women, and they constitute a serious threat to the health of many women; worldwide, 'at least one out of every three women has been beaten, coerced into sex or otherwise abused in her lifetime' (Abdool et al. 2010, p. 36). In 2013, the head of WHO described violence against women as 'a global health problem of epidemic proportions' (WHO 2013).

In the US, 'domestic violence is the leading cause of injury among women of reproductive age' (World Bank 1993, p. 50), and women appear to be at particularly high risk when they are pregnant (Stark & Flincraft 1991; Gazmararian et al. 1996). Despite uncertainty regarding exact numbers, the overall picture is similar in Australia and in many other developed societies (Taft et al. 2004). A woman is in more danger of being attacked (ABS 1996) or killed (Easteal 1993) by a man she knows—particularly by her partner or former partner—than by a stranger. For example, the Women's Safety Survey reported that 338,700 women were victims of physical violence, and 180,400 of these assaults were committed by the women's partners or former partners—nearly three times as many as those where the attacker was a stranger (67,300) (ABS 1996, p. 19). Australian research has found that 'intimate partner violence is responsible for more ill health and premature death in Victorian women under the age of 45 than any other of the well-known risk factors, including high blood pressure, obesity and smoking' (VicHealth 2004, p. 8). In summary, women's and men's vulnerability to violence is sharply differentiated and socially situated: 'violence against women is sustained by and helps to sustain women's unequal status in society' (Abdool et al. 2010, p. 36).

Recently, public health measures have been taken to address this major issue. The United Nations (UN) Secretary General has appointed a panel of men against violence against women (Abdool et al 2010) and in Australia, the Federal Labor Government's *National Plan to Reduce Violence Against Women and their Children 2010–2022* targets domestic and family violence and sexual assault, aiming 'to bring attitudinal and behavioural change at the cultural, institutional and individual levels, with a particular focus on young people' (COAG 2012, p. 12). The multimedia campaign 'Violence against Women: Australia Says "No"', which first ran in 2004, brought further attention to the issue and used a range of media to communicate a strong stance against violence against women.

Gendered experiences

The example of violence, discussed above, points directly to a consideration of how gender shapes the experience of health conditions. A particular injury, such as a concussion or laceration, may be physically the same, regardless of how one was injured; but the personal meaning and social consequences will be very different depending on whether the injury was sustained in a car accident, a mugging by a stranger, a pub fight with a drinking companion, or an attack by one's intimate partner. The first three of those sources of injury are likely to be singular or relatively rare events, to be publicly recognised, and to receive immediate assistance. By contrast, 'wife bashing' is apt to be repeated and escalating, shrouded in shame and secrecy, and often concealed from health care workers. Indeed, the source of injury is frequently undetected, even when injuries are so severe that the victim presents at an emergency service (Roberts 1994). While any injury can leave emotional scars, the psychological impact of being attacked by a loved and trusted partner is particularly devastating and personally debilitating. Because females are typically shorter and lighter than males, and are less likely to have learned skills of self-defence, women are often poorly equipped to protect themselves if their partner becomes violent. In the rare instance in which a man is attacked by a female partner, other elements of shame and denial may enter the picture because of the implicit insult to masculine power and strength. Thus, the experience of violent assault is highly variable and contains important gender dimensions. Even public violence among males is gendered insofar as displays of toughness and aggression are often considered markers of masculinity, so that men and boys who try to avoid violent behaviour may be victimised themselves (Plummer 1999).

Another area shaped by gender is the diagnosis and treatment of heart disease. Research in the US, the UK, and Australia suggests that cardiovascular symptoms may be investigated less thoroughly and treated less intensively in women than they are in men (Ayanian & Epstein 1991; Steingart et al. 1991). Sometimes the difference may reflect excessive intervention in the treatment of men (Bicknell et al. 1992), or morbidity before admission (Sonke et al. 1996), while other studies suggest that certain women may miss out on potentially beneficial therapies because of misdiagnosis (Tobin et al. 1987; Lawlor et al. 2001). Although some researchers believe that women's high mortality after a heart attack is accounted for by pre-existing risk factors (physiological and/or lifestyle), this does not fully explain the sex discrepancies (Feibach et al. 1990), and there is evidence of systematic under-diagnosis and under-treatment of women. The failure to pursue symptoms vigorously could be a result of the erroneous belief that women are less likely to get heart disease, or that they get it only in advanced old age. This might make doctors less likely to suspect heart disease in a woman, and hence less likely to investigate it thoroughly or manage it appropriately when it occurs (McKinlay 1996). It may also promote the belief among women and their families that heart disease is not a women's health problem, and therefore that their risk factors or symptoms are not important. Surprisingly, although these issues have been studied for two decades, research shows that doctors still tend to diagnose and manage patients with symptoms of heart attack differently, leading to the identification of a pattern the researchers called 'gendered ageism' (Arber et al. 2006).

Similar gender differences have been documented in admissions to intensive care units and in the treatment of a range of critical illnesses (Fowler et al. 2007). A popular impression prevails—perhaps shared by doctors—that men are prone to ignore symptoms, and that their elevated mortality is a consequence of their reluctance to seek medical care, but systematic research does not consistently confirm that idea (Macintyre 1999); on the contrary, American and British studies have found that women who have symptoms of a heart attack are more likely than men to delay seeking care (Meischke et al. 1993; Emslie et al. 2001; Martin et al. 2004). Researchers now suspect that heart disease (and perhaps other illnesses) may be characterised by different symptoms in females and males, so that clinical definitions of 'classic cases' derived from males could contribute to under-diagnosis of women. While such factors may account for delays and failures in diagnosing, they would not explain inadequate treatment of women once a diagnosis has been achieved.

Even such apparently trivial illnesses as colds and flus may be experienced in ways that are organised and given meaning by gender (Macintyre 1993). For example, because of women's responsibilities for unpaid domestic work (Bittman 1991) and their concentration in casual employment (with no paid sick leave), they may find it particularly difficult to stay in bed when they are ill. Married men are more likely to be in full-time employment and hence to be unavailable to supply domestic care to ailing family members, but when those same men get sick, they may have paid sick leave as well as a supportive wife. These patterns, and the lifelong habits and material circumstances to which they contribute, are particularly important with regard to the care of people with severe or **chronic illness**. Among older people, women are twice as likely as men to live alone and hence to have no co-resident who can care for them when they are sick or frail. Women are more likely to need care from outside the household at some time during their lives, and so have a different interest in state-funded services (Gibson & Allen 1993; OSW 1999).

Many of the patterns described above are inflected by other social variables such as **'race'**, and **ethnicity**, and **class**. For example, in some cultures, the expectation that health care will be supplied by members of the family (usually women) obstructs access to health and community services delivered by agencies or professionals. In Australia, when family members cannot supply needed support, ill and elderly migrants from such cultures can be disadvantaged by their reluctance to use the services they need.

Class has been found to correlate with most measures of health: better health is consistently associated with higher status. The relationship between health and socio-economic status prevails for both sexes, but the relative importance of various elements of social and material circumstances is, to an extent, distinctive for women and men (Arber 1991; Macintyre 1997; Broom 2008). It has, however, been difficult to establish appropriate measures of status for the whole population because of women's interrupted labour-force involvement and part-time employment to accommodate child rearing.

All these examples show how the experience of illness may be gendered in subtle and complex ways, even for conditions that are not sexually specific. They also illustrate how the relationship between health and gender can be complicated by other dimensions of social difference (see the other chapters in Part 2 of this book for further detail).

CHRONIC ILLNESS
A long-term or permanent illness condition that has no known cure (for example, diabetes).

'RACE'
A term without scientific basis that uses skin colour and facial features to describe what are alleged to be biologically distinct groups of humans. Race is actually a social construction used to categorise groups of people and sometimes implies assumed (and unproven) intellectual superiority or inferiority.

ETHNICITY
Sociologically, the term refers to a shared cultural background, which is a characteristic of all groups in society. As a policy term, it is used to identify migrants who share a culture that is markedly different from that of Anglo-Australians. In practice, it often refers only to migrants from non-English-speaking backgrounds (NESB migrants).

CLASS (OR SOCIAL CLASS)
A position in a system of structured inequality based on the unequal distribution of power, wealth, income, and status. People who share a class position typically share similar life chances.

Responding to gendered health and illness

For many years, it was commonly assumed that the gendered patterning of disease and death was a simple 'fact of nature' that humans could do little or nothing about. Culture and medicine constantly modify 'facts of nature', though, and in most societies health problems that could lead to severe illness, injury, or death if not treated are not allowed to run their course if they can be controlled. Notwithstanding, the best approaches to gendered health are less obvious than treating post-operative infection or catastrophic bleeding. It is one thing to describe the way gender interacts with health and illness; it is quite another to determine when those interactions are creating problems, and to discern how individuals, communities, and societies might respond constructively.

SEXISM IN MEDICINE
Doctors' discriminatory and harmful treatment of women by ignoring women's health concerns in medical research and intervention, not informing women of the availability of other treatments or the side effects of drugs/therapies, and labelling of women's problems as 'psychosomatic' rather than 'real'.

A problem identified over three decades ago has been referred to as **sexism in medicine**. Originally this term pointed to the sexual division of labour in medical care, where most doctors were men and nearly all nurses were women. Nursing is still mainly a female profession, but the medical workforce is now much more gender balanced, particularly among primary care doctors, although most medical specialties are still male-dominated (Chur-Hansen & Elliott 2007). The term 'sexism in medicine' later came to refer to the 'sexist' behaviour of some male doctors. Far from signalling a constructive sensitivity to the potential relevance of gender, sexism in medicine included behaviour that was at best objectionable and at worst dangerous. Anecdotal evidence was substantiated by systematic research showing that male doctors sometimes did not interact appropriately with their women patients (Broom-Darroch 1978). They failed to hear or accept women's accounts of their symptoms and did not inform women about unwanted effects of drugs and other therapies. Furthermore, doctors have been prone to label women's problems as psychiatric or psychosomatic rather than 'real' (Barrett & Roberts 1978).

Through the centuries, women's depression has often been labelled 'hysteria'—relating to the *hystera*, or womb—and 'initially viewed as a physical condition linked to the movement of the uterus' (Busfield 2010, p. 173). Women's depression was thus marginalised in comparison to the more 'legitimate' diagnoses of men's depression; for example, the binaries have included hysteria/melancholy and hysteria/shell shock: 'whatever the changing terms, hysteria has been constructed as a pejorative term for femininity in a duality that relegated the more honorable masculine form to another category' (Showalter 1993, p. 292).

The movement of substantial numbers of women into medicine does not automatically improve care for women, due to medical socialisation. Still, there is evidence that the changing sex ratio is also changing aspects of medical culture in ways that may diminish some of the most offensive and harmful aspects of sexism in medicine (Pringle 1998). The influx of women into medicine has prompted Riska (2010b, p. 398) to ask a series of vital questions: 'Does it make any difference whether there are more women doctors today? Is medicine practised differently if the doctor is a woman and not a man? To what extent do women physicians represent a vanguard within the profession, which will head the rest of the profession towards a substantial change in the way medicine is practised?'

Historically, women in Australia have had difficulty getting access to birth control services (Matthews 1984), especially if doctors felt that those women (young, unmarried, divorced, or disabled) should not be sexually active. The advent of family planning services and women's health centres has substantially alleviated the problem in most metropolitan areas, but it remains a significant health issue in some rural areas of Australia, as well as in many nations around the world.

RESEARCH

Service providers striving to give women the best possible care have been handicapped by limited medical research on women and their health problems. Until recently, men and other male animals have been the main, or only, subjects of most studies of disease, diagnostic procedures, management, therapy, and prevention (Melbourne District Health Council 1990). Often, even when women are included, no analysis by gender is reported (Greenberger & Marts 2000). One consequence has been the comparative neglect of many women's health concerns, except those that are directly relevant to fertility (Eckerman 1999), which is arguably the women's health domain of most interest to men. As a result, often relatively little is known about how non-reproductive disorders may manifest themselves differently in women and men, how risk factors may vary, or how the sexes may differ in their response to therapeutic interventions such as drugs (Woosley et al. 2000). This is due to a construction of the male body as normal, and, consequently, the female body becomes abnormal. The 'normal' body is not subject to hormonal cycling, lactation, or pregnancy, and women have thus been excluded from much medical research for these reasons. Not until the late 1980s did concerns arise that conducting research on white young men excluded the needs of not only women, but also children, ethnic minorities, and the elderly (Klinge 2010).

The women's health movement (see below) brought attention to the fact that the male body was considered standard and generic (Riska 2010a). When research was undertaken on men's and women's coronary heart disease (CHD) in a 10-year randomised double-blind placebo-controlled study in the US, it was found that men's risk of CHD was significantly reduced by a low dose of aspirin, but that this did not reduce the risk of stroke. In women, the drug had no impact on CHD, but reduced the risk of stroke by 17 per cent (Riska 2010a). This astonishing revelation also highlights how one-dimensional—and dangerous—it can be to translate research on men to women, and how further research needs to include subjects other than the young, white male.

While these deficiencies persist (Vidaver et al. 2000), they are gradually being addressed by the growth in gender-specific research, and by major longitudinal initiatives such as the 'Million Women' study in the UK and the 15-year Women's Health Initiative in the US (Finnegan 1996), which included **randomised control trials (RCTs)** of the effects of diet and hormone replacement therapy in preventing breast and colorectal cancer, heart disease, and osteoporosis. In the 1990s, the Australian Government sought to remedy the neglect of women's health research by funding a major longitudinal study, beginning data collection in 1996 (Brown et al. 1996). Known as the Australian Longitudinal Study on Women's Health, the ongoing study has recruited more than 40,000 respondents in three age cohorts (young, mid-age, and older-age women) to investigate health issues spanning social, psychological, and biomedical factors.

RANDOMISED CONTROL TRIALS (RCTs)
A biomedical research procedure used to evaluate the effectiveness of particular medications and therapeutic interventions. 'Random' refers to the equal chance of participants being in the experimental or control group, and 'trial' refers to the experimental nature of the method. RCTs tend to privilege biomedical over social responses to illness.

The exclusion of women from research has significant implications for population health. For example, a number of drugs originally approved for general use have later been found to affect men and women quite differently, as we have just seen, in some instances necessitating their withdrawal from the market—most frequently when they are belatedly found to be ineffective for or harmful to women (Woosley et al. 2000). Furthermore, a variety of non-lethal but difficult women's health conditions, such as endometriosis, remain poorly understood. Also, concerns that have been identified by women, such as poverty (Redman et al. 1988) and violence (Jones 1996), were for many years not considered as 'health' issues by researchers and largely escaped scrutiny.

GETTING MASCULINITY ON THE AGENDA

Perhaps a surprising aspect of the traditional perspective is that it has neglected masculinity—as well as femininity—in health and health research. This may seem paradoxical in light of the male domination of medicine, the focus on males in research, and the privileging of the male body as 'normal'; but it is less surprising when we note that these processes have occurred without being explicitly theorised. Hence, until recently, there was no conscious or thoughtful attention to masculinity per se. While men have featured in medical research and often in **health promotion** campaigns (Keleher 2004), there was little effort to consider how masculinity may figure in health and disease. The example of smoking has already been introduced. Although it was mainly a male activity for several decades, few people except advertisers have paid attention to its function as a means of confirming and displaying certain forms of masculinity. More interest in the gender—not to mention class—implications of smoking, and hence of quitting, might have reduced men's smoking sooner.

HEALTH PROMOTION
Any combination of education and related organisational, economic, and political interventions designed to promote behavioural and environmental changes conducive to good health, including legislation, community development, and advocacy. See also **primary health care** and **public health**.

Efforts to promote dietary change and exercise must also take gender seriously if they are to be effective. Tobacco use and drunkenness have been socially accepted behaviours for men, and are almost required in some circles of adolescent and young adult men. They are also becoming common among some young women. The similar prevalence of tobacco use or drunkenness should not be assumed to have the same meanings, social sources, or consequences for women and men, though (Broom 2008). For example, women were originally recruited to smoke when smoking prevalence was very high among men; and while prevalence has declined in both sexes, the decline has been much more rapid among males than females. Young people who take up smoking now do so in a very different social and symbolic environment. The social and sexual signification of smoking continues subtly to shape tobacco use in gender-specific ways (Nichter et al. 2006; Gilbert 2007). For example, it appears that young males have more alternative ways (such as sport) to establish attractive adolescent identities, whereas young females may risk appearing 'uptight' to their peers if they do not smoke (Plumridge et al. 2002).

In recent years, increased awareness of the pertinence of masculinity to health has stimulated a dramatic rise in research (Robertson 2003) and commentary on a wide range of issues, including policies (Smith 2007) and services (Bentley 2006). There are now many books devoted to the topic as well as several specialist journals, and new teaching and research programs have been established. These initiatives promise to enhance the basis on which fully elaborated approaches to gendered health can be developed.

Because gender is so much a part of the taken-for-granted world (Connell et al. 1999), it is easy to rely on anecdotes and stereotypes to interpret gendered patterns in health without realising that it is happening. For example, it is popular to refer to male risk-taking behaviour; but such generalised allusions are of much less value than information about which males take risks; which risks they take and in what circumstances; how their masculinity might be implicated in their behaviour; or how masculinity might be mobilised to diminish risk. A positive example is available in a study that investigated the culture surrounding particular sports, whose participants were more liable to engage in violent behaviour, as a way of understanding the specific dynamics involved in a stereotyped form of male health risk (Kreager 2007).

Another striking exception to the tendency to ignore or oversimplify masculinity has been the case of homosexual men dealing with HIV/AIDS. Their efforts have been distinguished by a focus on the lives of specific groups of men, and they have sought to transform prevention into a positive and pleasurable part of gay masculinity. Research into how HIV was originally controlled in Australia may supply valuable directions for the appropriate incorporation of gender in future research.

These examples point to the need for six major shifts in order to improve research (including applied research) on health:

1 the inclusion of women in clinical trials and epidemiological research;
2 routine analyses of health and medical data by gender;
3 the investigation of health issues to which women and men themselves give priority;
4 an understanding that 'women's health' and 'men's health' include conditions beyond reproduction;
5 the study of women's and men's health in their own right, and not simply in comparison with each other or when disease prevalence differs by sex;
6 the study of how particular forms or aspects of gender (specific masculinities and femininities) are distinctively related to health.

The women's health movement

By some accounts, contemporary sensitivity to the relationship between gender and health was initially created by the renascent women's movement, beginning in the late 1960s (Broom & Doyal 2004). Since that time, what might loosely be termed the **women's health movement** has worked to change the face of health services for women, and there is now substantial evidence of such change. Participants in this movement were the first to identify sexism in medicine (discussed above), and many of the movement's early activities were efforts to overcome sexism. Women have advocated innovations such as:

- improvements and expansion in health services;
- safer, cheaper, and more accessible contraceptives;
- better access to terminations of pregnancy;
- changes in medical education and increases in the number of women in medical practice;
- encouragement of multidisciplinary teams in the delivery of health care;
- fostering support groups to enable women to help one another.

WOMEN'S HEALTH MOVEMENT
A term broadly used to describe attempts to address sexism in medicine by highlighting the importance of gender in health research and services. Achievements include women's community health centres and Australia's 1989 National Women's Health Policy.

All of these are occurring, at least to an extent.

In contemporary Australia, perhaps the single most visible manifestation of the movement is the existence of several dozen predominantly community-based, feminist-influenced women's health centres. These centres are located in every state and territory, mostly in large urban areas, though some are in regional centres, country towns, and smaller cities. They have come into being largely as a result of community-based action that has sought to establish services that are controlled by women and more appropriate to women's needs, as defined by women themselves (Broom 1991). Because they are now such a familiar part of the Australian health care landscape, readers may be surprised to learn that their origins were highly contentious.

Despite the fact that most of the activities of women's health centres do not duplicate those supplied by mainstream medicine (Broom 1997), doctors in private practice feared that centres would compete for their clientele, or they objected to the employment of what they thought were 'unqualified' women's health workers. Several women's health centres were opened with minimal funding and relied heavily on volunteer labour and donations of money and materials. A few centres were notorious for their political radicalism, but almost all have sought to influence the mainstream, recognising that most women will obtain most health services from conventional sources. Reliance on government funding, a commitment to serving the most vulnerable clients, and the desire to encourage doctors and hospitals to become more 'woman friendly' are all challenges that have confronted women's health centres. They were partially legitimised as a strategy of the first National Women's Health Policy in 1989 (Gray 1998) and have become better established since the first centres opened in 1974. Nevertheless, and despite their long waiting lists, opposition persists and some commentators now claim that they have become obsolete. A recent detailed study of Australia's women's health movement would suggest that many of the underlying problems persist, though (Jamieson 2012).

GOVERNMENTS RESPOND

Governments—both state and Commonwealth—have responded to women's community-based action by developing women's health strategies, policies, and programs. Much of this activity took place during the 1980s and 1990s, with particular focus on the National Women's Health Policy launched in 1989 (CDCSH 1989) and the program for its implementation. Despite their apparent legitimacy, such developments have not been without their critics. During the early 1990s, considerable energy was expended defending a complaint against women's health initiatives and services brought by a male doctor (then employed by the Commonwealth Department of Health). The complaint used the *Sex Discrimination Act 1984* (Cth) to assert that women's health services discriminate against men. It was heard by the President of the Human Rights and Equal Opportunity Commission (HREOC) in 1991 and 1992, and the decision upheld the lawfulness of special women's health activities (Broom 1994). Nevertheless, by the mid-1990s, diminished resources for health, reallocation of previously targeted women's health funding, and an increasingly conservative political climate began to accomplish what the discrimination complaint could not: the partial winding-back of women's health services. The political pendulum swung back again in 2010, with the release of Australia's second National Women's Health Policy—recommitting the Federal Government to addressing women's health and well-being specifically (UN 2010a).

The 1995 Fourth World Congress on Women in Beijing brought women's health issues to an international forum (Van Wijk et al. 1996). Globally, a very broad range of common principles in health care (universal access, gender sensitivity, and appropriateness) were identified. The most urgent health needs, however, are nationally and locally specific. The emphasis in developing countries is on clean water, adequate fuel for cooking and heat, secure food supplies, and basic maternal and infant health. In developed countries, the focus tends to be more on dignity in medical treatment, participation in decision-making, better care for chronic conditions such as cancer, and reducing inequalities in access to services. Clearly, there can be overlap on many issues—such as access to safe means of fertility control and real choice about when to use them—but most priorities tend to be specific rather than universal. In 2010, the UN Commission on the Status of Women provided a 15-year review of the issues identified at the Beijing World Congress, noting considerable progress in many parts of the world (UN 2010b).

Men's health: progress or threat?

The focus on **men's health** in Australia and other English-speaking countries followed the women's health movement by about 20 years (Sabo & Gordon 1995; Primary Health Care Group 1996; Baker 2001). It has benefited from a number of the theoretical and political developments that resulted from the women's health movement, but identifies distinctive issues and strategies (Fletcher 1995). For example, goals such as reducing drink-driving and other highly risky behaviours are central elements on a men's health agenda, particularly for young men. Suicide is an urgent priority. Early detection of unhealthy weight, high blood pressure, and other lifestyle risk factors form the focus of relatively recent health promotion targeting middle-aged men, including screening checks at workplaces.

MEN'S HEALTH MOVEMENT
Running parallel to women's health initiatives, the men's health movement recognises that certain elements of masculine identity and behaviour can be hazardous to health.

Specific subgroups of men have particular needs, as is evident from the activities of gay men in relation to HIV/AIDS. Resonating with women's health initiatives, men's health advocates have identified the importance of investigating the role of masculinity in men's health, recognising that certain elements of masculine identity and behaviour can be hazardous to health. For Indigenous Australian men, the threats of morbidity and premature mortality from substance abuse, violence, and complications of diabetes loom very large (Rowley et al. 2008). These insights suggest that improving men's health will entail slow and careful shifts in understandings of what it means to be a man in contemporary society.

In Australia, Commonwealth-sponsored national men's health conferences have been held since 1995. A national centre of excellence in male reproductive health (called Andrology Australia) was established with Commonwealth funding in 1999. Initial steps towards a national men's health policy (Primary Health Care Group 1996) were taken in the mid-1990s at the direction of the then Commonwealth Health Minister, Carmen Lawrence. Although a change of government delayed the process (Lumb 1997; 2003), the return of the Federal Labor Government eventually led in 2010 to Australia's first National Male Health Policy; Australia is one of the few countries in the world to have such a policy. The policy builds upon a variety of school- and community-based health training, education, and health promotion programs that have targeted men's health issues in each state and territory since the 1990s. In addition, both the Australian Medical Association (AMA) and the Royal Australian College of General Practitioners (RACGP) have official statements on men's health.

Some women's health advocates are nervous about men's health initiatives. The anxiety is provoked in part by the stark realities of tiny budgets for community health activities and a perception that resources for men's health will be taken from hard-won, vulnerable, and poorly funded women's health programs. Such fears are inflamed by episodes such as the discrimination case brought before the HREOC, summarised previously, and by the rhetoric of a few individuals who assert that the accomplishments of women's health services have been made at the expense of men's health. Some commentators argue that women's health initiatives rely on feminist claims that women are 'victims' and that women are 'sicker' than men. These critics of women's health go on to assert that it is not women but men whose health is disadvantaged by sex, that attention to women's health is misplaced and the focus should be shifted to men. As we have seen above, such generalisations about which sex is 'sicker' are unlikely to be informative empirically, and still less likely to work to improve the health of men or women.

It is important to note that critics have pointed out that the conceptualisation of men's health is in itself flawed; while acknowledging that there are 'certainly groups of men with pressing health needs [it can be argued that] these are generally related to factors associated with men's class or socio-economic status, their indigeneity, ethnicity, sexuality and so on [and that] these differences are usually much greater than those identified between men and women' (Schofield 2010, p. 244).

Both laypeople and health professionals—female and male—are beginning to explore how various forms of masculinity may enhance or detract from men's health. Mothers and wives who become aware of neglected health problems in their sons and husbands have been among those who have stimulated the increased activity and awareness of diseases such as testicular cancer.

Several connections between men's health and masculinity can be noted, and these are influenced by dominant ideals of masculinity, especially for 'Anglo-Australian cultures, which deem it "unmanly" to publicly maintain health and voluntarily seek regular medical "check-ups"' (Oliffe 2009, p. 347). Risk-taking behaviours may also be a way to perform manhood, denial of illness can be a way to uphold masculinity, and the weakness and fragility that can come with illness can be seen as 'unmanly'.

In Anglo-Australian culture, men have traditionally worked physically, needing a strong and tough body, and have performed masculinity through sport and drinking (Oliffe 2009). This effectively perpetuates hegemonic masculinity: 'it is the daily "gendering" of behaviours that are constructed as masculine' and these are 'both habitual and defensive in order to protect men from being judged as less than masculine' (Rosenberg 2009, p. 418). In light of this, concerns have been raised with regards to men's **health literacy**—their understanding of health, health risks, and health behaviours (Peerson & Saunders 2009; Rosenberg 2009). Health promotion programs have attempted to address these issues, and 'men's sheds' have gone some way to engage men to talk about physical and mental health, as well as aspects directly related to health, such as bereavement and loss (Men's Sheds Australia 2012). The social construction of masculinity has clear impacts on men's health behaviours: 'Public health concerns across a range of men's health issues underpin the need for an increased focus on men's health policy

HEALTH LITERACY
The extent to which people are able to find, understand, and apply information about health issues and health services.

(or at the very least a policy incorporating a "gender mainstreaming" approach)' (Smith et al. 2009, p. 436). Equally importantly, attention to the relationship between gender and health stands to benefit both women and men.

THEORYLINK
See Chapter 24 for more on health literacy.

Intersectionality and gender mainstreaming

Intersectionality has its roots in the work of African American feminist scholars and aims to move beyond the favoured categories of analysis, which are often manifested in the three big areas of gender, 'race', and class (Hankivsky 2012; Connell 2012). Too often, gender—or other sociological categories—are added factors, rather than incorporated into a research design. The call for research that embeds categories is growing louder, and contemporary theorists such as Raewyn Connell (2012) state that '[p]olicy documents about gender usually take "women" and "men" as fixed, unproblematic categories' (p. 1657), and that '[c]ategorical thinking consistently underplays diversity *within* gender categories' (p. 1658). For these reasons, she recommends a relational approach that 'understands gender as multi-dimensional: embracing at the same time economic relations, power relations, affective relations and symbolic relations' (p. 1677).

Similarly, Olena Hankivksy (2012) comments that because intersectionality 'challenges practices that privilege any specific axis of inequality' (p. 1712), it is better equipped to examine 'how social locations and structural forces *interact* to shape and influence human experiences' (p. 1713). In order to address the negative impact on unequal gender relations on health care, an approach that aims to highlight the complexities of the debate rather than perpetuate a binary and simplified way to look at gendered health care is needed (Kuhlmann & Annandale 2010; Annandale & Riska 2009).

Answering the call for a larger focus on the institutional context, which some critics argue the intersectional approach has failed to overcome, is 'gender mainstreaming'—'an umbrella term for new approaches to both gender equality and policy-making' (Kuhlmann & Annandale 2010, p. 4). The World Health Organization (WHO) states that

> it is not enough simply to 'add in' a gender component late in a given project's development. Research, interventions, health system reforms, health education, health outreach, and health policies and programs must consider gender from the beginning ... All health professionals must have knowledge and awareness of the ways gender affects health, so that they may address gender issues wherever appropriate and thus make their work more effective. The process of creating this knowledge and awareness of—and responsibility for—gender among all health professionals is called 'gender mainstreaming'. (2012)

The aim to arrive at gender-sensitive health indicators means that gender needs to be a central component in any health conceptual framework (Lin & L'Orange 2010) and not just as an 'add-on' (Klinge 2010). For example, the disadvantage of health status and access to health care for gay and lesbian patients has been well established (Edwards 2010)—the health needs of homosexual men and women have often been marginalised. An intersectional perspective that rejects the dichotomous and categorical thinking that has dominated much of health care discourse is better equipped to address the specific health needs of homosexual men and women by taking into account the cultural and subcultural aspects that affect health needs. Since women's and men's health movements have focused on gender and not sexuality, they have 'inadvertently entrenched heterosexism, contributing to the ongoing obscurity of non-heterosexual women's [and men's] needs' (Edwards 2010, p. 257; see also Connell 2012).

Commentators have pointed out that a risk of speaking of 'gendered' health care is that it is often tacitly equated with women's health care, since men (white and heterosexual) have so long been the norm in health research (Connell 2012; Edwards 2010). The binaries of male and female have been seen as polar opposites and not as end-points on a fluid scale. Lesbian, gay, bisexual, transgender, and intersex (LGBTI) people challenge this categorical view and demonstrate that a more advanced intersectional perspective is necessary. Because a gendered social order influences the status of people—and in turn how they are treated and spoken to and about—non-heterosexual men and women's needs risk not being met in the heteronormative health care system. Research is rare on the physical health of non-heterosexual men and women (with the exception of research on HIV), often relying on small samples which cannot be generalised (Edwards 2010). Non-heterosexual men and women's self-reported health status is lower than that of straight men and women, and they also have higher levels of mental health problems and a higher risk of suicide. Health risks such as these, that are related to stigma and (lower) social status, warrant an intersectional perspective that takes the whole picture into account and steps away from the limited perspective of fixed notions of male and female.

Conclusion: towards a gendered understanding of health

In the future we may have to think of gender as a much more complicated concept than the simple dichotomous variable to which most of us are accustomed. Increasingly more writers now suggest that it is time to move towards gender-specific approaches that 'provide greater interpretive richness and give full voice to the complexity of the socially constructed meaning of gender' (Kunkel & Atchley 1996, p. 295). We must remember that such dimensions as 'race', ethnicity, and age are all implicated in gender in ways that cannot be reduced to binary thinking (Annandale & Riska 2009). A person is not black at one moment and male the next: he is always a black male (among many other things): 'A "gender-inclusive" agenda challenges dichotomous thinking about both the social and the biological, prompting us to think more in terms of continua of experience between women and men, both in terms of physical markers (such as hormone levels, body fat) and social markers (health-related attitudes and behaviours), rather than binary divides' (Annandale & Riska 2009, p. 125). The implications of such connections present challenges to accurate and constructive research about health and gender, and to the development and delivery of appropriate health promotion and medical care services.

Complex models may be awkward and more intellectually demanding than a simple bivariate model, but greater complexity promises more fruitful and ultimately more practical ways of thinking about contemporary social life and the health patterns with which it is inextricably entangled. A productive analysis of gender involves taking both masculinity and femininity seriously, and appreciating that gender is an aspect of every person's individual experience and social life. Femininity and masculinity are complex sources of risks and benefits, simultaneously—but differently—constraining and empowering.

Broad social, political, and economic change, the accomplishments of the women's health movement, and the emergence of activity regarding men's health have all altered the context in which health is created and managed. They have also effected subtle shifts in the meanings of gendered subject positions. For example, from the embattled beginnings of the women's health movement in the early 1970s, women's health has become more 'mainstream' and established, despite its continuing vulnerability, and the identities of all the actors (participants, supporters, and opponents) are modified by these developments (Singleton 1996). Approaches to funding health services and measuring their productivity are also in considerable flux throughout the developed world. All these and other changes have altered fundamental aspects of the way health and gender are understood, and therefore the way research, services, and advocacy will proceed in the future. While it is not clear how or by whom the next phase will be defined, it seems likely that revised assumptions and alliances will be necessary, and that attention to gender—not simply to women—will be a feature of developing understandings of health. If that is so, it will not be before time.

SUMMARY OF MAIN POINTS

- The typical way of life of each sex differs, and these differences can influence health. The statement that 'women get sick; men die' is a gross oversimplification. Men experience comparatively higher rates of life-threatening conditions, while women have a relatively high prevalence of some painful, but not lethal, conditions. Binary gender contrasts must be treated with caution since they can conceal as much as they disclose.
- A number of studies show that sexism in medicine has resulted in objectionable and harmful treatment of women by male doctors, such as male doctors ignoring women's accounts of their symptoms, not informing women about unwanted effects of drugs and other therapies, labelling women's problems as 'psychosomatic' rather than 'real', and failing to diagnose and treat serious illnesses in women.
- Until recently, men have been the main subjects of most medical research. Such bias is based on an assumption that the 'normal' body is not subject to such processes as hormonal cycling, pregnancy, lactation, or menopause, and that females can therefore be excluded from research.
- The women's health movement has advocated safer, cheaper, and more accessible contraceptives; better access to terminations of pregnancy; changes in medical education and increases in the number of women in medical practice; encouragement of multidisciplinary teams in the delivery of health care; women's health centres; and the National Women's Health Policy.
- Attention to gender and health stands to benefit both women and men, and as such both women's health services and men's health services are needed.
- Social change—including changes prompted by the advocacy of women's and men's health activists—are altering the environment in which health policy is developed, health services are delivered, and health and illness are experienced.
- An intersectional perspective recognises that 'male' and 'female' are not fixed categories and, through acknowledging the interplay between many social factors, encourages research and policy responses that move away from simplistic categorical thinking.

SOCIOLOGICAL REFLECTION

GENDER AND SMOKING

Smoking rates among teenaged women in Australia are very similar to those among similarly aged men. How therefore can gender still be relevant to understanding adolescent smoking? How is experimenting with cigarettes different for young women and young men? What about refusing offers to smoke? How does smoking operate to support certain gendered social relations and undermine others? What does smoking or sharing cigarettes symbolise to and say about young men and young women?

DISCUSSION QUESTIONS

1 In what ways is gender an important factor in determining the exposure to, and experience of, health and illness?
2 Why is the statement 'women get sick; men die' an oversimplification of the link between gender and health?
3 What are some examples of 'sexism in medicine' and how can it be addressed?
4 What do you think may be the impact on the practice of medicine of increasing numbers of women doctors? Have you experienced any difference in your medical treatment if the doctor is a woman and not a man?
5 Summarise some of the explanations of why sexual assault and domestic violence are overwhelmingly perpetrated by men against women.
6 What are the benefits of an intersectional approach to the study of gender and health? What are its drawbacks?

FURTHER INVESTIGATION

1 The rise in numbers of female doctors has made little impact on the practice of medicine. Discuss.
2 How successful has the women's health movement and the entry of increasing numbers of women into the medical profession been in addressing 'sexism in medicine'?
3 Examine the ways in which femininity and masculinity result in gendered exposures and gendered experiences of health and illness.

FURTHER READING

Annandale, E. 2009, *Women's Health and Social Change*, Routledge, London.

Australian Institute of Health and Welfare (AIHW) 2012, *The Health of Australia's Males: A Focus on Five Population Groups*, AIHW, Canberra: <www.aihw.gov.au/publication-detail/?id=10737421980&libID=10737421980>.

Broom, D.H. 1991, *Damned if We Do: Contradictions in Women's Health Care*, Allen & Unwin, Sydney.

Kuhlmann, E. & Annandale, E. (eds) 2012, *The Palgrave Handbook of Gender and Healthcare*, 2nd edn, Palgrave Macmillan, New York.

Mitchell, L. 2011, *Domestic Violence in Australia: An Overview of the Issues*, Department of Parliamentary Services, Canberra: <www.aph.gov.au/About_Parliament/Parliamentary_Departments/Parliamentary_Library/pubs/BN/2011-2012/DVAustralia>.

Robertson, S. 2007, *Understanding Men and Health: Masculinities, Identity and Well-being*, Open University Press/McGraw Hill, Berkshire.

Rosenfeld, D. & Faircloth, C.A. 2006, *Medicalized Masculinities*, Temple University Press, Philadelphia.

WEB RESOURCES

Australian Longitudinal Study on Women's Health: <www.alswh.org.au>.

Australian Women's Health Network: <www.awhn.org.au>.

International Journal of Men's Health: <www.mensstudies.com/content/120391>.

Journal of Men's Health: <www.jmhjournal.org>.

Mengage: The NSW Male Health Clearinghouse: <www.mengage.org.au/Home.aspx>.

The Men's Bibliography by Michael Flood: <http://mensbiblio.xyonline.net>.

National Male Health Policy: <www.health.gov.au/internet/main/publishing.nsf/Content/male-policy>.

National Women's Health Policy: <www.health.gov.au/internet/main/publishing.nsf/Content/national+womens+health-1>.

Women's Health Initiative (USA): <www.nhlbi.nih.gov/whi>.

DOCUMENTARIES/FILMS

Dance Me to My Song (1998): 101 minutes.

An Australian film directed by Rolf de Heer about a woman dealing with cerebral palsy and her belligerent carer.

The Shape of Water (2006): 70 minutes.

A documentary narrated by Susan Sarandon about five women striving for social justice in their developing countries. Information available online: <www.theshapeofwatermovie.com>.

REFERENCES

Abdool, S.N., García-Moreno, C. & Amin, A. 2010, 'Gender equity and international health policy planning', in E. Kuhlmann & E. Annandale (eds), *The Palgrave Handbook of Gender and Healthcare*, Palgrave Macmillan, New York, pp. 36–55.

Annandale, E. & Riska, A. 2009, 'Towards a gender-inclusive approach to women's and men's health', *Current Sociology*, vol. 57, no. 123, pp. 123–33.

Arber, S. 1991, 'Class, paid employment and family roles: making sense of structural disadvantage, gender and health status', *Social Science & Medicine*, vol. 32, no. 4, pp. 425–36.

Arber, S., McKinlay, J., Adams, A., Marceau, L., Link, C. & O'Donnell, A. 2006, 'Patient characteristics and inequalities in doctors' diagnostic and management strategies relating to CHD: a video-simulation experiment', *Social Science & Medicine*, vol. 62, no. 1, pp. 103–15.

Australian Bureau of Statistics (ABS) 1996, *Women's Safety Australia*, Cat. no. 4128.0, ABS, Canberra.

Australian Bureau of Statistics (ABS) 2006, *2004–05 National Health Survey: Summary of Results*, Cat. no. 4364.0, ABS, Canberra.

Australian Bureau of Statistics (ABS) 2009, *National Health Survey: Summary of Results, 2007–08 (Reissue)*, Cat. no. 4364.0, ABS, Canberra.

Australian Bureau of Statistics (ABS) 2012, *Year Book Australia*, Cat. no. 1301.0, ABS, Canberra.

Australian Government Office for Women 2009, *Women in Australia 2009*, Commonwealth of Australia, Canberra.

Australian Institute of Health and Welfare (AIHW) 2012, *Australia's Health 2012*, AIHW, Canberra: <www.aihw.gov.au/publication-detail/?id=10737422172>.

Ayanian, J.Z. & Epstein, A.M. 1991, 'Differences in the use of procedures between men and women', *National Men's Health Conference*, AGPS, Canberra, pp. 100–11.

Baker, P. 2001, 'The international men's health movement', *British Medical Journal*, vol. 323, no. 7320, pp. 1014–15.

Barrett, M. & Roberts, H. 1978, 'Doctors and their patients', in C. Smart & B. Smart (eds), *Women, Sexuality and Social Control*, Routledge, London, pp. 41–52.

Bentley, M. 2006, 'A primary care approach to men's health in community health settings: it's just better practice', *Australian Journal of Primary Health*, vol. 12, no. 1, pp. 21–6.

Bicknell, N.A., Pieper, K.S., Lee, K.L., Mark, D.B., Glower, D.D., Pryor, D.B. & Calif, R.M. 1992, 'Referral patterns for coronary artery disease treatment: gender bias or good clinical judgment?', *Annals of Internal Medicine*, vol. 116, no. 10, pp. 791–7.

Bittman, M. 1991, *Juggling Time: How Australian Families Use Time*, Office of the Status of Women, Canberra.

Bosma, H., Marmot, M.G., Hemingway, H., Nicholson, A.C., Brunner, E. & Stansfeld, S.A. 1997, 'Low job control and risk of coronary heart disease in *Whitehall II (Prospective Cohort) Study*', *British Medical Journal*, vol. 7080, pp. 558–65.

Broom, D. 1986, 'The occupational health of houseworkers', *Australian Feminist Studies*, vol. 1, no. 2, pp. 15–34.

Broom, D. 1991, *Damned if We Do: Contradictions in Women's Health Care*, Allen & Unwin, Sydney.

Broom, D. 1994, 'Taken down and used against us', in C. Waddell & A.R. Petersen (eds), *Just Health: Inequality in Illness, Care and Prevention*, Churchill Livingstone, Melbourne, pp. 397–405.

Broom, D. 1997, *There Should Be More: Women's Use of Community Health Facilities*, National Centre for Epidemiology and Population Health, Canberra.

Broom, D. 2008, 'Gender in/and/of health inequalities', *Australian Journal of Social Issues*, vol. 43, no. 1, pp. 11–28.

Broom, D. & Doyal, L. 2004, 'Sex and gender in health care and health policy', in J. Healy & M. McKee (eds), *Health Care: Responding to Diversity*, Oxford University Press, Oxford.

Broom-Darroch, D. 1978, *Power and Participation: The Dynamics of Medical Encounters*, PhD thesis, Australian National University, Canberra.

Brown, W., Bryson, L., Byles, J., Dobson, A., Manderson, L., Schofield, M. & Williams, G. 1996, 'Women's health Australia: establishment of the Australian longitudinal study on women's health', *Journal of Women's Health*, vol. 5, no. 5, pp. 467–72.

Busfield, J. 2010, 'Gender and mental health', in E. Kuhlmann & E. Annandale (eds), *The Palgrave Handbook of Gender and Healthcare,* Palgrave Macmillan, New York, pp. 172–88.

Chur-Hansen, A. & Elliott, T.E. 2007, 'Medical education and the medical workforce in Australia', *Journal of Continuing Education in the Health Professions*, vol. 272, no. 1, pp. 34–5.

Commonwealth Department of Community Services and Health (CDCSH) 1989, *National Women's Health Policy: Advancing Women's Health in Australia*, AGPS, Canberra.

Connell, R. 2012, 'Gender, health and theory: conceptualizing the issue, in local and world perspective', *Social Science & Medicine*, vol. 74, no. 11, pp. 1675–83.

Connell, R.W., Schofield, T., Walker, L., Wood, J., Butland, D., Fisher, J. & Bowyer, J. 1999, *Men's Health: A Research Agenda and Background Report*, Commonwealth Department of Health and Aged Care, Canberra.

Council of Australian Governments (COAG) 2012, *National Plan to Reduce Violence against Women and their Children 2010–2022*, COAG, Canberra: <www.fahcsia.gov.au/sites/default/files/documents/05_2012/national_plan.pdf>.

Doyal, L. 1995, *What Makes Women Sick: Gender and the Political Economy of Health*, Rutgers University Press, New Brunswick.

Easteal, P.W. 1993, *Killing the Beloved: Homicide Between Adult Sexual Intimates*, Australian Institute of Criminology, Canberra.

Eckerman, E. 1999, 'Towards a new gendered and "differentiated" social epidemiology', in L. Hancock (ed.), *Analysing Health Policy*, Allen & Unwin, Sydney.

Edwards, J., 2010, 'The healthcare needs of gay and lesbian patients', in E. Kuhlmann & E. Annandale (eds), *The Palgrave Handbook of Gender and Healthcare,* Palgrave Macmillan, New York, pp. 172–88.

Emslie, C., Hunt, K. & Watt, G. 2001, 'Invisible women? The importance of gender in lay beliefs about heart problems', *Sociology of Health & Illness*, vol. 23, no. 2, pp. 203–33.

Feibach, N.H., Viscoli, C.M. & Horwitz, R.I. 1990, 'Differences between women and men in survival after myocardial infarction', *Journal of the American Medical Association*, vol. 263, no. 8, pp. 1092–6.

Finnegan, L.P. 1996, 'The NIH women's health initiative: its evolution and expected contributions to women's health', *American Journal of Preventive Medicine*, vol. 12, no. 5, pp. 292–3.

Fletcher, R. 1995, *An Introduction to the New Men's Health*, University of Newcastle, Newcastle, NSW.

Fowler, R.A., Sabur, N., Li, P., Juurlink, D.N., Pinto, R., Hladunewich, M.A., Adhikari, N.K.J., Sibbald, W.J. & Martin, C.M. 2007, 'Sex- and age-based differences in the delivery and outcomes of critical care', *Canadian Medical Association Journal*, vol. 177, no. 11, pp. 1513–19.

Gatens, M. 1983, 'A critique of the sex/gender distinction', in J. Allen & P. Patton (eds), *Beyond Marxism? Interventions After Marx*, Intervention Publication, Leichhardt, pp. 139–57.

Gazmararian, J.A., Lazorick, S., Spitz, A.M., Ballard, T.J., Saltzman, L.E. & Marks, J.S. 1996, 'Prevalence of violence against pregnant women', *Journal of the American Medical Association*, vol. 275, no. 24, pp. 1915–20.

Gibson, D. & Allen, J. 1993, 'Phallocentrism and parasitism: social provision for the aged', *Policy Sciences*, vol. 26, pp. 79–98.

Gilbert, E. 2007, 'Constructing "fashionable" youth identities: Australian young women cigarette smokers', *Journal of Youth Studies*, vol. 10, no. 1, pp. 1–15.

Gray, G. 1998, 'How Australia came to have a National Women's Health Policy', *International Journal of Health Services*, vol. 28, no. 1, pp. 107–25.

Greenberger, P. & Marts, S.A. 2000, 'Women in NIH-funded research studies: there's good news, and there's bad news', *Journal of Women's Health & Gender-Based Medicine*, vol. 9, no. 5, pp. 463–4.

Hankivsky, O. 2012, 'Women's health, men's health, and gender and health: implications of intersectionality', *Social Science and Medicine*, vol. 74, no. 11, pp. 1712–20.

Hepworth, J. 2008, 'The social construction of eating disorders', in J. Germov & L. Williams (eds), *A Sociology of Food and Nutrition: The Social Appetite*, 3rd edn, Oxford University Press, Melbourne, pp. 368–82.

Hurst, D. 1996, 'Men's violence and men's health: some recent worldwide trends', in Commonwealth Department of Human Services and Health (ed.), *Proceedings of the National Men's Health Conference*, AGPS, Canberra, pp. 125–32.

Jamieson, G.G. 2012, *Reaching for Health: The Australian Women's Health Movement and Public Policy*, ANU E Press, Canberra.

Jones, W.K. 1996, 'Centers for disease control and prevention', *American Journal of Preventive Medicine*, vol. 12, no. 5, p. 410.

Keleher, H. 2004, 'Why build a health promotion evidence base about gender?', *Health Promotion International*, vol. 19, no. 3, pp. 277–9.

Klinge, I. 2010, 'Gender assessment: European health research policies', in E. Kuhlmann & E. Annandale (eds), *The Palgrave Handbook of Gender and Healthcare,* Palgrave Macmillan, New York, pp. 91–106.

Kreager, D.A. 2007, 'Unnecessary roughness? School sports, peer networks, and male adolescent violence', *American Sociological Review*, vol. 72 (October), no. 5, pp. 705–24.

Kuhlmann, E. & Annandale, E. 2010, 'Bringing gender to the heart of health policy, practice and research', in E. Kuhlmann & E. Annandale (eds), *The Palgrave Handbook of Gender and Healthcare,* Palgrave Macmillan, New York, pp. 1–18.

Kunkel, S.R. & Atchley, R.C. 1996, 'Why gender matters: being female is not the same as not being male', *American Journal of Preventive Medicine*, vol. 12, no. 5, pp. 294–6.

Lawlor, D.A., Ebrahim, S. & Davey Smith, G. 2001, 'Sex matters: secular and geographical trends in sex differences in coronary heart disease mortality', *British Medical Journal*, vol. 323, no. 7312, pp. 541–5.

Lin, V. & L'Orange, H., 2010, 'Gender-sensitive indicators for healthcare', in E. Kuhlmann & E. Annandale (eds), *The Palgrave Handbook of Gender and Healthcare,* Palgrave Macmillan, New York, pp. 72–90.

Lumb, P. 1997, 'An early death? Australian men's health policies', in A. Huggins (ed.), *Second National Men's Health Conference: Conference Proceedings*, Curtin University of Technology, Perth, pp. 194–200.

Lumb, P. 2003, 'Why is men's health and well-being policy not implemented in Australia?', *International Journal of Men's Health*, vol. 2, no. 1, pp. 73–88.

Macintyre, C. 1999, 'From entitlement to obligation in the Australian welfare state', *Australian Journal of Social Issues*, vol. 34, no. 2, pp. 103–29.

Macintyre, S. 1993, 'Gender differences in the perceptions of common cold symptoms', *Social Science & Medicine*, vol. 36, no. 1, pp. 15–20.

Macintyre, S. 1997, 'The *Black Report* and beyond: what are the issues?', *Social Science & Medicine*, vol. 44, no. 6, pp. 723–45.

Macintyre, S., Hunt, K. & Sweeting, H. 1996, 'Gender differences in health: are things really as simple as they seem?', *Social Science & Medicine*, vol. 42, no. 4, pp. 617–24.

Martin, R., Lemos, K., Rothrock, N., Bellman, S.B., Russell, D., Tripp-Reimer, T., Lounsbury, P. & Gordon, E. 2004, 'Gender disparities in commonsense models of illness among myocardial infarction victims', *Health Psychology*, vol. 23, no. 4, pp. 345–53.

Matthews, J.J. 1984, *Good and Mad Women: The Historical Construction of Femininity in Twentieth Century Australia*, Allen & Unwin, Sydney.

McKinlay, J.B. 1996, 'Some contributions from the social system to gender inequalities in heart disease', *Journal of Health and Social Behaviour*, vol. 37, no. 1, pp. 1–26.

Meischke, H., Eisenberg, M.S. & Larsen, M.P. 1993, 'Prehospital delay interval for patients who use emergency medical services', *Annals of Emergency Medicine*, vol. 22, no. 10, pp. 1597–601.

Melbourne District Health Council 1990, *A Sliver—Not Even a Slice*, District Health Councils of Victoria, Melbourne.

Men's Sheds Australia 2012: <www.mensheds.org.au>.

Nichter, M., Nichter, M., Lloyd-Richardson, E.E., Flaherty, B., Carkoglu, A. & Taylor, N. 2006, 'Gendered dimensions of smoking among college students', *Journal of Adolescent Research*, vol. 21, no. 3, pp. 215–43.

Oakley, A. 1972, *Sex, Gender and Society*, Sun Books, Melbourne.

Office of the Status of Women (OSW) 1999, *Women in Australia*, OSW, Canberra.

Oliffe, J. 2009, 'Health behaviors, prostate cancer, and masculinities: a life course perspective', *Men and Masculinities*, vol. 11, no. 3, pp. 346–66.

Peerson, A. & Saunders, M. 2009, 'Men's health literacy: advancing evidence and priorities', *Critical Public Health*, vol. 19, nos 3–4, pp. 441–56.

Plummer, D. 1999, *One of the Boys: Masculinity, Homophobia, and Modern Manhood*, Haworth Press, Binghamton.

Plumridge, E.W., Fitzgerald, L.J. & Abel, G.M. 2002, 'Performing coolness: smoking refusal and adolescent identities', *Health Education Research*, vol. 17, no. 2, pp. 167–79.

Primary Health Care Group 1996, *Draft National Men's Health Policy*, Commonwealth Department of Human Services and Health, Canberra.

Pringle, R. 1998, *Sex and Medicine: Gender, Power and Authority in the Medical Profession*, Cambridge University Press, Cambridge.

Redman, S., Hennrikus, D.J., Bowman, J.A. & Sanson-Fisher, R.W. 1988, 'Assessing women's health needs', *Medical Journal of Australia*, no. 148, vol. 3, pp. 123–7.

Riska, E. 2010a, 'Coronary heart disease: gendered public health discourses', in E. Kuhlmann & E. Annandale (eds), *The Palgrave Handbook of Gender and Healthcare,* Palgrave Macmillan, New York, pp. 158–71.

Riska, E. 2010b, 'Women in the medical profession: international trends', in E. Kuhlmann & E. Annandale (eds), *The Palgrave Handbook of Gender and Healthcare,* Palgrave Macmillan, New York, pp. 389–404.

Roberts, G.L. 1994, *Domestic Violence Victims in a Hospital Emergency Department*, Department of Psychiatry, University of Queensland, St Lucia.

Robertson, S. 2003, 'Men managing health', *Men's Health Journal*, vol. 2, no. 4, pp. 111–13.

Rosenberg, J.P. 2009, 'Circles in the surf: Australian masculinity, mortality and grief', *Critical Public Health*, vol. 19, nos 3–4, pp. 417–26.

Rowley, K.G., O'Dea, K., Anderson, I., McDermott, R., Saraswati, K., Tilmouth, R., Roberts, I., Fitz, J., Wang, Z., Jenkins, A., Best, J.D., Wang, Z. & Brown, A. 2008, 'Lower than expected morbidity and mortality for an Australian Aboriginal population: 10-year follow-up in a decentralised community', *Medical Journal of Australia*, vol. 188, no. 5, pp. 283–7.

Sabo, D. & Gordon, D.F. (eds) 1995, *Men's Health and Illness: Gender, Power and the Body*, Sage, Thousand Oaks.

Schofield, T. 2010, 'Men's health and well-being', in E. Kuhlmann & E. Annandale (eds), *The Palgrave Handbook of Gender and Healthcare*, Palgrave Macmillan, New York, pp. 239–55.

Sen, G., Ostlin, P. & George, A. 2007, *Unequal, Unfair, Ineffective and Inefficient: Gender Inequity in Health—Why it Exists and How We Can Change It* (Final Report to the WHO Commission on Social Determinants of Health: Women and Gender Equity Knowledge Network), Karolinska Institutet, Stockholm.

Sex Discrimination Act 1984 (Cth): <www.austlii.edu.au/au/legis/cth/consol_act/sda1984209>.

Showalter, E. 1993, 'Hysteria, feminism, and gender', in S. Gilman, H. King, R. Porter, G.S. Rousseau & E. Showalter (eds), *Hysteria Beyond Freud*, University of California Press, London, pp. 286–344.

Singleton, V. 1996, 'Feminism, sociology of scientific knowledge and postmodernism: politics, theory and me', *Social Studies of Science*, vol. 26, no. 2, pp. 445–68.

Smith, J.A. 2007, 'Addressing men's health policy concerns in Australia: what can be done?', *Australia & New Zealand Health Policy*, vol. 4, no. 20, pp. 1–4: <www.anzhealthpolicy.com/content/4/1/20>.

Smith, J.A., White, A.K., Richardson, N., Robertson, S. & Ward, M. 2009, 'The men's health policy contexts in Australia, the UK and Ireland: advancement or abandonment?', *Critical Public Health*, vol. 19, nos 3–4, pp. 427–40.

Sonke, G.S., Beaglehold, R., Stewart, A.W., Jackson, R. & Stewart, F.M. 1996, 'Sex differences in case fatality before and after admission to hospital after acute cardiac events: analysis of community based coronary heart disease register', *British Medical Journal*, vol. 313, no. 7061, pp. 853–5.

Stark, E. & Flincraft, A. 1991, 'Spouse abuse', in M. Rosenberg & A. Finley (eds), *Violence in America: A Public Health Approach*, Oxford University Press, New York, pp. 161–81.

Steingart, R.M., Packer, M., Hamm, P., Colianese, M.E., Gersh, B., Geltman, E.M. et al. 1991, 'Sex differences in the management of coronary artery disease', *New England Journal of Medicine*, vol. 325, no. 4, pp. 226–30.

Strazdins, L.M. & Broom, D.H. 2004, 'Acts of love (and work): gender imbalance in emotional work and women's psychological distress', *Journal of Family Issues*, vol. 25, no. 3, pp. 356–78.

Taft, A.J., Watson, L.F. & Lee, C. 2004, 'Violence against young Australian women and association with reproductive events: a cross-sectional analysis of a national population sample', *Australian and New Zealand Journal of Public Health*, vol. 28, no. 4, pp. 324–9.

Tobin, J.N., Wassertheil-Smoller, S., Wexler, J.P., Steingart, R.M., Budner, N., Lense, L. & Wachspress, J. 1987, 'Sex bias in considering coronary bypass surgery', *Annals of Internal Medicine*, vol. 107, no. 1, pp. 19–25.

United Nations (UN) 2010a, *Commission on the Status of Women: Report of the 54th Session of the Commission on the Status of Women*, UN, New York: <www.un.org/womenwatch/daw/beijing15/index.html>.

United Nations (UN) 2010b, *Review of the Implementation of the Beijing Declaration and Platform for Action, the Outcomes of the Twenty-third Special Session of the General Assembly and its Contribution to Shaping a Gender Perspective towards the Full Realization of the Millennium Development Goals: Report of the Secretary-General*, UN, Paris.

United Nations Development Programme (UNDP) 2013, *Human Development Report 2012: The Rise of the South: Human Progress in a Diverse World*, UNDP, New York.

Van Wijk, C.M.T.G., Van Vliet, K.P. & Kolk, A.M. 1996, 'Gender perspectives and quality of care: towards appropriate and adequate health care for women', *Social Science & Medicine*, vol. 43, no. 5, pp. 707–20.

VicHealth 2004, *The Health Costs of Violence: Measuring the Burden of Disease Caused by Intimate Partner Violence (Summary of Findings)*, Victorian Health Promotion Foundation, Melbourne.

Vidaver, R.M., Lafleur, B., Tong, C., Bradshaw, R. & Marts, S.A. 2000, 'Women subjects in NIH-funded clinical research literature: lack of progress in both representation and analysis by sex', *Journal of Women's Health & Gender-Based Medicine*, vol. 9, no. 5, pp. 495–504.

Waldron, I. 1995, 'Contributions of changing gender differences in behavior and social roles to changing gender differences in mortality', in D. Sabo & D.F. Gordon (eds), *Men's Health and Illness: Gender, Power and the Body*, Sage, Thousand Oaks, pp. 22–45.

Walsh, M. 2004, 'Twenty years since "A critique of the sex/gender distinction": a conversation with Moira Gatens', *Australian Feminist Studies*, vol. 19, no. 44, pp. 213–24.

Woosley, R.L., Anthony, M. & Peck, C.C. 2000, 'Biological sex analysis in clinical research', *Journal of Women's Health & Gender-Based Medicine*, vol. 9, no. 9, pp. 933–4.

World Bank 1993, *World Development Report 1993: Investing in Health*, Oxford University Press, New York.

World Health Organization (WHO) 2012, 'What is "gender mainstreaming"?', WHO, Geneva: <www.who.int/gender/mainstreaming/en>.

World Health Organization (WHO) 2013, *Global and Regional Estimates of Violence against Women: Prevalence and Health Effects of Intimate Partner Violence and Non-Partner Sexual Violence*, WHO, Geneva.

READING 9

Health throughout the life course

Christopher Fox

TOPICS COVERED

This chapter covers the following topics:

- definitions of life course, life course determinants, and social gradient
- life course determinants and their effects on health
- life course determinants and the social gradient
- life course determinants and policy

KEY TERMS

Cohort
Human agency
Life and historical times
Life course perspective
Life event
Linked lives
Social gradient
Timing of lives
Trajectory
Transition
Turning point

Introduction

Life course determinants are considered to be a relatively new approach to exploring health. Although such determinants have been around for about 50 years, as a concept, policymakers, academics, and researchers rarely draw on the approach. Glen Elder is recognised as one of the early developers of the life course approach and continues to be its key proponent (Hutchison 2010). Elder is a sociologist and was working in the 1960s on data from three early longitudinal studies of children when he identified patterns in the analysis (Elder 1974). These cohorts appeared to have been affected in similar ways when it came to individual and family trajectories. The common factor for the participants was they were children of the 1930s Great Depression. Elder became fascinated with the influence of history, or past events, on family, education, and work roles of individuals and communities (Elder 1974).

The life course approach to health draws on several disciplines: psychology, sociology, anthropology, epidemiology, and social history to name a few (Elder 1994). As an approach, or theory, it has developed key ideas and concepts. In this chapter readers will be introduced to the life course approach and explore how it can be applied to understanding the determinants of the health of an individual or social group.

Defining the life course perspective

The life course refers to the course of our lives from birth to death. One way of viewing the life course is as a path or road—definitely not straight, but with corners, turns, and twists (Hutchison 2010). The life course can be influenced by intra-generational and inter-generational events (Blane 2006); in other words, events that occur within your generation that affect you, or events that occurred in your parents'—even your grandparents'—generation that affect you.

Stop and Think

Why not draw a map of the key events that have affected you? Start at birth and then draw in the events. The events may not have happened in a straight line. Some events may have happened to someone else but affected you. Other events may have occurred simultaneously. Now connect these events. The path you would have drawn is not likely to be straight and is likely to have arms off it—more like a street directory. This is one way to capture the winding road concept of life course determinants.

Life course perspective The cumulative effects of events from earlier life on later life.

The **life course perspective** is also concerned with the impact of one stage of life on another. In this situation, we even consider events that occur while still in the womb. 'Events' that may have occured while you were in the womb can have an impact on your life today, or even in your older age. Or decisions, or events, that occur now could impact on your later life. For example, Delisle (2002), in her review of the relationship between birth weight and coronary heart disease (CHD), reported on studies which found that babies born with a low birth weight had an increased chance of developing CHD at a later stage in life.

The life course perspective is also interested in the roles that culture and social structures, or institutions, have on an individual's life. Culture here not only refers to ethnicity, but also the cultural groups we belong to and the society in which we live. Culture can refer to non-biological aspects of life: the aspects of life that are learnt and/or are symbolic, like the unwritten rules of society, customs, and use of language (Willis 2004). Social structures or institutions can refer to organised institutions like the law or education, or phenomena like gender, race, age, and sexuality. For example, children who have limited exposure to books and reading in early childhood may experience reading difficulties in later childhood (Baydar et al. 1993).

So far we know that life course determinants are about the paths our lives take, that each life stage impacts on a later life stage, and that culture and social institutions also have an influence. These three elements form part of the definition of life course determinants. Blane (2006) suggests that most chronic diseases which result in death result from cumulative developmental stresses, with adulthood health being influenced by circumstances in earlier life. The life course approach to health can also be viewed as the intersecting of socio-historical and cultural factors, with personal biological development. Elder (1994, p. 5) states: 'The life course can be viewed as a multilevel phenomen[on], ranging from structured pathways through social institutions and organisations to the social trajectories of individuals and their developmental pathways'. Elder's definition is considered to be the original formulation of the idea. Yet theory, like language, is dynamic; it is ever developing. Elder's definition is still relevant: the life course perspective can be applied to areas beyond physical and emotional health. The life course perspective, in accordance with its multidisciplinary origins, has been applied to other areas in the human services: individuals, families, groups, and organisations. Hutchison (2005, p. 144) suggests the life course approach could be viewed

> from the micro and macro advantage points. It has been studied from the perspective of the individual as *event history*, or the sequence of events, experiences, and transitions in a person's life from birth to death. It has also been studied from the perspective of the family, in terms of how family lives are synchronised across time. In addition, the life course has been studied as a property of cultures and social institutions that shape the pattern of individual and family lives. Some life course scholars have also conceptualised small groups, communities and formal organisations and social movements as having life courses marked by both continuity and change.

Hutchison's definition gives the approach broader perspective and a greater application beyond traditional ideas of health. In general, the life course is affected by historical, social, and cultural factors and the cumulative effects of circumstances and how these affect later events or outcomes. The life course approach can be applied to individuals, groups, communities, and organisations. In regard to health, the approach challenges the dominance of adult risk factors as causes of adult diseases.

Stop and Think

» The life course approach can be applied to more than individuals. Using your family as an example, how have earlier events affected later events in your family?

» You could also try the same exercise with an organisation (e.g. an AFL team).

Basic concepts

Cohorts

Cohort A group who share the same experiences, in the same time, in the same sequence.

Cohorts are groups of people who share the same time together in the same time period. A cohort could also be a group of people born in the same (historical) time, in the same culture, and who experience the same social changes in the same order (Hutchison 2005). For example, Elder's data analysis of people born in the USA during the Great Depression was the cohort he was studying when he noticed the effects of earlier life events on later life experiences (Elder 1974). Cohorts of people do not need to be born at the same time if we are talking about an organisation or group. In this instance, the cohort may be the people on a sporting team between 2008 and 2011. As a cohort on a sporting team, they share the same experiences in the same order with that team. A cohort could also be conceived as families who had their first child born in 1990. Cohorts can differ in size but face challenges in similar ways. For example, it is suggested that the baby boomer cohort faced the challenges of their demographic bubble by delaying marriage and childbirth, and having fewer children (Hutchison 2010).

Stop and Think

» People generally think of themselves as belonging to a birth cohort (e.g. Gen X, Gen Y, Gen Z, baby boomers), but we can also belong to other cohorts. Make a list of cohorts to which you belong. What experiences, in what time-frame and in what sequence, help define these cohorts?

Transitions

Transition Moving from one life stage to another, or from one life event to another.

Transitions can be viewed as stage changes in life. Transitions are often culturally bound, yet at a macro level may be similar to other groups of transitions. Transitions can be thought of as markers in life as we transit from one state (childhood) to another (adolescence). Transitions can revolve around family life: birth, marriage, divorce, death (Hutchison 2005). Transitions are about changes, exits, and entrances. In the workplace, transitions may be marked by the change of managers in a job, or the start of a new group of graduates in an organisation.

Case Study 13.1 Micro transitions and macro transitions: Markers of adulthood

The markers of entry into adulthood have changed, yet have not changed, since Dickens was chronicling life in the mid-1800s. Although on a micro level there are profound differences between Dickensian England and Australia in the 2010s, there are similarities on a macro level. When reading Dickens, we learn about some of the markers of the transition from childhood to adulthood, and one thing that is substantially different is the cultural idea of adolescence.

Adolescence is marked as the transition from childhood to adulthood. Biologically, it is defined by the development of secondary sex characteristics. Socio-culturally, it is marked by different experiences in different times and cultures. Adolescence is often referred to as a liminal state—not quite one state (childhood); not quite the other (adult). In contemporary Anglo-Australian culture, adolescence is (culturally) defined as the teenage years, where we experiment with adult identities and behaviours. Adolescence for most Australians begins at 13 and ends around 19. If we were to use biological markers for adolescence, it would begin somewhere around 9 or 10 years for girls, and 11 to 13 years for boys; and end at around 17 years for girls and 20 years for boys.

One of the markers of entering into adulthood in Anglo-Australian society is finishing school and beginning employment. Another possibility is moving out of home (although 'Dependults'—young people remaining in the family home until well into their twenties—challenge this notion), or getting married.

If we take adolescence as being culturally defined as the liminal state between childhood and adulthood, then in Dickensian England this lasted around two to three years. Childhood ended, as chronicled by Dickens, at around the age of 12. Dickens writes of young people entering employment in their early teenage years. In some cases, young people moved out of home to take up service (in the case of girls) or an apprenticeship (in the case of boys). If the same markers of entry into adulthood were applied in Dickensian England, then adulthood would have begun around the age of 14. Society in mid-1800s England managed this transition by delaying the onset of adulthood until the young person had completed their service or apprenticeship and could function as an independent person.

So, on a micro level the transitions are quite different, yet on a macro level there are similarities. The markers of entry into adulthood are about independence in both cases. This is how transitions can be similar and different at the same time.

Case Study 13.2 Life transitions

One of the key issues with working with transitions is how we define them. One model is proposed by Bartley and colleagues (1997). Another possible way of looking at critical transition periods is to use Erik Erikson's Psychosocial Stages of Development (1968). Erikson argues that at critical times in our lives we need to resolve a conflict in order to progress positively through life. It is not so much the 'conflict' to be resolved that this model offers; rather the age range represents critical periods of transitions. Erikson's model, like that of Bartley and colleagues, covers the life span.

Bartley and colleagues (1997)

Transition from primary to secondary school
School examinations
Entry to the labour market
Leaving parental home
Transition to parenthood
Job insecurity, change, or loss
Onset of chronic illness
Exit from the labour market [retire]

Erikson's Stages of Psychosocial Development (1968)

Infants, 0 to 1 year = Hope: Trust vs. Mistrust
Toddlers, 2 to 3 years Will: Autonomy vs. Shame & Doubt
Preschool, 3 to 5 years = Purpose: Initiative vs. Guilt
Childhood, 6 to 11 years = Competence: Industry vs. Inferiority
Adolescents, 12 to 19 years = Fidelity: Identity vs. Role Confusion
Young Adults, 20 to 40 years = Love: Intimacy vs. Isolation
Middle Adulthood, 45 to 65 years = Care: Generativity vs. Stagnation
Seniors, 65 years onwards = Wisdom: Ego Integrity vs. Despair

Stop and Think

» Bartley and colleagues (1997) and Erikson (1968) provide two potential lists of key transition periods in life. What would you list as key transitions in life?

» What do you consider to be key transitions you have experienced in your life? It might be turning 13, or starting secondary school or university.

» Draw two columns on a page. On one side write the transitions you have experienced. In the other column, write down the effects these had on you at the time.

Trajectory A stable path towards a life destination.

Transitions and **trajectories** are two key concepts in understanding life course determinants (Elder 1985). Where transitions are transitory, or moments in time, trajectories are more stable and follow a path towards a 'life destination' (Wheaton & Gotlieb 1997). Trajectories can consist of a number of transitions (Elder 1985; Macmillan & Elliason 2004). They can influence and be influenced by other trajectories. A change in trajectory results in a new 'life destination' (Wheaton & Gotlieb 1997). Trajectories, or 'careers', are multidimensional and interdependent (Elder 1985). Elder classes work, life, marriage, and parenthood as trajectories one might face in one's life. As one can see, these trajectories are interdependent or interrelated. Macmillan and Elliason (2004, p. 2) define trajectories as the 'stable component of a direction toward a life destination [which] is given by the probability of occurrence'.

Life events

Life events can be defined as unexpected and sudden with an outcome markedly different from what was previously expected (Settersten & Mayer 1997; Wheaton & Gotlieb 1997). Life events require the individual to change and can result in experiences of great stress (Hutchison 2005). Some events in our lives are expected, for example, marriage after an extended period of dating. If one of these events happens out of normative sequence and this results in significant change—marriage at a younger age because of an unplanned pregnancy and so not completing university—then this is a life event. The change is unexpected, significant, and has consequences for our trajectory.

Life event Abrupt and sudden change in life resulting in significant change in trajectory and stress.

Turning points

Turning points are classed as significant changes or change of direction in life (Rutter 1996) and result in crucially important moments in life (Wheaton & Gotlieb 1997). A turning point may not become apparent at the time, and to identify turning points we need a baseline that is stable over time. Turning points, unlike life events, may not be abrupt single events, unusual events, or anything dramatic (Wheaton & Gotlieb 1997). Rutter (1996) identifies three types of life events that can also be turning points:

Turning point A crucial point in time that leads to significant change of direction.

1. An opportunity is closed off or opened up.
2. A change in the individual's personal environment (e.g. marriage) results in a change in social networks.
3. Changes in the individual's self-concept, beliefs, values, and views.

Trajectories are made up of transitions and life events. A change of trajectory results from a turning point in an individual's life. Turning points are not mere detours but result in a significant change of direction.

Stop and Think

» So far you thought about the cohorts you belong to and transitions you have experienced. Now consider what trajectories you have been on in your life. What life events have resulted in detours? When did these trajectories change? What turning points occurred for the change in trajectory?

» Now what possible impacts will these phenomena have on your later life?

Elder's four themes of the life course

Elder (1994) posits four central themes in the life course approach. These overarching themes account for the interaction between the social and developmental trajectories. He argues that the link between our lives and historical events (times) accounts for some dynamic features of the life course, while the timing of events, the interdependence of our lives (with others), and our agency are all avenues that influence the paths we take (Elder 1994). Below is a summary of each of the four central themes.

Lives and historical times

Life and historical times A way of accounting for cohort effects and how they affect the individual now and in the future.

Elder's phrase '**life and historical times**' refers to the intersection of our lives with the (historical) events that occur around us, for example, a cohort affected by the Vietnam War. Different birth cohorts experience a different social world. Elder (1994) suggests that historical effects are cohort effects. Yet, these effects not only affect us at the point at which they occur but will affect our future and therefore indirectly affect the next generation. When applying a life course approach, we also need to consider how the historical event and its effects, and how we embody these effects, become part of our life course. For example, does the event result in a transition, a life event, or a turning point? Does the historical event effect a change in trajectories? For the people of Queensland in late 2010 and early 2011, who were hit by floods or cyclones, how will this historical event affect their lives and how will they embody the changes? What will be the outcome of these events on their health, in ten or 15 years' time? A life course approach can account for this question.

In exploring life and times, we also need to consider the individual's agency: what they contribute and how significant the event is to them and the subsequent change (Elder 1994). The impact of technological growth on young people is minimal and they have the skills to cope with a technological change in the workplace, whereas an older person might not have the skills and could therefore experience a greater impact of the change. In this example, the lack of skills in the older person will possibly lead to the introduction of new technology as having greater significance and therefore the subsequent change may also have greater impact.

Stop and Think

- In developing the map of your life course, ask yourself what significant historical events have occurred in your life? Are these events unique to you or your family? If so, maybe these are life events or turning points. Remember, we are talking about events that affect cohorts.
- Make a list of historical events and then describe how they affected your cohort.

The timing of lives

In developed nations, especially, there are parallels between chronological and social ageing (Elder 1994). In other words, the social events and transitions associated with marking periods of life are now prescribed for the individual according to their chronological age. Adulthood in Australia is marked by an 18th birthday party. The party is the social marker of the legal definition of adulthood. Social timing is the defining of values and beliefs of a role, alongside the incidence, duration, and sequence of roles (Elder 1994). So, a childbirth in a marriage at a 'planned stage' has minimal impact, yet parenthood in adolescence is costly. The importance of **timing of lives** is that the impact of an event is moderated by where

Timing of lives An account for the age-graded perspective of social markers, roles, and events.

the person is in their life stage. Elder (1994) cites his exploration of the service of men in the Second World War: men who entered service young with no family had minimal social disruption, while men in later life with families felt the full brunt of social disruption.

Case Study 13.3 Understanding age: How old are you?

Age is not universally defined. It is a dynamic concept. The author can recall working with a colleague, who was an anthropologist, on a survey. The author wanted to ask respondents the question, 'how old are you?' He was quickly informed that the question had different meaning to different people—how age is defined is culturally bound. He needed to ask, 'In what year were you born?' in order to calculate the age he needed for analysis.

Think of how in the past we have described our age. When we were children, we might have said, 'I am nearly 4', when in fact we had not long turned 3. Or during our late adolescence when we were trying to convince our parents we were old enough to make a decision, we might have said, 'I am nearly an adult', or believing that our physical maturity allowed us to look adult enough in order to purchase alcohol. And we hear older people say, 'I'm only 40.' All of these statements mark age differently. Earlier, we looked at the markers of childhood, adulthood, and adolescence. Now we can consider the different ways we can define age.

Chronological age is the age according to our birth year. This is how many of us think of age when we talk about it. If you were born in 1990, then in 2011 you will be 21 years old. Hutchison (2010) argues that chronological age is not the only aspect in the timing of our lives, but differences in roles and behaviours are also the result of biological, social, and psychological processes. For example, being able to drive is a widely recognised marker of adulthood in many societies. Permisson to engage in this adult behaviour is arbitrarily determined by law in various localities to occur at the age of 15, 16, 17, or 18, depending largely on social need and perception of the biological and psychological state of young people.

Biological age is when we use biological development as an indicator of age, for example, when a paediatrician uses the Tanner Stages of Puberty (Marshall & Tanner 1969, 1970) to define where a person is at in development. Biological age can also be defined according to our health and how well our organs function.

Psychological age is when age is defined according to the stages of psychological and cognitive development, for example, where an individual's cognitive or motor skills are in the developmental stages, or how well the individual copes with certain life crises (e.g. Erickson's Stages of Psychosocial Development).

Social age is the expected age-graded role and behaviours. For example, a society may have expectations of when it is okay for young people to begin romantic lives, or when it is appropriate for children to begin household chores. Social age is often defined by markers and events as recognition. Social age could also be defined by asking how old do you feel? Our perception of age is often based on social markers, or engagement with age-grade roles/behaviours.

Stop and Think

» Since age is dynamic and fluid and not easily defined, using the four examples of defining age above, write down how you fit into each category. Is there a difference in how you could perceive your age?

Linked lives

Linked lives The interdependence we have with others in our social networks and relationships and how these affect our life course.

Linked lives is Elder's (1994) recognition of the interdependence of our lives. We are all embedded in social relationships and networks. We are interdependent. We live in a family network with multiple social relationships. We study or work in a network with multiple social relationships. Sometimes our networks even overlap. The life course approach recognises that relationships and networks are structures of socialisation and management, and these relationships also provide us with necessary interaction. These relationships and networks influence our decisions, and therefore our transitions, life events, and turning points—if not directly, then in reaction to them, which is of equal importance. Our parents can influence us in our immediate world and can also affect us in our later life. For example, parental socio-economic level can have an impact on our infancy and childhood health and can also impact on health in later life.

Elder's (1974) work on the longitudinal data of the Great Depression children highlights the interdependence between parents and children over the life course. The parents expressed high levels of stress, depression, and marital discord which in turn affected their ability to care for and nurture their children. This too was to have an effect on the children's later lives. Linked lives are the interaction of our social worlds over the duration of our life (Elder 1994).

Stop and Think

» How is your life linked?

» Using a large piece of paper, draw the networks in which you are a member. What networks are interdependent? How are these networks part of the multiple trajectories along which you might be travelling?

» Consider the role these networks have in your life and what impact they might have in the future.

Mythbuster

Consider whether you see the following as questionable. What does this tell you about your own values?

A life course approach to addictions, whether smoking, gambling, or alcohol and other drugs, highlights the importance of past events and transitions in determining current experiences. Current health promotion campaigns to address addictions tend to focus on the individual to make a choice. To reorient our campaigns would mean greater interventions at earlier life stages. This is a costly exercise to govern and would lead to greater intrusions into people's lives, especially at the lower end of the social gradient.

Human agency

Human agency Our ability to negotiate the social structures and a way to account for individual differences in the life course.

Human agency refers to our free will, or our ability to act independently of social constraints or structures (Abercrombie et al. 1994). In the life course approach, human agency is how we as actors in our social world make choices in relation to the world and events around us (Elder 1994). Elder believes that although we are influenced by the social structures around us, we can make decisions within and around the influences of the social structures. Human agency can account for some individual differences identified through the life course approach to exploring health issues.

Social structures, on the other hand, can be conceived of as key social institutions in society. These institutions can be constituted (e.g. school and education or the justice system) or can be more symbolic (e.g. gender, age, sexuality). Social theorists such as Durkheim and Marx argued that our lives are governed by social structures, while others, such as Weber and Habermas, suggested that life is about agency. There is a third school of thought which argues that our lives are influenced by our agency engaging with social structures (e.g. Bourdieu). For example, social structures can be used to account for successes in life. Children from high socio-economic groups are more likely to succeed at school; more likely to have professional jobs with higher salaries, therefore better superannuation savings, and resulting in a better quality of old age than someone of low socio-economic status (Blane 2006).

Health effects and the life course

Hertzman (2000) sees life course effects as a gradient that increases in time and with age. These gradual effects provide one way for us to understand how life course events affect our health. According to Hertzman, there are three types of outcome effects to the life course approach when looking at health: latent effects, pathway effects, and cumulative effects. *Latent effects* are biologically or developmentally based and result in effects in later life, regardless of future experiences. They result from events occurring during foetal and infant development stages which program organ systems, for example, low birth weight and the increased likelihood of coronary heart disease (Delisle 2002). *Pathway effects* result from experiences which set us on particular trajectories that can later influence our health or well-being. Limited exposure to literacy in early childhood can lead to poor reading in early schooling (Baydar et al. 1993), in turn affecting educational outcomes and therefore later life experiences. Hertzman and Power (2004) suggest that children who are not prepared for school (emotionally, cognitively, and behaviourally) are more likely to experience 'education failure' and people with poor educational outcomes are less likely to engage in health-enhancing behaviours. *Cumulative effects* are a combination of latent and pathway effects (Hertzman 2000) and can refer to an accumulation of either disadvantage or advantage. Hertzman argues that these effects could be risks or protective factors. He cites the study by Power and colleagues (1999) of the effect of socio-economic class on adult health where low socio-economics status in early life may lead to cumulative effects on health outcomes in later adulthood. Cumulative effects are also affected by the social gradient.

The social gradient and the life course

Social gradient Life expectancy is shorter and most diseases are more common further down the social ladder.

When we consider the effects thesis put forward by Hertzman (2000), we can also discuss the effects of the life course in terms of the social gradient. When we apply the **social gradient** to life course determinants and health, we note that the health of people is better towards the top of the gradient. Most diseases, especially chronic diseases, are concentrated at the bottom of the gradient and at earlier stages.

Case Study 13.4 The social gradient and mortality

As we have just seen, people at the lower end of the SES scale have on average poorer health for a longer time than do people at the upper end of the scale. These differences also affect not only when but also where people die.

The social gradient in health was first recognised through the relationship between age of death and social class: the lower people's SES, the lower their average age of death in comparison with higher SES groups. Further, people with lower SES have a higher average number of years of disability before their earlier deaths (Marmot 2010).

The most detailed studies of causes and place of death as a function of deprivation have been carried out in the UK (National Audit Office 2008; National End of Life Intelligence Network 2010). These show higher rates of death from cancer and respiratory diseases, and more deaths in hospital, in more deprived (lower SES) groups. The available Australian data is consistent with this. For example, male mortality in Victoria is lower than average in most rural areas and the western suburbs (Victorian Department of Human Services 1999; Draper et al. 2004). Tobacco- and alcohol-related diseases contribute more to deaths in lower SES groups, while accidents and suicide further reduce the average age of death for men in rural areas.

Surveys consistently show that the majority of people would prefer not to die in hospital but, as indicated above, people with lower SES are more likely to do so. The reasons for this are not yet clearly established, but it has been shown that a combination of informal care (from family and friends) with formal care in the community significantly increases the odds that a person will be able to die at home. A recent study in Western Australia found that people who accessed community-based specialist palliative care had a seven times higher chance of dying in their usual place of residence (McNamara & Rosenwax 2007). Studies in Australia and overseas show that many people die in hospital when there is no clinical reason for them to be there. Not only is this contrary to their wishes in many cases, but it also contributes to increased healthcare expenditure in the last days of life. Governments have recently endorsed Advance Care Planning (ACP) as a means by which people can document their wishes about end-of-life care, but evidence to date indicates that the options available may not be able to deliver on people's choices. The National Health and Hospitals Reform Commission even suggested that ACP could become a consumer tool for shaping end-of-life services—but these services are inextricably linked with health service provision in general.

The policy implication seems clear. Providing more community services that are more accessible—that is, shaped by local needs and demand—should both meet dying people's expressed wishes to die at home (or in a 'homelike' environment such as a residential aged care facility) and reduce demand on expensive acute hospital services. It is clear that in the coming decades Australia will need to accommodate a large increase of ageing and deaths. A health service focus on providing primary care services that allows not only ageing in place, but also dying in place, is imperative.

This case study is contributed by Bruce Rumbold

According to Blane (2006), dis/advantage accumulates cross-sectionally and longitudinally, with dis/advantage in one stage of life affecting other phases of life. To accommodate this idea of accumulation of positive or negative impacts, Blane uses three processes: social accumulation, social mobility, and social protection. *Social accumulation* is used to explain the continuity of parental socio-economic status to conditions throughout the life course (infancy, childhood, adolescence, adulthood) (Blane 2006). It also accounts for the intersection between biological programming and social conditions of life. Two possible disruptions to the cumulative role of social disadvantage are, first, when a person shifts social class and, second, when a socio-economic system evolves or changes. For example, in Australia we have moved from a production economy to a service economy. A similar effect is felt when economic events like the global financial crisis occur.

Social mobility accounts for the accumulation of health and social factors that can lead to better or poorer health in later stages of life (Blane 2006). Parental socio-economic status can influence whether their offspring move up the social ladder, down the social ladder, or remain in the same position. If a person moves up the social ladder (i.e. increases in status), they will add 'advantage' to their life course; they will have less advantage than those of already equal footing, but more advantage than those left behind. The corollary is also true. Downward mobility adds disadvantage, with the individual experiencing less advantage than those left behind and more advantage than those they have joined (Blane 2006).

Social protection also explores the interaction between health and life course events. Social protection moderates the experience of impact of new disadvantage (Blane 2006). New disadvantage has minimal impact on previous advantage—this is positive social protection. A new disadvantage, however, will have an increased impact on previous disadvantage. Blane (2006) explains the idea of social protection by using examples from the Analysis of General Household Survey in the UK (Bartley & Owen 1996). Working men with a restrictive chronic illness were more likely to be unemployed compared with men who reported good health. Blane argues that people of low socio-economic status with a chronic illness were more likely to experience disadvantage from the chronic illness, as it affects life choices like employment, whereas people of high socio-economic status are likely to be protected from further disadvantage.

Policy implications

Little has been undertaken in Australia in using life course determinants as a basis for developing social and economic policy. The UK Government made moves to include life course determinants in social and economic policy development in 1994 with the establishment of an interdepartmental working group (Dorozynski 1994; Bartley et al. 1997). One of the first acts of the working party was to set a research agenda which explored factors that accumulate over the life course (Bartley et al. 1997). The Queensland Government acknowledged the significance of life course determinants in health (Queensland Health 2001), yet this has not to date been explicitly articulated in policy development.

Bartley and colleagues (1997, p. 1194) recommend that policy development should focus on key transitional periods in life which could have material effects and psychosocial effects by 'preventing dramatic falls in living standards and by a wider effect on the degree to which citizens experience a sense of control over their lives'. Policy that builds resilience will strengthen individual and community health and well-being (Queensland Health n.d.). The Queensland Government suggested key transitional periods (e.g. birth, school, adolescence, changes in employment, and ageing). One of the problems with this idea is knowing how to define key transitional periods in life that can accommodate the differences in population—though it can be argued that we all experience some critical points in the life course.

See Case Study 13.2 for a discussion of critical periods in the life course.

Summary

Points in the life course are one of the social determinants of health and well-being. When we consider the causes of illness and disease we need to look beyond the individual and explore their history (and possibly that of their families and communities) to gain a better understanding of the effects their past has had on them. What we now know is that effects accumulate over the life course and when combined with the social gradient we see greater impact. The utility of life course determinants has also moved beyond health and can focus on other areas of well-being such as families (Hutchison 2005).

Although the early history of life course determinants focuses on foetal and early childhood development, researchers have acknowledged that events that happen at any time in our lives can have an impact (Lynch & Smith 2005). The challenge for us as health and well-being practitioners is to advocate for acknowledgment of life course determinants and to advocate for policy change that addresses these determinants in the policy response.

Tutorial exercises

1. Throughout this chapter you have undertaken a number of exercises. You now need to bring this information together and explore how your life course is affecting or could affect your health.
2. Many people confuse life course determinants with the life span approach to development. How are each of these terms defined? How can life span approaches be integrated into life course approaches?
3. What is the role of life course determinants in young women living with HIV in sub-Saharan Africa?
4. What policy action could we take to address the issues of life course determinants in the experiences of women living with HIV in sub-Saharan Africa?
5. Which critical periods in life would impact on domestic violence? How can we address this issue at those critical periods?

Further reading

Bartley, M., Blane, D., & Montgomery, S. (1997). Socioeconomic determinants of health: Health and the life course: Why safety nets matter. *British Medical Journal*, 314, 1194–95.

Blane, D. (2006). The life course, social gradient and health. In M. Marmot & R.G. Wilkinson (eds), *Social determinants of health*. Oxford: Oxford University Press, 64–80.

Elder, G.J. (1985). *Life course dynamics: Trajectories and transitions, 1968-1980*. Ithaca, NY: Cornell University Press.

Elder, G.J. (1994). Time, human agency, and social change: Perspectives on the life course. *Social Psychology Quarterly*, 57(1), 4–15.

Hertzman, C., & Power, C. (2004). Child development as a determinant of health across the life course. *Current Paediatrics*, 14(5), 438–43.

Hutchison, E. (2010). A life course perspective. In E. Hutchison (ed.), *Dimensions of human behavior: The changing life course*. London: Sage Publications, 3–38.

Liu, S., Jones, R.N., & Glymour, M.M. (2010). Implications of lifecourse epidemiology for research on determinants of adult disease. *Public Health Reviews*, 32. <www.publichealthreviews.eu/upload/pdf_files/8/Glymour_for_website.pdf>.

Mayer, K.U. (2009). New directions in life course research. *Annual Review of Sociology*, 35, 413–33.

Mortimer, J.T., & Shananhan, M.J. (2004). *Handbook of the life course*. New York: Springer.

Power, C., Manor, O., & Matthews, S. (1999). The duration and timing of exposure: Effects of socio-economic environment on adult health. *American Journal of Public Health*, 89(7), 1059–66.

World Health Organization Commission on Social Determinants of Health (2007). *A conceptual framework for action on the social determinants of health*. Geneva: WHO. <www.who.int/social_determinants/resources/csdh_framework_action_05_07.pdf>.

Websites

<www.who.int/social_determinants/en>

This is the website of the WHO's Commission on Social Determinants of Health. It is a good source of discussions on social determinants and provides crucial background papers and reports as well as examples of actions in relation to social determinants.

<www.longstudies.longviewuk.com/index.shtm>

The Society for Longitudinal and Life Course Studies is an international, multidisciplinary society. It aims to increase the visibility and influence of life course studies. The website has access to publications and links, including to the *Longitudinal and Life Course Studies: An International Journal.*

<http://aging.utoronto.ca>

The Institute for Life Course and Aging is based at the University of Toronto. It focuses on ageing research from a life course perspective.

<www.sfb186.uni-bremen.de/frames/main.htm>

The Special Collaborative Centre 186: Status Passages and Risks in the Life Course is a research centre based at the University of Bremen. The website provides a link to an extensive bibliography and links to other organisations.

<www.lebenslaufarchiv.uni-bremen.de/index.php?id=567&no_cache=1&L=>

The Archive for Life Course Research is an archive for qualitative social science research and is available for life course researchers.

<www.ucl.ac.uk/icls>

The International Centre for Life Course Studies in Society and Health is a UK-based centre with a focus on the UK birth cohort studies. The Centre is under the directorship of Mel Bartley and David Blane, two leading researchers in life course determinants.

<www.journal.longviewuk.com/index.php/llcs>

Longitudinal and Life Course Studies: An International Journal's website has archived copies of past issues.

<http://caepr.anu.edu.au/population/lectures2011.php>

The Centre for Aboriginal Economic Policy and Research at the Australian National University, 2011 Online Lecture Series is on 'Measures of Indigenous wellbeing and their determinants across the life course'. There are 14 lectures, with a transcript, a copy of the presentation, and an audio file.

Acknowledgment

The author would like to thank Dr Bruce Rumbold for his assistance in writing this chapter and for providing the text on which *The Social Gradient and Ageing* is based.

READING 10

Social determinants of health: Historical developments and global implications

Bruce Rumbold and Virginia Dickson-Swift

TOPICS COVERED

This chapter covers the following topics:

- social determinants of health
- an introduction to health promotion
- how individual risk factors can determine health status
- key principles of public health
- how healthcare reform may address the social determinants of health

KEY TERMS

Equity
Social determinants
Social epidemiology
Social exclusion
Social gradient
Social inclusion
Socially inclusive society
Socio-economic status

Introduction

In every society, the health status of the population is fundamentally determined by social and cultural factors. However, national healthcare systems, particularly in developed nations, are devoted to delivering clinical services that respond to immediate health problems confronting individual citizens. The underlying social and cultural determinants, the causes of these health problems, are neglected, either because they are seen as secondary to meeting immediate needs or because they raise issues too difficult to address through the short-term policy agendas of governments driven by election cycles. These asocial clinical models also influence the healthcare systems of most developing nations through the support provided by overseas aid programs and the developed-world training given to their healthcare workforce.

This chapter traces the growth in understanding of the roles played by social factors in health, and the development of a body of evidence that identifies the factors and strategies through which

Figure 11.1 The Social Skeleton: Health, illness, and structure energy

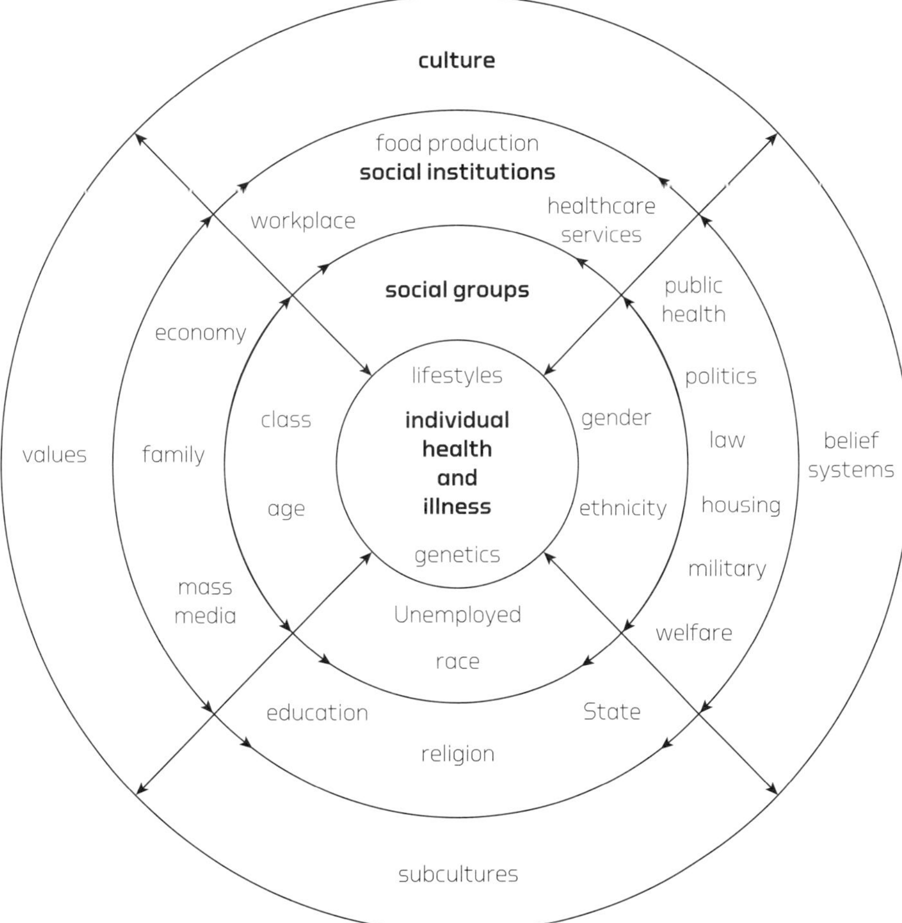

Source: Germov 2005

they might be addressed. The findings and recommendations of the WHO Commission on Social Determinants of Health, currently the most comprehensive repository of global information on social determinants, will be outlined. Findings and recommendations will be applied to Australian society and current debates about reforming the health system.

Social determinants mediate between the individual and environmental determinants dealt with in the previous ten chapters. Social experience and social structures shape both our individual capacities and the way the environment supports and challenges us. These interactions between human biology, lifestyle, and the physical and social environment all influence how we experience health and illness.

Social determinants involve much more than interpersonal support, which is often the limited meaning given to 'social' in a biopsychosocial framework. Rather, 'social determinants of health are the circumstances in which [we] are born, grow up, live, work, and age, and the systems put in place to deal with illness. These circumstances are in turn shaped by a wider set of forces: economics, social policies, and politics' (WHO CSDH 2008a, p. 1). In experiencing these determinants, we find a tension between structure and agency, between constraints (circumstances and forces) that we cannot immediately influence, and initiatives that we can take despite those constraints. Bauman (1999) observes that individual choices in *all* circumstances are limited by two sets of constraints: choosing from among what is available; and social roles or codes that tell the individual the rank order and appropriateness of preferences. People can act independently of the social structures in their lives, but the occasions on which they do so appear to be rare.

Social determinants
Social, cultural, economic, environmental, and political factors that can impact on the health of individuals.

Stop and Think

Tristan is 9 years old and he lives with his mum and his brother in a public housing flat in a high-rise inner-city housing estate. They have recently moved to the city and most of their family live in a rural town some four hours away. The flats are in quite good condition but his mum worries about the smell of the carpet and the fact that there are not many places for the boys to play. Tristan and his brother attend the local primary school, about a 15-minute walk away. They do not have a car and public transport costs are high so mum walks Tristan and his brother to school. Tristan is happy at school but lately he has been complaining of feeling he cannot breathe at times during the day and he has been coughing quite a lot at night. Tristan was diagnosed with asthma when he was 4 and has had a number of hospital admissions for asthma over the years. He takes a reliever medication when he feels wheezy and has also had a preventer prescribed some time ago but he does not use it as often as he should.

» Based on the information provided above, explore some of the social determinants of health for Tristan. Why is it that we treat people without changing what makes them sick?

Stop and Think

Often children like Tristan end up in the Accident and Emergency room of the local hospital. Frequently this leads to a hospital admission and further forms of treatment. When we take a social determinants approach to examining conditions like asthma we can begin to see that the issues that impact on Tristan's asthma can come from several places: his housing environment, the stress of moving to a new school, air pollution, lack of asthma education, just to name a few. We can treat kids like Tristan with the latest asthma drugs to get them through the acute episodes but if we do not address the social determinants (housing, transport, education, environment, etc.) then it will be difficult for Tristan to feel healthy.

Obviously, asthmatics need to follow a medication regime, but health professionals also need to be aware of those social issues that can determine a person's health. If we continue just to treat the Tristans and send them home to an environment that may be polluted, into a house that may be damp, to a family that lacks the education to follow the asthma plans, then we are actually achieving very little (and adding to the health budget quite a lot).

Often initiatives to respond to social determinants have had to run ahead of conclusive evidence, but in recent years much greater coherence has emerged, and a global consensus is taking shape. Much of the impetus for this has grown from the classic publication *The solid facts* (Wilkinson & Marmot 2003). The contributors reviewed thousands of publications and condensed their findings into ten key propositions about social determinants of health, intentionally packaged to be accessible to policymakers. The propositions are:

- *The social gradient*: Life expectancy is shorter and most diseases are more common further down the social ladder in each society.
- *Stress*: Stressful circumstances, making people feel worried, anxious, and unable to cope, are damaging to health and may lead to premature death.
- *Early life*: A good start in life means supporting mothers and young children.
- *Social exclusion*: Life is short where its quality is poor. By causing hardship and resentment, poverty, social exclusion, and discrimination cost lives.
- *Work*: Stress in the workplace increases the risk of disease. People who have more control over their work have better health.
- *Unemployment*: Job security increases health, well-being, and job satisfaction. Higher rates of unemployment cause more illness and premature death.
- *Social support*: Friendship, good social relations, and strong supportive networks improve health at home, at work, and in the community.
- *Addiction*: Individuals turn to alcohol, drugs, and tobacco and suffer from their use; but use is influenced by the wider social setting.
- *Food*: Because global market forces control the food supply, healthy food is a political issue.
- *Transport*: Healthy transport means less driving and more walking and cycling, backed up by better public transport.

These ten solid facts are key social determinants of health.

Social factors in illness

In urging policymakers to attend to social determinants of health, Wilkinson and Marmot (2003) are not introducing a new idea. Human societies have for millennia managed illness through a variety of forms of social organisation. Nomadic groups, for example, kept on the move not only to maintain an adequate and varied diet but also to maintain equilibrium with their environment. Their moving on minimised their impact on the land and ensured that food supplies would be replenished. Their life span rituals were correlated with their cyclic movement through the landscape, so that birth, growth, illness, and death were integrated into the journey. Human settlement, taking up permanent quarters, raised new problems, particularly concerning hygiene. These were handled by strategies that ranged from religious prescription (as, for example, in Judaism's rules for food preparation and for conducting social relationships) through quarantine (the social exclusion of 'infectious' people, lepers in particular) to town planning and engineering (the Romans' separation of water supply from sewage disposal, construction of public bath houses, and so forth).

Older town planning strategies broke down as new manufacturing technologies changed the use of waterways and led to the rapid construction of cheap housing as well as the overuse of older dwellings as cities expanded. Concerns about hygiene drove reforms necessitated by the Industrial Revolution, culminating in the Public Health Acts of the 1850s. An explanation of why these Acts were effective in reducing the incidence of disease came decades later with the development of germ theory. This theory led in rapid succession to the population-wide initiatives of vaccination and immunisation, a huge social experiment in its own right, and an indication of the ascendancy of scientific knowledge at the end of the 19th century. The new theory of infectious disease, reinforced by each citizen's personal experience of an immunisation needle in the arm, focused credit for the growing control of infectious illness upon clinical advances and obscured the foundation that had been laid in the hygiene acts. In many respects, this love affair of Western society with clinical practice has continued: the care of individuals is elevated, and the social context is played down. Only now at the beginning of the 21st century are we starting to understand some of the less desirable outcomes of our medical advances and to consider both their social preconditions and social impact.

In Western societies, the requirements of adequate hygiene are now assumed. They remain the responsibility of health departments, but seldom does the public see them as the core business they are—except when they fail under extreme circumstances such as the impact of cyclone, earthquake, fire, or flood. Our society's health focus continues to be on hospitals, places where health problems arrive once they become critical. Strategies to deal with potential problems earlier, through prevention or earlier intervention, are less developed and minimally funded. Our social mindset has moved away from prevention or containment to elimination or cure as a first-line response. We seem to be questioning whether we still need prevention when we can now effect cures. But increasingly we are finding that these cures often come with unwanted side effects, are not necessarily complete fixes, and are ultimately not affordable as people live longer and the costs of medical technology spiral upwards. The 'triumphal progress of medicine' stories in today's popular media tend to ignore many of these limitations, including the fact that in the end mortality remains 100%: we must all die from something.

In developing nations, the fundamental health problems caused by inadequate water supply and poor sanitation are more obvious. Western influence, however, still skews interest towards clinical approaches, and has too often created situations where a poor country's health budget has been devoted to developed-world hospital-based strategies that can benefit only a few, rather than primary

Social epidemiology
The systematic and comprehensive study of health, well-being, social conditions or problems, and diseases and their determinants, using epidemiology and social science methods to develop interventions, programs, policies, and institutions that may reduce the extent, adverse impact, or incidence of a health or social problem and promote health.

care resources or community infrastructure development that have the potential to improve the health of many.

In the latter part of the 20th century, **social epidemiology** has identified and mapped social patterns in prevalence and incidence of disease (Cwikel 2006). This evidence itself is shaped by social and cultural factors, such as the UK's interest in the effect of social class, and the USA's interest in the effect of race and gender upon health. Such divergent interests complicate comparison of the data; but nevertheless an increasing number of multinational studies and meta-analyses are identifying global themes in health and illness.

Stop and Think

- » Has medical intervention in the form of immunisation been unambiguously good?
- » What, if anything, might be the downside of such interventions?

Social factors in health

The heroic narrative of medical progress has dominated much of the 20th century, and it is unquestionable that the increasing effectiveness of medical treatments has rendered treatable or curable many conditions that earlier might have led to premature death. The removal of these causes has, however, resulted in a larger ageing population, placing an increased burden on the health system as death often follows upon years of disability or degenerative illness. While health planners gauge the effectiveness of healthcare by a society's increasing life expectancy, the same planners are now beginning to see it as a looming problem for the future (see e.g. the Intergenerational Report 2010 on Ageing in Australia [Australian Treasury 2010]).

As noted above, the first great social health intervention of the modern era was the Public Health Acts, and arguably the second was universal immunisation. Immunisation has certainly contained, and in some instances eliminated, infectious disease, although its preventive power was quickly challenged by its inability to respond to the great influenza pandemic of 1919–20 during which, depending on the estimate preferred, between 40 and 100 million people died worldwide. (Ten million men perished in the Great War; our continued social memory of these deaths contrasts strangely with the lost memory of many more deaths in half the time during the pandemic.)

A further major social intervention midway through the century was exemplified by the UK's National Health Service (NHS), an attempt to improve the nation's health by providing accessible clinical services funded not through an insurance scheme but by taxation revenue. It was one manifestation of the post-Second World War interest in nation-building expressed variously through the renewal of war-ravaged Europe and the emerging prosperity of the USA. The aim of the NHS was, by providing universal access to health services, to improve the health of the population to an extent where expenditure might decrease. This particular outcome was certainly not achieved, as the Black Report (1980) showed with devastating clarity—although it should be said that the NHS has achieved better population health outcomes for a much lower per capita expenditure than many other health systems, most notably that of the USA.

The NHS experiment did at least raise the question 'what is health?' as distinct from 'how can we cure illness?' This question about health became important globally. Colonialism ended, expanding global awareness brought questions about development to the fore, and emerging nations began to take responsibility for services that to this point had been an uneasy mix of traditional medicine and institutions set up by the colonisers.

In the climate of optimism and expansion that marked the postwar period, there was as yet little or no sense that resources might be finite, that wealth creation might have actual, if not ethical, limits, or that a century of industrialised progress might have consequences for the environment. (Warning voices on all these issues began to emerge in the 1970s, but had little impact on political and economic leaders who were, as today, largely immersed in their own immediate concerns.)

It is not possible in the space of a single chapter to review the huge body of evidence for social and cultural determinants of health that has been compiled in recent decades. However, there are several key studies that have established new directions in research and become models for many others. Similarly, there are a number of key documents that have given rise to many other similar national reports and policy documents. These are available in the WHO collection *Milestones in Health Promotion* (2009c), and provide the backbone of what follows here.

Health promotion as a response to the emerging evidence

Irwin and Scali (2007) identify four phases in social approaches to health after the Second World War:

- 1950s: emphasis on technology and disease-specific campaigns
- 1960s and early 1970s: rise of community-based approaches
- 1980s: neoliberalism dominates the political economic context
- 1990s and beyond: contested paradigms and shifting power relations.

1950s

The focus of public health in the postwar decade was on supporting the new clinical services that were emerging. Unlike today's public health advertisements that encourage individuals to make behavioural and lifestyle changes, the advertisements in the 1950s educated individuals about the symptoms for which they should seek expert medical advice. Another major focus was on immunisation for baby boomer children (children born 1946 64).

1960s and early 1970s

The baby boomers' entry into adulthood led to social change, with a particular interest in community. Health workers and community organisers joined forces to explore new approaches to community health. One Australian expression of this in the early 1970s was the community health movement initiated by the Whitlam Government. The focus was on creating health, not just combating illness; on community participation, not just professional activities. Australia was at this time a world leader in health promotion.

1980s

The 1980s saw the rise of neoliberal governments and a corresponding concern for economic management of the burgeoning healthcare sector. The new managerialism introduced in that decade arose to contain the healthcare costs that resulted from myriad confidential consultations between healthcare practitioners and clients. By identifying and assigning costs to various clinical interventions, and requiring practitioners to report their activities in terms of these services, managers were able to monitor and influence clinical decision-making. The new public health movement that was developing in this decade found itself caught between its social reformist vision and the realities of governance in the health sector from which funding was sought. Community health found itself reporting not in terms of community development but according to frameworks set up for health service delivery. The resulting compromise caused health promotion to lose its reforming edge and focus more on changing individual health behaviours.

1990s

The evidence-based medicine movement in the 1990s reasserted some professional control of territory by mandating best practice interventions, but clinical practice continued to balance best practice with cost-effective practice. The effect on health promotion was to intensify further the pressure to adapt to its healthcare environment—that is, to describe its work in terms of interventions and its outcomes in terms of services delivered, if not to individuals then to identifiable groups in the community, evaluated by short-term outcomes. It led inevitably to a focus on agency—what individuals could be instructed or persuaded to do—more than upon the structures that shaped or constrained those choices.

Case Study 11.1 The problem with tobacco

The first clue that smoking might be harmful came from studies that showed an exponential rise in cancer of the lung in UK men (Kenneway & Kenneway 1936, 1947). Various interpretations of this increase were put forward, until Doll and Hill (1950) concluded, on the basis of a retrospective epidemiological study, that smoking was an important factor in the production of carcinoma of the lung.

Their paper was criticised severely, so they embarked on a prospective study (Doll & Hill 1954). Their inspired choice was to investigate smoking in medical practitioners. All 59,600 men and women on the UK Medical Register were contacted, and 40,637 enrolled in the trial—34,445 men and 6192 women. All respondents were classified as current smokers, ex-smokers, or non-smokers. The group was followed for 50 years: the study closed in 2004 once all participating smokers had died and some 6000 non-smokers were still living. Doll himself was involved in the study from start to finish.

As early as 1957 the Medical Research Council endorsed the hypothesis of a cause-and-effect relationship between smoking and lung cancer. Doll and Hill's ten-year follow-up (1964) associated smoking with seven causes of death, coronary disease among them. The 20-year follow-up consolidated and extended these findings (Doll & Peto 1976), while at 22 years the pattern of mortality among the women doctors matched that of the men

(Doll et al. 1980). The 40-year review, with over 20,000 of the group having now died, found 25 causes of death associated with cigarette smoking, only one of them (Parkinson's Disease) positively (Doll et al. 1994). These findings were confirmed in the 50-year final review (Doll et al. 2004). Numerous other studies supported this longitudinal study, but no other has followed a smoking epidemic to its conclusion.

Responses to the evidence for cigarette smoking as a health determinant show strategies evolving according to the pattern outlined by Irwin and Scali (2007), beginning in the 1960s with health information encouraging young people not to start smoking and older smokers to moderate consumption. In the 1970s health promotion campaigns began advocating actively for smoking cessation. By the 1980s pressure on governments to introduce tobacco control was increasing, and restrictions on labelling, availability, and use of tobacco products were introduced. In the 1990s the focus turned to passive smoking, and controls were extended to include this aspect of health threat. At every step these strategies were resisted, both overtly and covertly, by the tobacco industry. While tobacco use has declined in developed nations, an epidemic of smoking among young women continues to cause concern. The tobacco industry has now turned its attention to increasing markets in developing countries.

While smoking among men in the USA peaked in the 1950s, the peak of tobacco-related deaths was not reached until the 1990s. Thus, in a country like China, where the smoking epidemic peaked in the 1990s, tobacco-related deaths, which are already increasing rapidly, can be expected not to peak until around 2030 (Boyle et al. 2006).

The key issues shown by this history are both the time involved in developing epidemiological evidence and the social process of reception. Only through sustained political process has regulation of tobacco products become possible. The right of the state to legislate arises from the responsibility of the state to fund the consequences of having legalised and benefited from taxation on tobacco products.

Individual risk factors and social determinants

The thrust of a great deal of epidemiological research has been to identify risk factors that relate to particular illnesses. Many of these risk factors overlap or coincide to identify a series of social behaviours that adversely affect health. Chief among these is cigarette smoking, accompanied by others such as obesity, substance abuse, and risky sexual behaviours. Health education programs seek to raise individual awareness and modify or eliminate risky behaviour. But the social underpinning of many of the risk factors is not adequately addressed. Identifying the risk factor 'poverty', for example, may not adequately represent the complex picture of deprivation that excludes people from constructive participation in their society (Harris et al. 2001, p. 259).

Identifying social determinants of health and disease is important to highlight pathways in the social production of health. The health iceberg model can help us examine the determinants of health and explore how those determinants relate to health outcomes (Talbot & Verrinder 2009). The iceberg is divided into three sections. Only the small section at the top that is visible above the waterline refers to observable states of health. These can be positive or negative and can include morbidity and mortality measures or prevalence of risk factors (e.g. cardiovascular disease [CVD]).

Figure 11.2 The iceberg

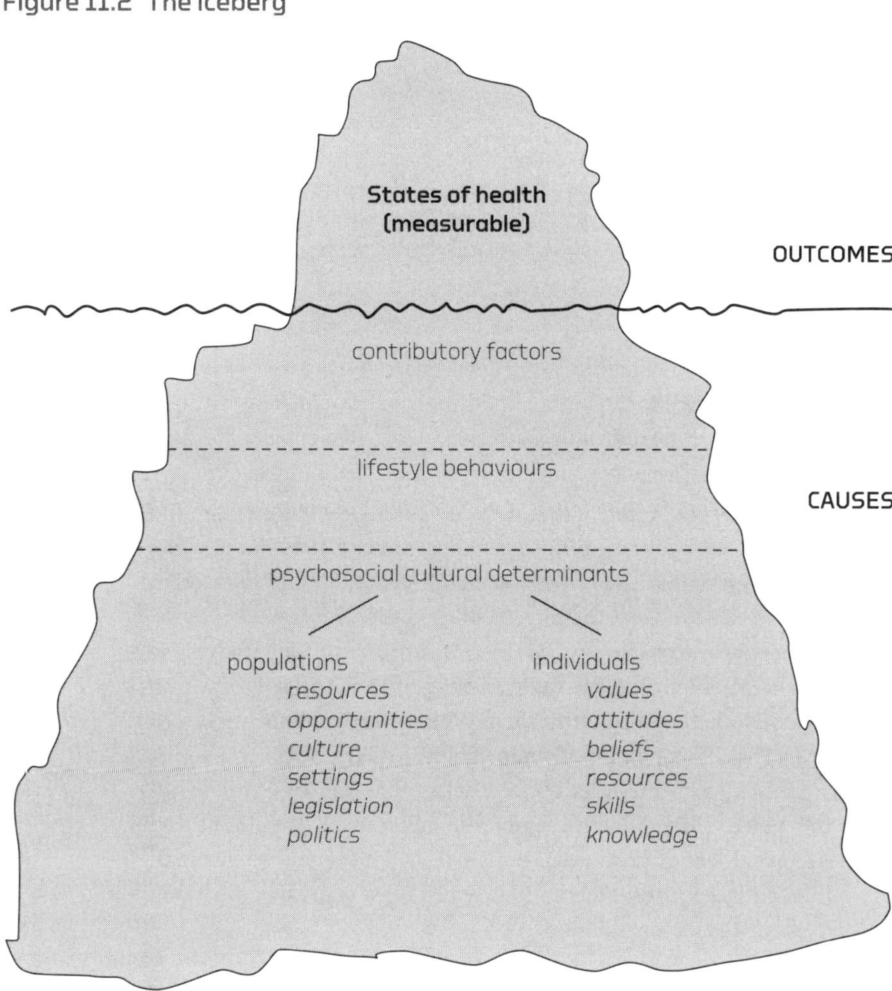

Source: Talbot and Verrinder 2009

The second section of the iceberg (just below the waterline) relates to easily identifiable individual lifestyle choices and behavioural risk factors (e.g. the link between lack of physical activity and CVD). In the next section of the iceberg lie the major psycho-socio-cultural factors that influence individual and population health. At the very bottom of the iceberg are ecological and environmental factors that underpin our future health status (Talbot & Verrinder 2009).

The social gradient

The changing statistics on morbidity and mortality at population level are only part of the story. We often speak of differences in life expectancy that correspond to variations in health and disease across societies. These differences are evident between nations, and are variously attributed to differences in standard of living, in national infrastructure, and the quality of health services available. Figures like these are familiar to us.

Table 11.1 Men's life expectancy at birth in 2008

India	61
Philippines	65
Korea	65
Lithuania	66
Poland	71
Mexico	72
Cuba	75
USA	75
UK	76

Source: WHO 2008

A further important part of the story is that there are differences in morbidity and mortality within each society, and those differences appear to be a function of social position: those towards the bottom end of the social scale are on average more often sick and die earlier than those towards the top end of the scale. This is known as the **social gradient** in health. The classic example of this is the Whitehall Study II, so called because it was a major longitudinal study of mortality and social class within the British public service, whose headquarters are in Whitehall in London. It followed Whitehall I, which had been a study of men's vulnerability to CVD. Michael Marmot, who headed both studies, used categories of social class that had appeared in UK censuses since the 1930s. Class I includes professionals, class II is intermediate (managerial and technical) occupations, class IIIN is skilled non-manual occupations, class IIIM is skilled manual occupations, class IV is semi-skilled manual occupations, and class V unskilled manual occupations.

Social gradient Life expectancy is shorter and most diseases are more common further down the social ladder in each society.

Table 11.2 Life expectancy by social class 1972-76 and 1992-96, England and Wales

Social Class	Men 1972-76	Men 1992-96	Women 1972-76	Women 1996
I	72.0	77.7	79.2	83.4
II	71.7	75.8	77.0	81.1
IIIN	69.5	75.0	78.0	80.4
IIIM	69.8	73.5	75.1	78.8
IV	68.4	72.6	75.0	77.7
V	66.5	68.2	73.9	77.0
Difference	5.5	9.5	5.3	6.4

Source: Marmot 2003

Mythbuster

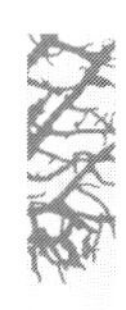

Providing health services to all will ensure equal health outcomes for all.

Consider Glasgow's figures for male life expectancy. These are 54 years in an inner-city suburb (well below India's average) and 82 years in an affluent suburb (well above UK's average). These differences occur in the same city, in the same country, for people potentially able to access the same health services, under the same universal insurance scheme (Hanlon et al. 2006).

Case Study 11.2 The health of 2000 San Francisco bus drivers

Among drivers over the age of 60, workplace medical examinations found the prevalence of hypertension to be 90%. A study was launched. This found that drivers complained of back pain, and then gastrointestinal and respiratory difficulties. High rates of alcohol use after work were also observed. More funding was secured and more interventions designed, but this did not solve the essential problem.

The researchers were so focused on specific diseases that they failed to recognise the fundamental problem: the job. They then investigated why the job caused so many problems. Computers devised a rigid bus schedule that allocated time depending on the number of buses available, but the computers were allocating time in a city with a bus shortage. Drivers had to get from Mission and Army Street to Mission and Geneva Street, for example, in 2 minutes. A fast trip in a Ferrari on Sunday morning would take longer. In addition, because drivers were penalised when they arrived late, they gave up rest stops and dashed into fast-food restaurants instead. And since the drivers were almost always late, the passengers were almost always angry. Drivers lacked control over a host of variables such as traffic and terrible shift arrangements, and drove during both morning and evening rush hours without enough time to go home in between shifts. At the end of a long day, many visited the local tavern. When they got home, they did not often socialise with family, but went to bed, only to get up at 4 a.m. to begin another gruelling day. They had health problems that needed attention, but obviously it was the job that had to be fixed to allow drivers some control of destiny and sense of empowerment (Syme 2004).

In addition to the social gradient in mortality across social classes for both males and females, it is evident that the gradient has become steeper over the period: that is, while life expectancy for all classes has increased, the rate of increase is much higher for class I than for class V, so that the gap between classes is greater.

Explanations for the gradient in health continue to be debated. Clearly it cannot be understood merely in terms of deprivation, or access to health services, or health literacy, for these differences between adjacent social classes are not substantial. The hypothesis put forward by Marmot (2004), Syme (2004), and others is that differences arise from factors such as self-esteem, status differences, self-direction in work, control over one's environment, social capital, and sense of social support—all variables that decline in strength as one descends the social ladder (Cockerham 2007, p. 94).

Social inequality and social exclusion

The Whitehall studies' finding of a social gradient in health status and life expectancy has been replicated around the world. Direct comparisons between countries are, however, made difficult by different measures of social class and **socio-economic status** (SES). Wilkinson and Pickett (2009) have developed comparisons for developed nations using per capita income as an indicator of SES, and a ratio of the per capita income of the top 20% to that of the bottom 20% as a measure of social inequality. Their findings can be summarised in two key graphs:

Further, they are able to show that health is related to the differences in income *within* societies, but not to differences *between* societies. It is inequality within a society, not that society's overall prosperity, which predicts the level of problems (Pickett & Wilkinson 2009).

Income is only a rough indicator of SES or deprivation, and more sensitive measures are now being developed. In Europe, social exclusion is increasingly used as an indicator of social inequality to reflect the complexity of the processes creating

Socio-economic status Represents how individuals and groups are 'placed' in a society, and how social and economic factors interact to affect health. These factors include social prestige, education, occupation, material resources, housing, and working conditions.

Figure 11.3 Health and social problems are worse in more unequal countries

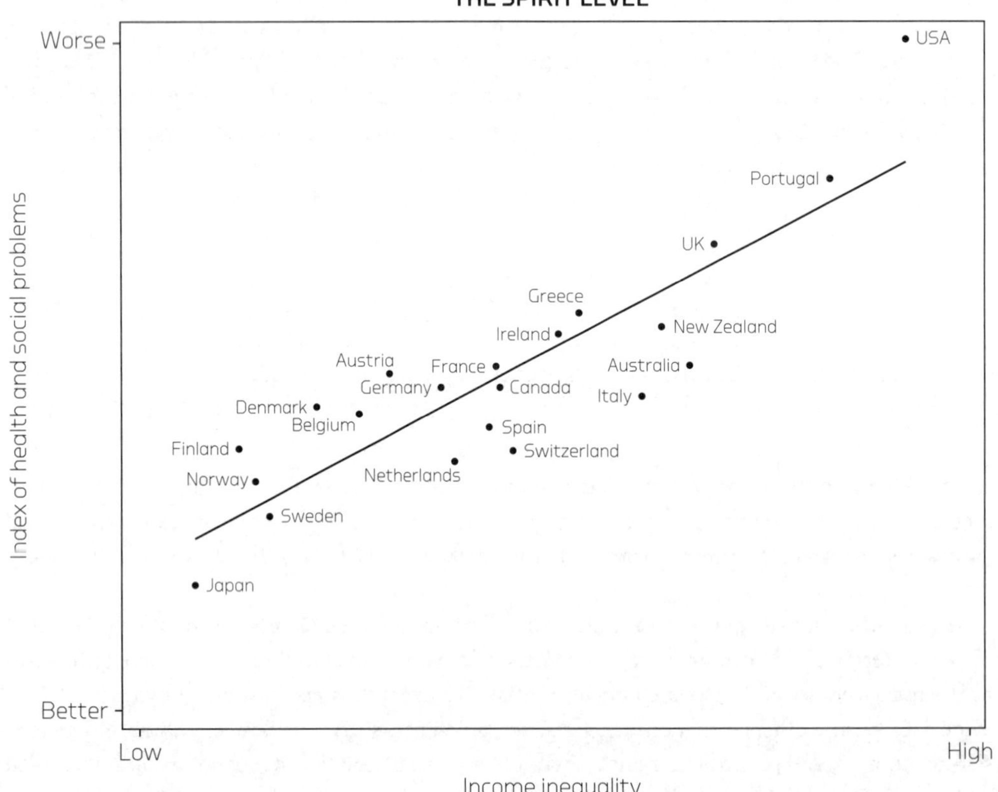

Source: From The Spirit Level by Richard Wilkinson & Kate Pickett, Allen & Lane. © Wilkinson and Pickett 2009

Figure 11.4 Life expectancy is longer in more equal rich countries

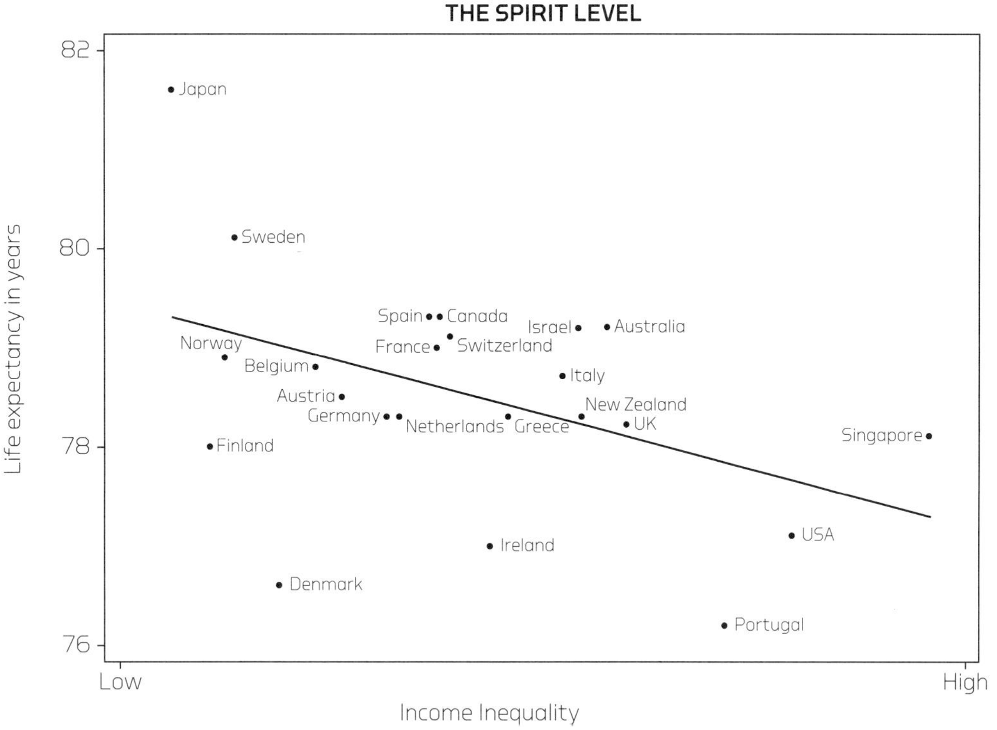

THE SPIRIT LEVEL

82
80
78
76
Life expectancy in years
Japan
Sweden
Spain
Canada
Israel
Australia
Norway
France
Switzerland
Belgium
Italy
Austria
New Zealand
Germany
Netherlands
Greece
UK
Singapore
Finland
USA
Ireland
Denmark
Portugal
Low
High
Income Inequality

Source: From The Spirit Level by Richard Wilkinson & Kate Pickett, Allen & Lane. © Wilkinson and Pickett 2009

Social exclusion A shorthand label for what can happen when individuals or areas suffer from a combination of linked problems such as unemployment, poor skills, low incomes, poor housing, high crime environments, bad health, and family breakdown.

Equity In healthcare can be defined as the absence of systematic disparities in health (or in the major social determinants of health) between social groups who have different levels of underlying social advantage/disadvantage.

inequality and provide a basis for addressing inequality. **Social exclusion** is a complex and multidimensional process. It involves the denial of resources, rights, goods, and services, and the inability to participate in normal relationships and activities available to the majority of people in a society, whether in economic, social, cultural, or political arenas. It affects both the quality of life of individuals and the **equity** and cohesion of society as a whole (Levitas et al. 2007). The Bristol Exclusion Matrix (Figure 11.5) provides an overview and summary.

Social exclusion is one of the most serious consequences of poverty and inequity. There are strong interconnections between the many social determinants of health, and the construct of social exclusion holds these multiple contributions together, demonstrating that social exclusion is an active process within societies. Being socially included means that people have the resources (skills and assets, including good health), opportunities, and capabilities they need to learn, work, engage, and have a voice (Social Inclusion Unit 2009, p. 3). Australia's **social inclusion** policy and strategy has been designed as a whole-of-government tool to be used in evaluating all policy initiatives in all sectors. The policy contains both aspirational and practical principles as follows:

Aspirational principles

- Reducing disadvantage
- Increasing social, civil and economic participation
- A greater voice, combined with greater responsibility

Figure 11.5 Bristol Exclusion Matrix

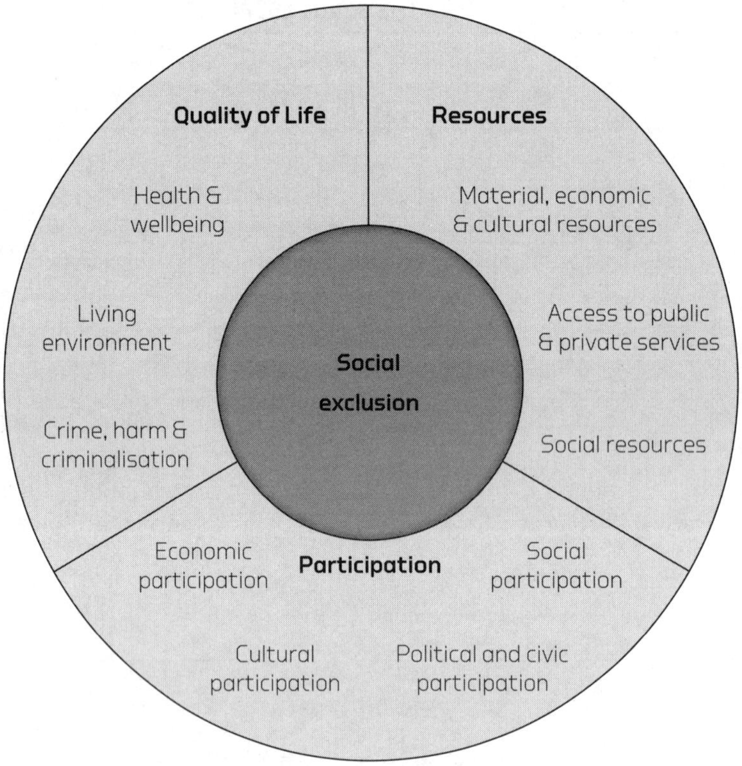

Source: Reproduced by permission from Professor Ruth Levitas and Dr Eldin Fahmy, Copyright University of Bristol.

Principles of approach

- Building on individual and community strengths
- Building partnerships with key stakeholders
- Developing tailored services
- Giving a high priority to early intervention and prevention
- Building joined-up services and whole of government(s) solutions
- Using evidence and integrated data to inform policy
- Using locational approaches
- Planning for sustainability

Social Inclusion Unit 2009, p. 21

A primary aim of such policies is to remedy the mechanisms of social exclusion, identified principally as stereotyping, discrimination, and stigma.

A major influence upon social exclusion theory is the capabilities model devised by Sen (1984) and developed with Nussbaum (2001, 2005). This approach recognises the relationship between personal agency and social structure. Each nation has the responsibility, through its governance of social life, to ensure that individuals have the capacity to make choices about key aspects of their lives; each individual must take responsibility for their choices. A number of lists of capabilities exist, but

Social inclusion Used to describe strategies and policies designed to create a **socially inclusive society**, and also the experience of belonging to such a society.

Socially inclusive society One where all people feel valued, their differences are respected, and their basic needs are met, so they can live in dignity.

Nussbaum's (see tutorial exercise) is indicative. The reforms called for in the *World health report 2008* (WHO 2008) and *Closing the Gap* (WHO CSDH 2008b) outline structural changes that are needed to nurture capabilities.

Health as a global concern

Wilkinson and Pickett (2009) show that health status is dependent on the degree of social inequality of a nation, not the overall average income. Obviously, income matters—some income is required to sustain life—but as the following graph, the Preston curve, shows, life expectancy effectively plateaus once a relatively low per capita income has been reached. From there, increasing the overall wealth of a nation may have less effect on health (as reflected in increasing life expectancy) than will reducing social inequality.

A major current initiative that aims at improving the health status of developing nations, in particular those at the leading edge of the Preston curve, is the WHO's Millennium Development Goals. These goals are strongly linked with the WHO's assertion that health is a human right. They are an immediate precursor to the work of the Commission on Social Determinants of Health (CSDH), which was given a global brief by the WHO to examine the evidence for social determinants of health in developing and developed nations.

In 2005 the WHO established the CSDH to provide advice on ways of reducing the widening inequalities in health. The CSDH made it clear from the very beginning that health equity was to be the cornerstone of their work. The Commission's final report, *Closing the gap in a generation: Health equity through action on the social determinants of health*, was released in 2008 (WHO CSDH 2008) and contained three overarching recommendations:

- Improve daily living conditions.
- Tackle the inequitable distribution of power, money and resources.
- Measure and understand the problem and assess the impact of action.

The work of the Commission provides guidelines for practitioners and policymakers alike and provides the evidence for how action on these recommendations will improve health status for the most vulnerable members of our society. Of necessity, it does not commit itself to specific strategies for radical social reform (Green 2010; Lee 2010); rather, it enunciates principles and values to guide implementation in particular contexts. It is worth noting, however, that the CSDH implications for health system reform have been taken up in the *World health report 2008*, which asserts the central importance of primary care and critiques the structure and leadership of individualistic and medicalised health systems (WHO 2008).

Already the report has provided an important foundation for further national policy documents, among them *A healthier future for all Australians* (NHHRC 2009b,c) and *Fair society, healthy lives: The Marmot review* (Strategic Review of Health Inequalities in England post-2010 2010). Further major collections of evidence also continue to be published, such as *Equity, social determinants and public health programmes* (Blas & Kurup 2010). These reports reinforce Beauchamp's contention that 'the historic dream of public health...is a dream of social justice' (Beauchamp 1996, p. 105).

Figure 11.6 Preston curve

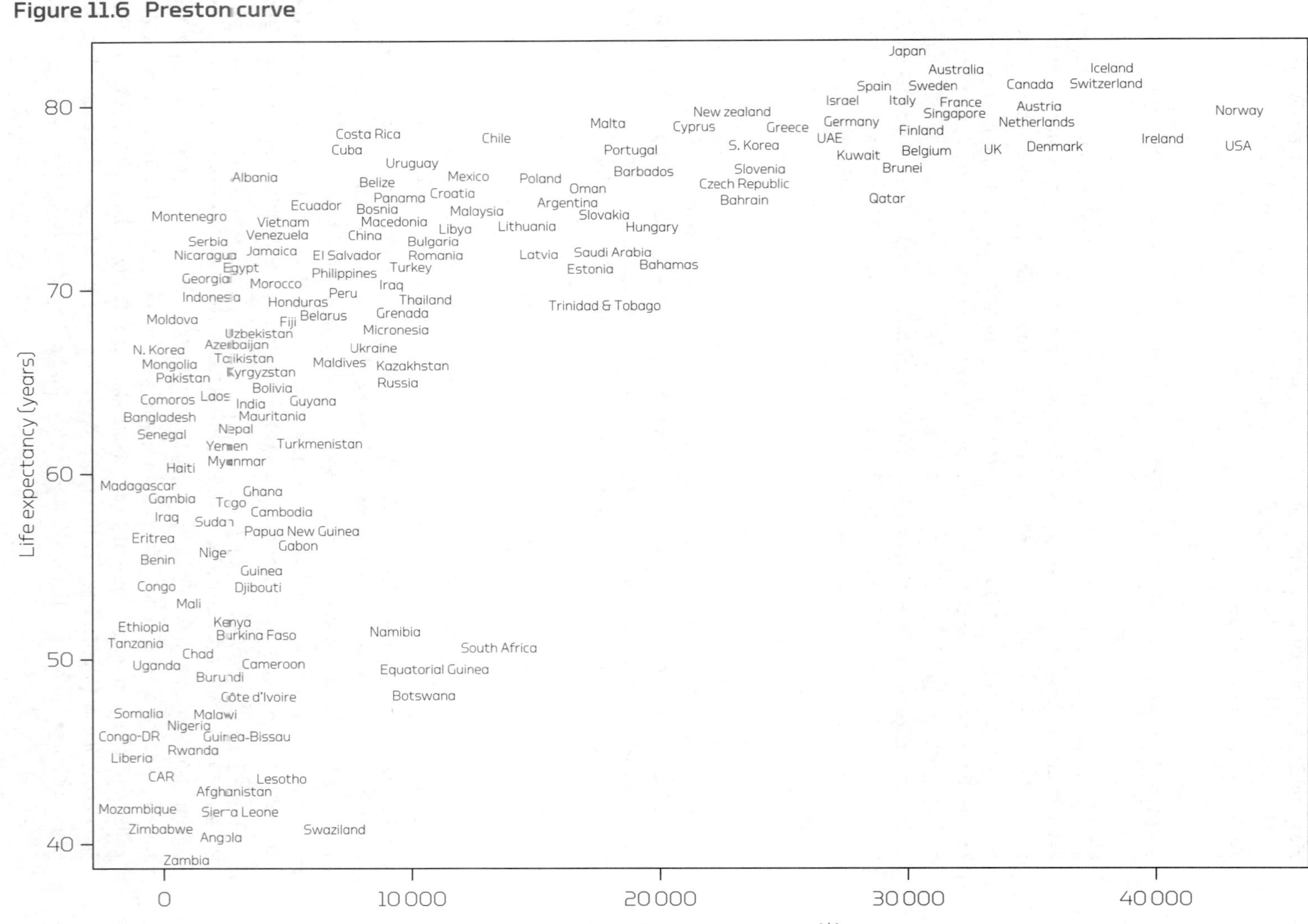

Source: From The Spirit Level by Richard Wilkinson & Kate Pickett, Allen & Lane. © Wilkinson and Pickett 2009

Getting the balance right

Because this chapter has been arguing the case for taking social determinants of health seriously, it may have conveyed an impression that we are playing down or even questioning the contribution of clinical science to a population's health. This is certainly not our intention. What we are arguing is that clinical advancements need to be seen in their social and global contexts, and that we need as societies to work out how the illness-management strategies of the clinical disciplines can best serve each nation's health. It is becoming abundantly clear that the largest proportion of national health budgets around the world is devoted to resolving or ameliorating health problems that could have been avoided, or reduced, or at the very least delayed in their onset. It is also clear that a significant proportion of these health budgets is spent on investigations and interventions that are, at best, of marginal benefit, at worst futile. But we seem unable to reorient our approach to health expenditure to accommodate the wider view, with the result that our expenditure on prevention and health education is still around 5% of the total budget.

Summary

The variation in health status between different societies and different groups within societies has always hinted that social and cultural factors contribute to illness, disability, and reduced life expectancy. The extent of this contribution has, however, not been clear, and some have suggested that differences are largely attributable to variations in the level and quality of healthcare services. Now that the primary causes of disability and death for most nations are found in so-called lifestyle illnesses—cancer, cardiovascular disease, diabetes—that are in turn linked with particular behaviours—smoking, alcohol abuse, obesity—and specific social contexts—unemployment, abusive relationships, social exclusion—it is becoming clear that social and cultural factors have a profound influence on health status both within and between nations.

Solid evidence from many epidemiological studies shows that health is shaped by social determinants, in particular social inequity and social exclusion, which produce a social gradient in health. As this evidence has emerged, so has a range of strategic responses. Most are strategies within the health system designed to address and enhance citizens' health knowledge and improve their agency to change unhealthy behaviours. A fundamental dilemma, however, is that action to address the social determinants of health also involves factors outside the control of the health system. Better health depends on changing settings and social structures that produce inequity and exclusion.

Healthcare reform thus involves not only a focus on preventive measures and primary healthcare, but also on social inclusion. Social justice is the key to building healthy societies that promote the well-being of the whole population.

Tutorial exercises

1 Return to the story of Samantha (Case Study 1.2). From the various contributions to her death that you identified then, list the social determinants. Consider where Samantha or her mother has agency, and where they are constrained by these determinants.
2 The suggestion has been made that some food companies are promoting some of their products in terms of their health benefits (high fibre, added vitamins, reduced fat...) while ignoring

dangerously high levels of sugar or sodium in those same products. Check this claim by a field trip to the supermarket during which you inspect the list of ingredients of some of these products. What strategies are needed to ensure that an accurate depiction of health benefits and risks is available to the public?

3 Go to the United Nations website <www.un.org/millenniumgoals> and look up the eight Millenium Development Goals. Choose one goal and examine any fact sheets that go with that goal. What has been achieved? What is still to be done? How might health workers ensure that this goal is met?
4 What are some of the main shifts in conceptualising and addressing social determinants that you see in comparing 2003's *The Solid Facts* with 2008's *Closing the Gap?*
5 What are some of the obstacles to implementing social inclusion strategies in Australia? In the light of this, what do you see as the benefits and risks of Australia's social inclusion policy?
6 Martha Nussbaum (2005) suggests that the core capabilities for living a good life are that each person should be able to
   a live a life of normal length
   b have bodily health
   c maintain bodily integrity
   d exercise the senses, imagination, and thought
   e experience and express emotions
   f develop practical reason (a conception of the good)
   g affiliate with others
   h have respect for other species
   i play
   j have appropriate control over their environment (political and material).

   Are there capabilities you would add to, or omit from, Nussbaum's list?

Further reading

Baum, F. (2008). *The new public health*, 3rd edn. Melbourne: Oxford University Press.

Blas, E., & Kurup, A. (eds) (2010). *Equity, social determinants and public health programmes*. Geneva: WHO Press.

Keleher, H., & MacDougall, C. (eds) (2009). *Understanding health: A determinants' approach*, 2nd edn. Melbourne: Oxford University Press.

Lin, V., Smith, J., & Fawkes, S. (2007). *Public health practice in Australia: The organised effort*. Sydney: Allen & Unwin.

Marmot, M. (2004). *Status syndrome: How your social standing directly affects your health and life expectancy*. London: Bloomsbury.

Marmot, M., & Wilkinson, R. (eds) (2006). *Social determinants of health*, 2nd edn. Oxford: Oxford University Press.

National Health and Hospitals Reform Commission (2009). *A healthier future for all Australians: Final report, May 2009*. Canberra: Commonwealth of Australia.

Wilkinson, R., & Pickett, K. (2009). *The spirit level: Why more equal societies almost always do better*. London: Allen-Lane (Penguin).

World Health Organization Commission on Social Determinants of Health (2008b). *Closing the gap in a generation: Health equity through action on the social determinants of health. Final Report of the Commission on Social Determinants of Health*. Geneva: WHO.

Websites

<http://aihw.gov.au/>

This is the website of the Australian Institute of Health and Welfare. It provides data on the health of Australians.

<www.marmotreview.org>

The 2010 Marmot Review *Fair Society, Healthy Lives* was an independent review into health inequalities in the UK. The site continues to report on many developments based on the approach advocated in the review, and provides links to other related European studies.

<www.equalitytrust.org.uk/resource/the-spirit-level>

The Equality Trust conducts a program of public and political education designed to improve the understanding of, and create action on, income inequality. It is non-partisan, and draws heavily on the research of Wilkinson, Pickett and colleagues.

<www.socialinclusion.gov.au/Pages/default.aspx>

This is the Australian Government website on social inclusion policy and strategy. It provides resources, regular reports from the Australian Social Inclusion Board, and research papers.

<www.un.org/millenniumgoals>

The UN Millennium Development Goals (MDG) website gives an overview of the global action plan implementing the millennium goals. It provides a wealth of resources and current information concerning a range of MDG initiatives.

<www.who.int/social_determinants/en>

This is the central global resource for data on the social determinants of health. The Commission's website contains a wealth of documents supporting the *Closing the Gap* report, and continues to be updated with fresh material on program developments and publications arising from the CSDH Report.

READING 11

Deviance, difference, and stigma as social determinants of health

Pranee Liamputtong and
Somsri Kitisriworapan

TOPICS COVERED

This chapter covers the following topics:

- definitions of deviance, difference, stigma, and discrimination
- impact of deviance and stigma on health
- stigma and HIV/AIDS
- what has been done to combat HIV-related stigma

KEY TERMS

Deviance
Difference
Discrimination
HIV/AIDS
Labelling theory
Moral career
Social exclusion
Social norms
Stigma
Stigmatisation

Introduction

Sciologist Emile Durkheim (1895/1982) suggested that deviance is a universal feature of all societies because it implies the values and norms of a culture. Moral interpretation exists in all societies, and some qualities and conduct are perceived as more desirable than others, so deviance is always present in every society. By identifying what is deviant, societies identify what is not. This in turn creates shared standards within a society (Clinard & Meier 2008, p. 10).

Often, the notion that some people are different in an unacceptable way leads to stigma, which refers to certain traits and behaviours that are devalued by others. The word 'stigma' is derived from an ancient Greek word meaning 'mark'. Marks were impressed on slaves as a way to identify their position in the social structure, which was one of inferiority (Whitehead et al. 2001a; Sherman 2007). Although deviance, difference, and stigma are socially constructed concepts, they are often thought of as somehow intrinsic, and so have a negative impact on the life and well-being of the individuals and groups who are so labelled. As such, they form an important component of the **social determinants** of health.

Social determinants A number of factors, including social, cultural, economic, and political, which can impact on the health of individuals.

This chapter will bring readers through several important issues relevant to deviance, difference, and stigma. The chapter will first introduce these notions, then discuss the impact they have on the health and well-being of those who are stigmatised. It also discusses stigma and HIV/AIDS and what has been done to combat HIV-related stigma as a case study.

Deviance and difference

Deviance constitutes a universal aspect of our everyday social life (Roach Anleu 2006, 2009). Indeed, the ideas of conformity, rule observation, and correct conduct can only be comprehended because of the existence of deviance. Even a simple question like 'Why did you do it?' could suggest that the person has violated some social rule. Questions like this usually elicit unease or awkwardness and may eventually discourage individuals from violating those particular rules. As such, it is a form of informal social control that stops people from engaging in deviant behaviour (Roach Anleu 2006, 2009).

Deviance Behaviour that transgresses social expectations and is likely to attract sanctions from other members of the society.

At the simplest level, Clinard and Meier (2008, p. 8) suggest, deviance marks out those who are **different**. Deviant people behave differently, and hence they are different from us. However, the concept of deviance goes beyond a simple examination of differences between individuals and their behaviour. Often, when we refer to the notion of deviance, we tend to think about some things we devalue or evaluate negatively (Clinard & Meier 2008). A common definition of deviance refers to 'behaviour which violates social norms' (Roach Anleu 2006, p. 420). Deviance symbolises nonconfomity to a norm or set of norms that is approved or observed by the majority of people in a particular society or culture (Scambler 2003). Deviant behaviour signifies behaviour which, 'once it has become public knowledge, is routinely subject to sanctions—to punishment, correction or treatment' (Scambler 2003, p. 192).

Difference Used when an individual possesses characteristics that are dissimilar to or behaves differently from the majority of people within a society.

Social norms Rules or standards that guide or constrain individuals' actions or behaviour.

Social norms are rules or standards that guide or constrain individuals' actions or behaviour (Stuber et al. 2008; Roach Anleu 2009). A norm is a social rule indicating what individuals ought to or ought not say, think, or do in a given situation (Blake & Davis 1964). Transgressions of norms usually elicit negative responses or sanctions from others in the society. These responses or sanctions put pressure on people to conform to social norms (Clinard & Meier 2008). Relevant to the concept of normatic deviance is social control—the use of strategies that attempt to compel comformity, or at least to deal with or deflect deviant behaviour (Roach Anleu 2006, 2009).

Although norms are shaped, encouraged, and sustained by the social and situational contexts within the society (Becker 1963a; Clinard & Meier 2008), most concepts of deviance are created by some segments of society who strive to harden their positions about what is proper and improper and what is right and wrong into norms (Clinard & Meier 2008). They tend to be those who have more power because of their social status (Roach Anleu 2009). When these groups sense threats to their interests from particular conditions or acts, they might try to advance those interests by convincing others of the authority of their concern (Clinard & Meier 2008). These processes have shaped criteria for many forms of deviance, for example, drink driving, consumption of illegal drugs, abortion, prostitution, and homosexuality.

Stop and Think

Emma, who is in her late thirties, has a great career path. She does not have any children, and has recently got a divorce. Because of a promotion, she moved to Melbourne. As she meets new colleagues and friends, Emma starts to feel that she is somehow being treated differently. In a number of conversations with them, it becomes clear to her that some of her new network regard her 'family situation' as unusual. Emma begins to feel that she is excluded from social gatherings where couples with children are welcomed. This makes Emma think that she is in some sense deviant. *But is she?* (adapted from Clinard & Meier 2008, p. 2).

Stop and Think

Consider the case of Emma presented above. Nowadays, more couples choose not to have children and divorce is common. There are no absolute standards which dictate that adults should have children or that one should not be divorced. But Emma feels uncomfortable around her social network because she is excluded from social occasions, and this is due to her social status as childless and a divorcee. But why would her colleagues and new friends see her as deviant? Clinard and Meier (2008, p. 7) contend that an answer might be that 'the norms of their groups suggest that couples and parents are statuses that are valued'. Emma might be feeling deviant because her new social network groups who have partners and children think that this is the way things *should* be in our society.

» What is your view about this theory? Is there any other theory that you can use to explain this case?

Concepts of deviance ebb and flow over time and can change in different situations (Roach Anleu 2006; Clinard & Meier 2008). For example, in most Western societies there is no longer much moral disapproval of premarital sexual intercourse, so it is no longer seen as deviant behaviour. Masturbation has also been increasingly accepted. Some may even perceive the practice as an essential part of 'normal sexual development' (Janus & Janus 1993, p. 106; Clinard & Meier 2008, p. 297). Homosexuality was once seen as an extremely deviant and morally wrong behaviour. However, it is now more tolerated by many people, and also seen merely as an example of difference (Roach Anleu 2006, p. 3).

Looking through the daily newspapers in Australia reveals that the kinds of deviance seen as requiring social control nowadays tend to include abortion, domestic violence, bottle-feeding practices, homelessness, drug trafficking, juvenile delinquency, sex work, environmental pollution, and tobacco consumption. These activities have always gone on in Australian society, but they have not always been labelled as deviant (Roach Anleu 2006). Cohen (1974) uses the term 'elasticity of evil' as the title of his book to suggest that activities and behaviour which are interpreted as deviance are always evolving. Hence, what is deviant at one point of time or situation might not be perceived as such in another (Roach Anleu 2006).

As we have suggested, some particular groups in society have more power to elicit, change, and sustain specific concepts of deviance. There are constant movements to abandon the perception of practices such as personal drug consumption, public drunkenness, and prostitution as 'deviant'. There have also been some attempts to make some activities sanctioned by law as deviant and hence criminal. A good example of this is the prevailing categorising of cigarette smoking as deviant, which has occurred in a number of nations including Australia and the USA. Up to the 1970s, cigarette smoking was an acceptable behaviour; nowadays, it is viewed as deviant. This can be seen through the 'no smoking' signs that appear in numerous public places, including restaurants, planes, and in Australia, all Commonwealth Government offices and buildings. Smoking is forbidden by law in these locations. There are penalties if this statute is violated (Roach Anleu 2006).

What is deviant in one culture, however, may be normal or acceptable in another. For example, in many Western societies, smoking marijuana is deviant but consuming alcohol is not. In some Middle Eastern cultures the reverse is true (Scambler 2003). Belching loudly when eating is acceptable in Japanese or Chinese culture (it is a form of food appreciation), but this is seen as rude by most people in Australia. Traditional practices regarding painful initiation ceremonies, arranged marriages, or the confinement of women during childbirth and menstruation, for instance, may seem highly deviant, if not barbaric, to Australian and other Western societies, but these practices are normal in some cultures and form an important part of their ways of life (Roach Anleu 2006).

Case Study 15.1 Breast and bottle-feeding: Moral and deviant mothers

Notions of deviance always elicit a strong moral stance. Even everyday conduct can have this moral tone. The argument on whether mothers should breastfeed or bottle-feed babies embodies a moral attitude of this kind. Murphy's (1999) study of first-time mothers in England and Liamputtong and Kitisriworapan's research with working mothers in Thailand (see Liamputtong & Kitisriworapan 2011) reveal that whether the mothers intend to breastfeed or bottle-feed, they face tremendous challenges from those who disagree with them. Clinard and Meier (2008, p. 2) put it succinctly, that 'not even the time-honoured institution of motherhood is immune from allegations of deviance'.

The dominant idea that 'breast is best' is pervasive in literature on infant feeding patterns and in policy and health promotion material which attempt to educate women about their infant feeding practices. Within the lay population, this idea is also promulgated. Due to the societal perception of the superiority of breastfeeding, mothers' intention not to breastfeed their babies may tarnish the 'moral status' of motherhood. By choosing to bottle-feed, a mother is subjected to the accusation that she is a 'bad' mother who 'places her own needs, preferences or conveniences above her baby's welfare'. On the contrary, the 'good mother' is 'deemed to be one who prioritises her child's needs, even (or perhaps especially) where this entails personal inconvenience or distress' (Murphy 1999, pp. 187–8), such as trying to breastfeed in the face of many obstacles.

Motherhood is 'often represented as the ultimate expression of womanhood while breast-feeding is represented as the ultimate experience of motherhood' (Nadesan & Sotirin 1998, p. 221). Because of this, the decision to bottle-feed 'leaves women open to the charge of being a poor mother, in short, of maternal deviance' (Murphy 1999, p. 188). The intention to formula-feed threatens women's claims to qualities such as selflessness, wisdom, responsibility, and far-sightedness, all of which are widely seen as evidence of being a 'good mother' (Murphy 1999, p. 188).

The discourses on motherhood have created this moral image of breastfeeding (Guttman & Zimmerman 2000). In Earle's study (2000, p. 327) with women in Coventry, England, women perceived breastfeeding as natural. A woman who did not breastfeed was perceived as a 'horrible mother' (Liamputtong 2006).

Deviance, according to Murphy (1999, p. 189), 'involves a charge that public morality is being violated' and in the case of infant feeding, mothers break the rules of infant feeding. But more than that, as Murphy (1999, p. 188) theorises, 'the moral mother is not simply one who follows the rules. Rather, she is one who follows the rules *knowingly*'. Hence, simply breaking the rules does not make the mother deviant. Rather, 'her deviance rests upon a judgement that she has broken the rules *knowingly*' (McHugh 1970, p. 188, original emphasis). In the case of infant feeding, mothers who choose not to breastfeed their infants despite knowing very well the likely impact on their infant's health are potentially subjected to the charge of deviance, or being stigmatised as 'immoral mothers'.

However, there appear to be some possibilities for women who intend to bottle-feed to 'challenge or resist the interpretation of their behaviour as morally sanctionable' (Murphy 1999, pp. 189–90). To do so, women who intend to bottle-feed must prove that, while it breaks the rule, it is nonetheless justified. When the decision to formula-feed her baby is questioned, a mother must justify that her intention is 'non-conventional'; that is, 'she could not have done otherwise' (Murphy 1999, p. 190). As she has no other choice, her intention is justified and therefore should not be sanctioned. When breastfeeding is socially valued in societies, women choosing not to breastfeed may use socially and culturally acceptable grounds for their actions, such as the need to work in a paid job or having insufficient milk. This will help them to escape being seen as 'bad mothers'.

Stigma, stigmatisation, and discrimination

Closely related to deviance is the concept of **stigma**. The foundation of stigma lies in 'differences'. These differences can be in physical appearance, personality, age, gender, sexuality, illness, disability, and specific behaviour which evoke discontent, abhorence, panic, or sympathy from others (Mason et al. 2001).

Stigma An attribute or characteristic that separates people from one another. It is used by individuals to interpret specific attributes of others as 'discreditable or unworthy' and this results in the stigmatised person becoming devalued.

Stigma, according to Goffman (1963, p. 3) is a 'devaluation' process that links with stereotyping and prejudice. It is used by individuals to interpret specific traits of others as 'discreditable or unworthy' and this results in the person stigmatised becoming 'discounted' or 'tainted' (Thomas 2006, p. 3175). Those who are stigmatised will then be 'disqualified from full social acceptance' (Goffman 1963, preface). Following Goffman's theory of stigma as an attribute, Jones and colleagues (1984) used 'mark' to indicate stigma, which would eventually lead to the definition of someone as 'flawed' or 'spoiled' (Yang et al. 2007, p. 1525). On the basis of a social position which dictates that some individuals are 'tainted' and 'less than', stigma is a mark that separates people from one another (Pescosolido et al. 2008, p. 431).

According to Mason and colleagues (2001, p. 4), the main element of the stigmatising strategy is to create the 'them and us' principle (see also Foucault 1973). Its aim is to lay a foundation which could separate individuals who are perceived as 'good and in favour' from those who are 'bad and out of favour' within a given social norm (Foucault 1973). Once this principle is initiated, **stigmatisation** and **social exclusion** are permitted. This process is then established and confirmed by the prejudiced position that accentuates the difference between 'them' and 'us'. As Sontag (1991) suggests, HIV/AIDS symbolises 'sinful' and 'evil'. Hence, people living with HIV/AIDS tend to be perceived as discredited individuals who have immoral characters. As a consequence, they are socially conditioned as not 'one of us' (Mason et al. 2001, p. 4). Often, this leads to **discrimination** against the discredited persons.

Stigmatisation The process of stigmatising a person.

Social exclusion The exclusion of individuals from social networks and resources because of their different and stigmatised status.

Discrimination The idea that someone is of less value and should be excluded from social networks and the benefits of society.

Goffman (1963) suggests that there are three kinds of stigmatising conditions. The first is 'tribal identities', which include such characteristics as gender, race, religion, and nationality. Second is the 'blemishes of individual character', which may include having mental illness, having a history of addiction or imprisonment, and living with HIV/AIDS. Third is 'abominations of the body' which include such bodily conditions as deformities and physical disabilities (LeBel 2008, p. 411). Based on Goffman's stigmatising conditions, there are many individuals who would be stigmatised because of their social and health status in many societies. More recently, Falk (2001) proposes two types of stigmatising states which are based on the 'cause' of stigma. First, 'existential stigma' occurs when an individual does not create stigma or has very little control over it. These include being old, having a certain race and ethnicity, and having a mental illness. Second, 'achieved stigma', which happens when an individual has acquired a stigma because of their own action and behaviour and/or because they have personally cultivated it. These may include such actions as becoming a refugee, immigrant, prisoner, homeless, or living with HIV/AIDS (LeBel 2008).

Similar to the concept of deviance presented above, stigma theorists have focused more on the position of social norms in the process of constructing stigma (Stuber et al. 2008, p. 422). Goffman (1963), for instance, contends that because deviations from social rules are inescapable, stigmatisation is a common characteristic of any society. Others suggest that stigmatisation is a characteristic of all socio-cultural groups and that it is employed to elicit conformity with the social standings of society so that law and order can be enforced. From this perspective, stigmatisation is the result of deviating from social rules that attempt to make the deviant individual conform. It is also used to illustrate to other group members the behaviours that are not condoned, and the effects that will be felt by those who engage in such actions. However, it can only be used in these ways to enforce conformity around voluntary behaviours, for example, illicit drug consumption and cigarette smoking (Stuber et al. 2008). Stigma has also now been defined by scholars in terms of a person's social identity, and their unique social contexts has been more emphasised. According to Crocker and colleagues (1998), the central feature of social stigma is that stigmatised persons have, or are believed to have, some characteristics that are associated with a devalued social identity in a particular social situation.

How does stigma occur? Goffman (1963) contends that stigma is a process grounded within the 'construction of social identity' (Yang et al. 2007, p. 1527). Stigma eventuates through what Goffman (1963, p. 32) refers to as a '**moral career**': when a stigmatised individual initially makes sense of their social position in society and later acquires a set idea of what it would be like to have a specific stigma. The person will then pass from 'normal' to a 'discreditable' status, and through social interaction, they will eventually obtain a 'discredited' status. In Goffman's term, when an individual's new identity is 'assumed through interaction (i.e., "re-identifying") with socially constructed categories', stigma will occur (Yang et al. 2007, p. 1527). A good example is the case of mental illness. A person with mental illness (a non-visible stigma) passes from a 'normal' status to a 'discredited' one. Their 'discredited' status is gained when they disclose the mental illness condition to others.

Moral career A process when a stigmatised individual initially makes sense of their social position within the society and later acquires a set idea of what it would be like to hold a specific characteristic.

Stigma also occurs through the process of 'labelling'. Scheff (1966) posits a **labelling theory** and applies it to the case of mental illness. He suggests that when an individual living with mental illness is given a deviant label, it will eventually lead them to change their self-perception and lose social opportunity (Yang et al. 2007). Scheff argues that individuals learn about the stereotypes of mental illness through the process of socialisation and daily reinforcement. Because of its highly discrediting status, once the stereotype is fully formed, the person's 'patient' role will appear as a 'master status' (Markowitz 2005). Consistent reactions from others, particularly the application of social exclusion, will prevent the person from reclaiming their former ('normal') social functions (Yang et al. 2007).

Labelling theory The process of labelling a person with stigma, which through the process of social interaction will eventually lead the person to change their self-perception and lose social opportunity.

The impact of deviance and stigma on health

> For the stigmatized, stigma compounds suffering. (Yang et al. 2007, p. 1528)

The greatest suffering inflicted by stigma in modern times can be seen in what is now called 'ethnic cleansing'. The mass killing of harmless people occurs simply because they are of different race, ethnicity, religion, or culture, or merely because they are different. This is proof of what humans can do to others if the reactions to stigma are not taken seriously (Whitehead et al. 2001b).

Health and illness conditions that tend to produce stigma are those connected with negative characteristics, those that have uncertain or unknown causes and limited treatment, and those that produce intense reactions such as fear and disgust (Sontag 1991; LeBel 2008). Historically, leprosy and tuberculosis were met with revulsion and later on we witnessed the same emotional responses towards cancer, mental illness, and, more recently, HIV/AIDS (Sontag 1991; LeBel 2008) (see later section on stigma and HIV/AIDS). Currently, we still see numerous health-related issues which have attracted stigma: abortion, infertility, being overweight, obesity, bottle-feeding, and cigarette smoking. Those who belong to stigmatised classifications (or the deviants as we outlined earlier), such as poor people, homeless people, gays and lesbians, refugees, indigenous people, and ethnic minority groups, are also likely to have to deal with the negative repercussions of stigma-related health issues (Pescosolido et al. 2008).

The effect of stigma on the stigmatised individuals can differ in its manifestation and magnitude (Link & Phelan 2001; Mason et al. 2001; Corrigan et al. 2003a,b). Often, stigma generates negative credibilities, in other words stereotypes. It then gives legitimacy to the negative credibilities; this is referred to as prejudice. This prejudice then leads to a wish to shun individuals who possess stigmatised status; this is discrimination (Pescosolido et al. 2008, p. 431; see also Link & Phelan 2001; Williams et al. 2008). Any form of discrimination and prejudice may lead to social exclusion as it functions to disconnect stigmatised persons from society and prohibits them from having societal benefits such as access to education, housing, social support, and healthcare (Mason et al. 2001; LeBel 2008).

Individually, the effects of stigma and social exclusion can be very destructive. They can result in isolation, low self-esteem, depression, self-harm, poor academic achievement and social relationships, and poor physical and mental health (Mason et al. 2001; Major & O'Brien 2005; Yang et al. 2007). For stigmatised individuals with major health problems, the stigma they carry can 'intensify the sense that life is uncertain, dangerous, and hazardous' (Yang et al. 2007, p. 1528). Therefore, it is clear that stigma and discrimination are harmful to the quality of life of stigmatised persons (Pescosolido et al. 2008).

Importantly, an emphasis on the association between a person's behaviour and health has created a 'new morality' (Becker 1993, p. 4). 'Being ill' is reinterpreted as 'being guilty'. For example, people with obesity are stigmatised because they let themselves go and smokers are stigmatised because they 'have no willpower' to stop (Bayer 2008, p. 468). Guilt is used as a prompter, and it might be successful in certain situations. However, guilt itself has tremendous ability to produce adverse physical and emotional effects on health (Becker 1993). It may be worth noting that the idea that health conditions, poverty, non-standard lifestyles, and so forth have long been considered a failure of will and evidence of lack of moral fibre. The reconstruction of alcoholism as a disease, for example, was an attempt to shift the focus from a moral problem to a physiological one.

The impact of stigma on the public health of the stigmatised individuals and groups is huge. Herek (2002, p. 604) states bluntly that 'stigma and discrimination are the enemies of public health'. The fact that stigma has a damaging effect on people's health has led public health officials and advocates to notice the powerfully negative results of stigmatisation for public health. In the area of HIV/AIDS, for example, it is now clear that the stigmatisation of certain groups such as commercial sex workers, injecting drug users, and gay men would only make them more susceptible to HIV infection and push them out of reach of those who attempt to help them to modify the behaviours that put them and others at risk (Stuber et al. 2008).

Within healthcare settings, Whitehead and colleagues (2001b, p. 29) contend that perceptions of difference may 'become professionalised'. Within a medical framework, it may be acceptable to treat someone differently because they are seen, in some ways, to be too 'dis-ordered'. For example, because of the lack of an interpreter, healthcare providers might be reluctant or refuse to provide care to individuals living with mental illness who are from ethnic minorities. This is simply because healthcare providers think that these people cannot or do not speak English and would not understand what they are told. This means that these individuals could be excluded from healthcare services to which others in the society have access. This is what we have referred to as 'social exclusion', which can have a negative impact on the lives of many marginalised people.

Stop and Think

» An injecting drug user who has no history of HIV infection is not allowed to donate blood at a local blood donation event. What do you think may explain this?

» A new mother who has been living in her local residence for a number of years is told not to bring her newborn baby to a play group in her local area because the baby has a visible physical malformation. What impact will this have on her and her newborn?

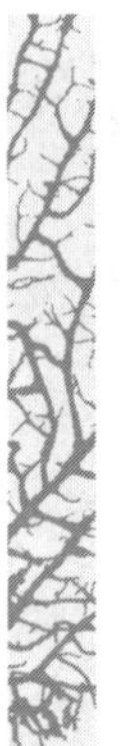

Mythbuster

Consider whether you see the following as questionable. What does this tell you about our societal values?

- A nurse refuses to provide care to a female patient who lives with HIV/AIDS because of her own ideas about the cause of HIV/AIDS. She believes that the woman acquired the disease through promiscuity, which she does not approve of.
- A mother of an autistic boy has difficulty placing him in the local school because the school thinks he would not be able to learn or fit in with others, and his condition may lead to discrimination against him.
- An overweight young woman who works at a local business office is told to lose a substantial amount of weight or she will be sacked from her work, even though such an action is illegal.

Stigma, discrimination, and HIV/AIDS

HIV/AIDS Human Immunodeficiency Virus (HIV) and Acquired Immunodeficiency Syndrome (AIDS) emerged as a major public health issue in 1981 in North America. It is a highly stigmatised illness because it is seen to be associated with individuals who engage in deviant sexual behaviour or anti-social behaviour of other kinds.

Globally and locally, the **HIV/AIDS** epidemic has offered the circumstance for a powerful argument that connects stigmatisation and public health (Bayer & Stuber 2006). From the onset of the epidemic, HIV/AIDS has been seen not only as a medical condition, but also as a stigmatised state (Herek & Glunt 1993; Letteney & LaPorte 2004). Scambler (2003, p. 199), states clearly that HIV/AIDS 'has been both medicalized as "disease" and moralized as "stigma"'. HIV/AIDS was first recognised in 1981 and since then it has provoked forceful reactions from others (Scambler 2003). HIV/AIDS uniquely combined 'sex, drugs, death and contagion' (Scambler 2003, p. 199). This unique combination made HIV/AIDS a powerfully stigmatising disease. It is also prevalent among those who are already members of stigmatised groups, initially gay men, and later injecting drug users (Parker & Aggleton 2003; Scambler 2003). Globally, in countries where HIV/AIDS is predominantly heterosexually transmitted, stigmatisation and discrimination are also pervasive. Those who are from marginalised groups such as poor people, women, mothers, sex workers, and injecting drug users heavily bear the brunt of the impact of HIV/AIDS. Some have suggested that the stigmatisation and discrimination of these people have violated human rights. Mann and Tarantola (1998, pp. 4–5) put it succinctly: 'Those who—before the arrival of HIV/AIDS—were societally marginalized, stigmatized or discriminated against, were found gradually and increasingly to bear the brunt of the HIV/AIDS epidemic. Human rights violations are now recognized to be primordial root causes of vulnerability to the epidemic.'

Despite the fact that society now has better understanding of the causes and impacts of HIV/AIDS, the burden of prejudice continues to exist (Carlisle 2001; Liamputtong et al. 2009; Vlassoff & Ali 2011). Goffman (1963, p. 70) warns that 'familiarity need not reduce contempt'. Research continues to reveal the ways in which society neglects the need for healthcare for those living with HIV/AIDS (Carlisle 2001; Deng et al. 2007; Anderson et al. 2008).

It is suggested that HIV and AIDS have particular traits which initiate a high level of stigma (Parker & Aggleton 2003). As stigma is socially constructed and is attributable to cultural, social, historical, and situational factors, stigmatised individuals can be beset by feelings of shame and guilt. As discussed earlier, a major consequence of stigmatisation is discrimination and it occurs when an individual 'is treated unfairly and unjustly' because of the perception that the individual has deviated from a norm observed by others (Deng et al. 2007, p. 1561). As such, the HIV/AIDS stigma is perceived as 'an individual's deviance from socially accepted standards of normality' and these can include such deviance as 'immorality', 'promiscuity', 'perversion', 'contagiousness', and 'death'. Hence, people living with HIV/AIDS (PLWHA) are socially constructed as the 'other' who are 'disgracefully different from and threatening to the general public' (Zhou 2007, p. 2856).

The HIV/AIDS stigma continues to manifest inequalities in class, race, and gender (Parker & Aggleton 2003; Reidpath & Chan 2005; Simbayi et al. 2007). Those who are seen to be associated with sexual promiscuity, homosexuality, and drug use are particularly vulnerable to stigma. Women are more vulnerable to the stigma associated with HIV/AIDS as a sexually transmitted disease (Lawless et al. 1996; Cullinane 2007; Ndinda et al. 2007). In African and Asian countries, women living with HIV/AIDS are frequently referred to as 'vectors', 'diseased', and 'prostitutes', but these terms are seldom used about infected men (Ndinda et al. 2007, p. 93). Clearly, discrimination against PLWHA is not simply about HIV/AIDS as a disease. Rather, it intersects with other social prejudices and these include homophobia, racism, and sexism (Parker & Aggleton 2003). Hence, when women living with HIV/AIDS feel stigma, it is not 'only their internalization of the AIDS stigma, but also an effect of their interactions with others or actual experiences with public attitudes through which AIDS-related social standards are manifested' (Zhou 2007, p. 2856).

Often, stigma is multidimensional. There are three broad types of HIV/AIDS-related stigma. First is self-stigma which occurs through 'self blame and self-deprecation' in those living with HIV/AIDS. Second is perceived stigma, which is related to a person's fear that if they disclose their HIV positive status, they may be stigmatised. Third is enacted stigma, which occurs when individuals are actually discriminated against because of their HIV status—actual or perceived (Thomas 2006, p. 3175).

Stigma may be manifested in actions such as gossip, verbal abuse, and distancing from people living with HIV/AIDS. It ranges from subtle actions to 'extreme degradation, rejection and abandonment' (Thomas 2006, p. 3175). These manifestations may change over time (Thomas 2006).

Case Study 15.2 Stigma and Thai women living with HIV/AIDS

There is currently a high prevalence of HIV and AIDS among Thai women. Despite the fact that Thailand has a progressive national approach to dealing with HIV and AIDS, the stigma of HIV/AIDS and the fear of the infection remains. Liamputtong and colleagues (2009) suggest that stigma and discrimination towards PLWHA in Thailand, as experienced by the women in their study, still exists, although it was not as marked as others found earlier. Thai people, even family members of the women in their study, still have fears about HIV and AIDS. This fear is created by the AIDS campaigns in the nation (Lyttleton 2000). Although the initial mass media campaigns in Thailand acted as an 'effective buffer against high rates of transmission' (Lyttleton 2000, p. 224), the aggressive campaigns have also created fear of AIDS among Thai people and a continuing sense of the stigma that people attach to HIV and AIDS. Although there is more local acceptance in some parts of Thailand, such as in the north and in rural areas because of the common presence of HIV/AIDS (Lyttleton 2004; VanLandingham et al. 2005), PLWHA are still rejected by their family, close kin, and particularly others in the community (Lyttleton 2004; Maneesriwongul et al. 2004; Sringernyuang et al. 2005; Apinundecha et al. 2007). The advancement of HIV treatments such as antiretroviral vaccine (ARV) has prolonged the lives of many PLWHA as well as reduced AIDS to a manageable chronic condition (Lyttleton et al. 2007). This has, however, also increased the disclosure of HIV/AIDS and many PLWHA are now subjected to stigma and discrimination in the community (Apinundecha et al. 2007).

Often, ignorance, a lack of accurate information about HIV and AIDS, and misunderstanding about HIV transmission are the common sources of HIV/AIDS stigma (Apinundecha et al. 2007; Zhou 2007; Vlassoff & Ali 2011).

However, as Parker and Aggleton (2003, p. 17) warn, it is crucial to recognise that stigma occurs 'within specific contexts of culture and power'. They also suggest that 'discrimination is characterized by cross-cultural diversity and complexity' (p. 14). Hence, socio-cultural beliefs, values, and morals within local contexts have played a major role in constructing stigma and discrimination (Zhou 2007). Stigma also changes over time. What was stigmatised in older times may not be seen as carrying too much of a stigma now. The HIV/AIDS stigma may also appear far more transparent to some groups of people, but not so to others (Reidpath & Chan 2005; LeBel 2008). Some individuals or groups are more likely to be perceived by society as 'innocent victims of HIV' (Sontag 1991), for example, infants who have contracted HIV through maternal transmission or infected blood. The label of 'innocence' is applied because they are perceived as 'blameless' (Katz 1981). On the contrary, those who have contracted HIV/AIDS through homosexual activities and drug use tend to carry an extra stigma because of their own 'deviant behavior' (LeBel 2008, p. 411).

What has been done to manage stigma

According to LeBel (2008), in order to entirely reshape public perceptions and reactions towards stigmatised people, there is a need for more organised and structural attempts that include both policy and legal action. The results of these attempts may produce a long-term effect on our anti-stigma efforts (see Link et al. 2002; Parker & Aggleton 2003; Puhl & Brownell 2003; Heijnders & Van Der Miej 2006). It has been suggested that through contact with the stigmatised persons and educational campaigns, the stigmatising attitudes of the public could be improved. It has been shown that when the general public have a direct interaction with individuals from stigmatised groups, public attitudes towards the stigmatised have improved (Corrigan & Penn 1999; Brown et al. 2003). Similarly, involving stigmatised individuals as speakers in educational sessions to educate the general public is effective in promoting favourable perceptions and responses of the target audiences as these people can give more accurate information and debunk many misconceptions about them (see Corrigan et al. 2002; Couture & Penn 2003).

Additionally, LeBel (2008) suggests that protest and advocacy can work effectively as a strategy to reduce stigma. Collective tactics such as 'social activism' have proved to be valuable. Thus far, we have witnessed these collective tactics among several stigmatised groups including gays/lesbians, individuals with physical disabilities, people living with mental illness, and other stigmatised groups, and they have been successful in changing official policies and laws. It is argued that this strategy is the most powerful and long-lasting way of reducing and eradicating prejudice and discrimination (Major et al. 2000; see also Sayce 2000; Corrigan & Lundin 2001; Parker & Aggleton 2003; Shih 2004).

The motive and ability to resist or deny the label of deviance among stigmatised groups is an interesting aspect of stigma-related reduction and eradication. In Foucault's term (1981), these people would employ 'reverse discourse' as a way to resist the label of deviance and hence avoid being stigmatised. This discourse allows individuals and groups to 'present a positive affirmation of their identity and perspectives rather than a deviance designation' (Roach Anleu 2006, p. 422). Collectively, the stigmatised groups can generate a strategy that can be used to reject the standard social values and norms (Anspach 1979). In the HIV/AIDS area, according to Taylor (2001, pp. 795–6), there have been many strategies that individuals and groups have used to combat and abolish stigma. Gay men have adopted such symbols as the pink triangle, which is a symbol that the Nazis used in the Holocaust to mark out homosexuals before slaughtering them, to counteract their stigmatisation (Gilmore & Somerville 1994). Two UK voluntary organisations, 'Gay Men Fighting AIDS' and 'ACT UP' (AIDS Coalition to Unleash Power) are good examples of political activation which make use of power as a response to combat stigma. See also Case Study 15.3 below about a stance that Thai women living with HIV/AIDS adopt as a way to resist the stigmatisation of their condition.

Case Study 15.3 AIDS support group and women living with HIV/AIDS in Thailand

Because of stigma and discrimination, many people living with HIV/AIDS attempt to find strategies to deal with or fight against it. A study by Liamputtong and colleagues (2009) revealed that joining AIDS support groups was a strategy used by some Thai women to counteract the stigma of their conditions and lives. As Lyttleton and colleagues (2007, S49) contend, PLWHA support groups act as 'a panacea for stigma and alienation', hence it is not too surprising to see many women in this study joining and participating in group activities regardless of their physical condition.

Support groups offered women more knowledge about the illness and how to deal with it better. As Foucault (1980) theorises, with more knowledge, individuals feel that they have more power to deal with their situations. Support groups also provided women with a sense of belonging. The Thai women got to know more about others who were in the same situation as themselves. Joining the group made them realise that they were not alone in the lonely world of living with HIV and AIDS. With more knowledge and an increased sense of belonging from being part of the support groups, the women attained greater emotional strength to deal with their health condition and the stigma associated with it. Joining support groups created collective power for all women, and this collective power allowed the women to defend their conditions and see their situations in a more positive light.

The most powerful way to fight against stigma and discrimination against HIV and AIDS occurs when the communities are able to mobilise themselves to do so (Parker & Aggleton 2003). Several studies have clearly demonstrated empowerment and social mobilisation in response to HIV and AIDS in various societies (see Daniel & Parker 1993; Altman 1994; Epstein 1996; Parker 1996; Liamputtong et al. 2009). Parker and Aggleton (2003) advocate that it is time for us to begin thinking more seriously about using new models for advocacy and social change in our response to HIV/AIDS-related stigma and discrimination, and building community strength is one of these models. The development of AIDS support groups in Thailand as presented by Liamputtong and colleagues (2009) and elsewhere is a good example of community strength.

Summary

Deviance is a common characteristic of all societies because it signifies the values and norms of a culture. It is based on the idea that some individuals are unacceptably different and this often leads to stigma. Although deviance and stigma are socially constructed, they can impact on the lived experiences of many individuals and groups, particularly those who are already vulnerable to ill health such as individuals with mental health concerns or living with HIV/AIDS. In order to eradicate deviance and stigma, the authors agree with Scambler (2003, p. 201) who contends that there should no longer be any sanction to 'mark' some individuals as deviant and stigmatised and then treat them as 'outsiders'. Instead of treating difference as a basis for discrimination and rejection, it should be credited as 'a source of celebration'. As primary deliverers of healthcare, health professionals are in the best position to embark on local and global dialogue, which can influence the creation of new policies and laws that would make the experiences of stigmatised individuals and groups more positive. This will inevitably enhance their health and well-being and make the lives of marginalised and vulnerable people better in many ways.

Tutorial exercises

1 Watch the Australian film *The Black Balloon* (Film Finance Corporation Australia Limited 2007) which portrays the lives of the parents and a brother of an autistic child. It is accessible in most university libraries and DVD shops. How can the film help you make sense of the concepts that are included in this chapter, particularly in terms of difference, deviance, and stigma?

2 Gay and bisexual men and injecting drug users have been labelled 'guilty HIV/AIDS carriers' by the media (Scambler 2003). What is your opinion of this accusation? How has this label come about? What can we explain about this accusation?
3 Cigarette smoking used to be a norm in society, but recently it has been seen as 'deviant behaviour'. As a result, there have been many bans on smoking in offices and public places such as restaurants. What are the main reasons for this change in societal norms? What arguments have people put in place to make the behaviour deviant? Is there any benefit in making cigarette smoking a deviant behaviour?

Further reading

Bayer, R. (2008). Stigma and the ethics of public health: Not can we but should we. *Social Science & Medicine*, 67, 463–72.

Becker, H.S. (1963b). *Outsiders: Studies in the sociology of deviance*. New York: Free Press.

Falk, G. (2001). *Stigma: How we treat outsiders*. Amherst, NY: Prometheus Books.

Goffman, E. (1990). *Stigma: Notes on the management of spoiled identity*. Harmondsworth: Penguin.

Liamputtong, P., Haritavorn, N., & Kiatying-Angsulee, N. (2009). HIV and AIDS, stigma and AIDS support groups: Perspectives from women living with HIV and AIDS in central Thailand. *Social Science and Medicine*, special issue on Women, Motherhood and AIDS Care in Resource Poor Settings, 69(6), 862–8.

Link, B.G., & Phelan, J.C. (2001). Conceptualizing stigma. *Annual Review of Sociology*, 27, 363–85.

Mason, T., Carlisle, C., Watkins, C., & Whitehead, E. (eds) (2001). *Stigma and social exclusion in healthcare*. London: Routledge.

Roach Anleu, S.L. (2006). *Deviance, conformity and control*, 4th edn. Sydney: Pearson Education Australia.

Scambler, G. (2009). Health-related stigma. *Sociology of Health and Illness*, 31(3), 441–55.

Stuber, J., Galea, S., & Link, B.G. (2008). Smoking and the emergence of a stigmatized social status. *Social Science and Medicine*, 67, 420–30.

Yang, L.H., Kleinman, A., Link, B.G., Phelan, J.C., Lee, S., & Good, B. (2007). Culture and stigma: Adding moral experience to stigma theory. *Social Science and Medicine*, 64, 1524–35.

Websites

<http://community-2.webtv.net/stigmanet/LINKSAntiStigma>

This website is maintained by the National Stigma Clearinghouse and provides information on anti-stigma programs, resources, and research.

<www.sdsmt.edu/online-courses/is/soc00/Deviance.htm>

This website includes a collection of different sites that discuss issues relevant to deviance and criminology.

<www.avert.org/hiv-aids-stigma.htm>

The website provides good discussions on the impact of stigma and discrimination on people living with HIV/AIDS.

<www.stampoutstigma.org>

This is a good website that provides information on news, research, and other material. It aims to provide information about how to combat and eradicate HIV/AIDS-related stigma.

<http://nortonbooks.typepad.com/everydaysociology/2010/03/rethinking-nudity-and-deviance.htm>

This is an interesting blog that discusses deviance in the context of cosmetic surgery, which has been a popular trend among celebrities and movie stars and many others.

<www.positivedeviance.org>

This website explores the notion of positive deviance, which is an interesting concept that readers might like to explore further.

THE CLASS ORIGINS OF HEALTH INEQUALITY

John Germov

Overview

- What is class and how can it help to explain health inequality?
- What is the social gradient of health?
- What can be done to address class-based health inequality?

CLASS MATTERS

We all have some basic notion of class—we see it every day in the differences between low-priced and expensive cars, takeaway shops and fine-dining restaurants, public and private schools, and overcrowded and exclusive suburbs. In surveys over the years, Australians have regularly reported they believe that classes exist and have no trouble placing themselves into a class—only 5 per cent claim they have no class affiliation (Western & Baxter 2011). Debates over the importance of class focus on the extent to which it determines your life chances; that is, your chances of social mobility, of gaining an education, and of getting a certain type of job. While most people acknowledge the existence of class, few recognise that health status is one of the clearest indicators of class inequality in Australia. Despite access to free public health services in Australia, working-class people have higher rates of death, illness, and disability as a result of their living and working conditions.

Key terms

class (or social class)
economic rationalism/ economic liberalism
empirical
epidemiology/social epidemiology
ethnicity
gender/sex
gross domestic product (GDP)
individualism/ individualisation
life chances
public health infrastructure
'race'
risk factors
risk society
ruling class
social capital
social Darwinism
social exclusion
social gradient of health
social justice
social structure
social wage
socio-economic status (SES)
structure–agency debate
victim-blaming

Introducing class

CLASS (OR SOCIAL CLASS)
A position in a system of structured inequality based on the unequal distribution of power, wealth, income and status. People who share a class position typically share similar **life chances**.

LIFE CHANCES
Derived from Max Weber, the term refers to people's opportunity to realise their lifestyle choices, which are often assumed to differ according to their **social class**.

THEORYLINK
See Chapter 2 for more on theoretical perspectives.

Popular notions of **class** tend to focus on lifestyle differences and consumption patterns, particularly regarding fashion, as a social marker of status. While these may indicate class membership in a general sense, they shed little light on how class differences are generated in the first place. This chapter discusses the concept of class, provides up-to-date evidence of class-based health inequality, and examines five main explanations of health inequality:

1 artefact
2 natural/social selection
3 cultural/behavioural
4 materialist/structural, and
5 psycho-social/social capital.

The chapter ends with a discussion of a number of ways of tackling health inequality, with the aim of achieving equity in health outcomes.

Sociological analyses of class tend to focus on the underlying factors that produce and reproduce class differences. It is important to note that different theoretical perspectives used by sociologists have resulted in continuing debate over appropriate definitions and theories of class, most of which focus on Erik Olin Wright's neo-Marxist and John Goldthorpe's neo-Weberian class models, but these debates are not addressed here (see Baxter et al. 1991; Goldthorpe 1996; Wright 1997; 2005; Crompton 1998; Crompton et al. 2000). To help clarify the concept of class, we will consider a three-class model based on a hybrid of Marxist and Weberian perspectives, in which classes—upper class, middle class, and working class—are defined according to the following characteristics: ownership and control of scarce economic resources; ownership of marketable skills and qualifications; and wage labour. It is important to note that this is a simplified model, and that contemporary class analyses tend to support a more complex seven-class model (compare Savage et al. 2013; Western & Baxter 2011).

The 'upper class' refers to those who own and/or manage economic resources (capital), such as raw materials, technology, and workplaces, and employ others to create profit for them. This group includes many senior executives who may not own a company, but nevertheless have access to the company's profit through share ownership, profit-sharing arrangements, and high incomes. Therefore, they control how work is organised and carried out, including the power to hire and fire. The 'middle class' represents a diverse group of people who possess some form of qualification and skill that allows them to attract higher wages and better working conditions than unskilled workers, and includes health professionals and teachers. This group can also include small-business owners and the self-employed. The 'working class' consists of unskilled manual and non-manual (blue- and white-collar) workers who gain employment solely by selling their labour power. Based on 2003 data from the Australian Survey of Social Attitudes (Western & Baxter 2007) we can construct the following three-class model of Australian society:

- upper class: 15 per cent
- middle class: 47 per cent
- working class: 38 per cent.

All class models have 'grey areas'. For example, whether a plumber is considered working class or middle class will depend on the particular class model used.

While it is relatively easy to divide the population into a class model statistically, it is important to remember that the concept of class is meant to reflect real-life groups of people who share similar living and working conditions. At this point, we need to clarify the difference between the terms 'class' and '**socio-economic status**' **(SES)**. These terms are often used interchangeably, but they do not mean the same thing. SES is determined by ranking people usually according to income, education, and occupation levels, and grouping them into corresponding high, medium, and low-SES groups. It is a relatively straightforward process to categorise people into SES groups, which is why most of the **empirical** evidence of class inequality tends to be based on SES; this is often where the confusion arises between the two terms (see Connell 1977 and 1983 for more discussion of this issue). Measures of SES can only indicate levels of inequality in a society. It is a descriptive classification system and offers little insight into analysing how and why such inequality exists, effectively ignoring such questions by transforming 'the lived reality of class ... to an abstraction for the purpose of statistical treatment' (Connell 1977, p. 33). The 'lived reality' of class refers to people who are class conscious, have class-based values, lifestyles, and identities, and who mobilise politically as a class on certain issues (Connell & Irving 1992). To substitute SES for class ignores the key insight of class analysis—that the unequal distribution of wealth and power is embedded in the **social structure**, and thus that class is not simply a label or status easily acquired or discarded.

SOCIO-ECONOMIC STATUS (SES)
A statistical measure of relative inequality that classifies individuals, households, or families into one of three categories—low SES, middle SES, or high SES—derived from a combination of income, occupation, and education.

EMPIRICAL
Describes observations or research that is based on evidence drawn from experience. It is therefore distinguished from something based only on theoretical knowledge or on some other kind of abstract thinking process.

SOCIAL STRUCTURE
The recurring patterns of social interaction through which people are related to each other, such as institutions and social groups.

Class inequality in Australia

One of the key indicators of class inequality is the distribution of wealth in a country. Figure 5.1 depicts the distribution of household wealth in Australia and shows that the average (mean) in 2009–10 was $720,000, but this figure is skewed by the relatively few high-wealth households. The better indicator of wealth distribution is the median figure (the mid-point at

FIGURE 5.1 DISTRIBUTION OF HOUSEHOLD WEALTH IN AUSTRALIA, 2009-10

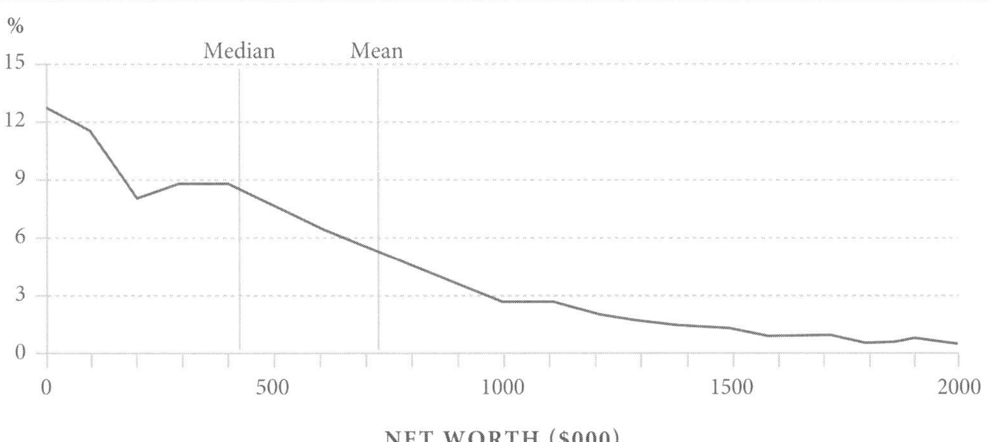

Note: Households with net worth between $150,000 and $2,050,000 are shown in $100,000 increments

Source: ABS 2011, p. 5

which half the population is either above or below). As shown in Figure 5.1, the median-wealth figure was much lower: $426,000 (ABS 2011).

Figure 5.2 shows the wealth distribution for Australia in 2009–10 by dividing the population into quintiles (fifths of the population). Quintile 1 represents the bottom 20 per cent of households (the poorest or most disadvantaged), and quintile 5 refers to the top 20 per cent of households (the wealthiest or most advantaged). As Figure 5.2 indicates, the top 20 per cent (quintile 5) own 62 per cent of the nation's wealth, the top 40 per cent (quintiles 4 and 5) own 82 per cent, and the remaining 60 per cent (quintiles 1 to 3) own 18 per cent. This means that the bottom 40 per cent account for only 6.7 per cent of all the known wealth in Australia. Such figures indicate that Australia is among the most unequal of countries and challenges the view that we live in a classless society.

FIGURE 5.2 WEALTH DISTRIBUTION IN AUSTRALIA, 2009–10

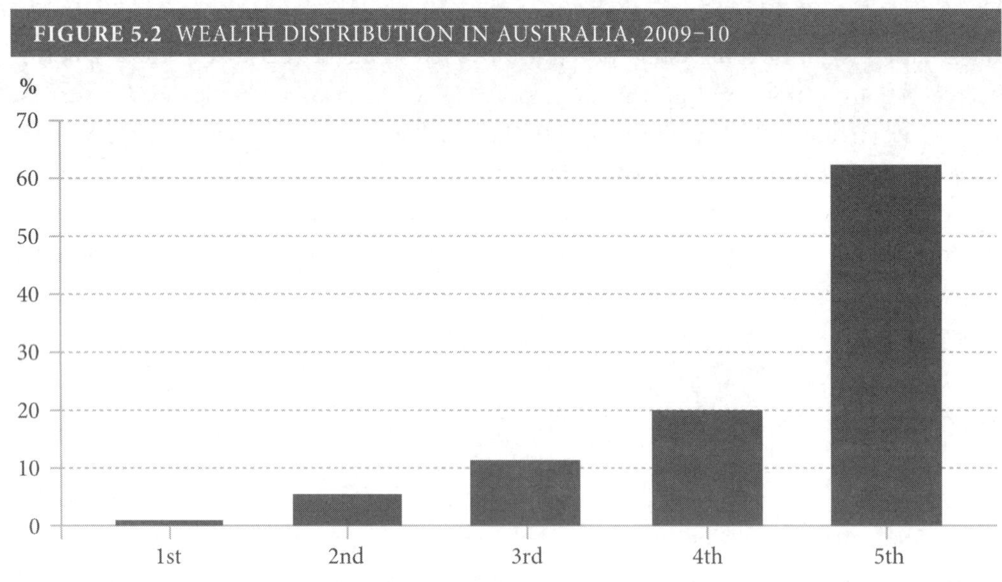

1st Quintile = Poorest 20%; 5th Quintile = Wealthiest 20%

Source: ABS 2011, p. 5

UPPER CLASS OR RULING CLASS?

Each year, the *Business Review Weekly* (BRW) publishes a list of the richest 200 people and families in Australia. The cut-off point for entry to the top 200 has increased markedly over the years, rising from $10 million in 1984, to $45 million in 1995, to $210 million in 2012, indicating how well the rich have been doing in the past two decades. The 2012 Top 10 are shown in Table 5.1. Between 1984 and 2012, the aggregate wealth of the richest 200 increased from $7.3 billion to $181.2 billion (almost a 25-fold increase). Of the 200 richest people in Australia in 2012, 32 were billionaires, headed by Gina Rinehart, and while by far the richest, she was only one of 16 women in the top 200 (BRW 2012, p. 66). It is worth noting that these figures are 'guesstimates', based on the officially declared assets and earnings of the wealthy, and as such are likely significantly to under-report the full extent of wealth.

TABLE 5.1 THE TOP 10 RICHEST PEOPLE IN AUSTRALIA, 2012

INDIVIDUAL OR FAMILY	ESTIMATED WEALTH ($ BILLION)
Gina Rinehart	29.2
Ivan Glasenberg	7.4
Frank Lowy	6.5
Andrew Forrest	5.9
Anthony Pratt & family	5.4
James Packer	5.2
Harry Triguboff	4.8
Clive Palmer	3.8
Chris Wallin	3.8
John Gandel	3.3

Source: Adapted from BRW 2012, p. 70

According to the *World Wealth Report 2012,* the combined wealth of 'high net worth' individuals around the world was US$42 trillion (Capgemini 2012). The wealth of the super rich is difficult to fathom and the exponential rise in their wealth in the past two decades is historically without parallel.

Debates about the upper class concern not only its wealth but also its influence—whether it acts as a **ruling class**. While few theorists would argue that the upper class rules in a direct way, there is also little dispute that through their companies, the members of the upper class can affect investment, employment, and the stock market. In this way, their economic power provides them with significant political influence. The upper class may not pull the strings directly, but its members share similar interests. For example, they may pressure governments to adopt policies of low taxation and deregulation to aid the pursuit of profit maximisation, which tend to benefit those already well off. That said, there is no natural law of profit and wealth, and as recent history teaches us, social policies and taxation rates can work either to consolidate or redistribute wealth.

INTERSECTING STRUCTURES OF INEQUALITY AND THE 'DEATH OF CLASS'

Class has been a central feature of sociological analysis, particularly the role that class plays in shaping individuals' beliefs, behaviour, and access to social rewards such as employment, education, and health (Western 2000). Some authors, though—notably notably Jan Pakulski and Malcolm Waters (1996)—argue that 'class is dead' in terms of its influence over individuals' lives and as the basis of the distribution of wealth and power. Others criticise studies of class for ignoring or marginalising key social groups, such as the disabled, retirees, welfare recipients, the unemployed, and women not in paid work. Instead, they argue that class has been replaced by social inequalities and power struggles based in **gender**, **'race'**, or **ethnicity**, and new social movements, such as gay rights, grey power, and environmental groups

RULING CLASS
A hotly debated term used to highlight the point that the upper class in society has political power as a result of its economic wealth. The term is often used interchangeably with 'upper class'.

GENDER/SEX
This pair of terms refers to the socially constructed categories of feminine and masculine (the cultural identities and values that prescribe how men and women should behave), and the social power relations based on those categories, as distinct from the categories of biological sex (female or male).

'RACE'
A term without scientific basis that uses skin colour and facial features to describe what are alleged to be biologically distinct groups of humans. Race is actually a social construction used to categorise groups of people and sometimes implies assumed (and unproven) intellectual superiority or inferiority.

ETHNICITY
Sociologically, the term refers to a shared cultural background, which is a characteristic of all groups in society. As a policy term, it is used to identify migrants who share a culture that is markedly different from that of Anglo-Australians. In practice, it often refers only to migrants from non-English-speaking backgrounds (NESB migrants).

(for more on this debate, see Eder 1993; Westergaard 1995; Pakulski & Waters 1996; Crompton 1998; Pakulski 2005; Wright 2005).

INDIVIDUALISM/ INDIVIDUALISATION
A belief or process supporting the primacy of individual choice, freedom, and self-responsibility.

Ulrich Beck (1992) suggests that a process of **individualisation** has overtaken class as the dominant marker of social distinction, whereby individual identity is now an outcome of lifestyle choice and consumption patterns (admittedly based on the ability to pay). According to Beck (1992, p. 131), tradition and family ties are no longer dominant in a 'post-class' society, so that individuals are free to construct their identity from a variety of lifestyle choices that are increasingly reflective of and 'dependent upon fashions, social policy, economic cycles and markets'. Therefore, class has lost its subcultural distinctiveness in the age of consumption as 'forms of perception become private and ahistorical' (Beck 1992, p. 235) and people actively construct their self-identity. The argument here is not that social inequality has decreased, but that class as a major determinant of social groups and individual identity has declined.

Pakulski and Waters (1996, p. 10) identify the following four key features of class analysis, arguing that each has diminished in importance in recent times:

1 *Economism*: class structure is an economic phenomenon, based on the unequal ownership of productive capital and marketable skills, that allows a minority to accumulate wealth.
2 *Groupness*: classes are real social groupings of people; these groupings result from conflict over social and economic rewards.
3 *Behavioural and cultural linkage*: members of a class share 'class consciousness', political preferences, similar interests, and lifestyles.
4 *Transformational capacity*: classes allow for collective action and can transform the social structure; class conflict is the central dynamic that shapes social life.

Given the huge increase in wealth among the rich in recent decades, it may appear curious that some authors are declaring the death of class. One way to accommodate the insights of the 'death of class' argument is to reinvoke the distinction between objective and subjective notions of class, or, following Karl Marx (1818–83) among others, the difference between a class 'in itself' and a class 'for itself' (Crompton 1998). A class 'in itself' refers to the objective dimension of class as the basis of social inequality. The unequal distribution of wealth, income, occupation, and education means that any population can be readily categorised into a social hierarchy of distinct classes.

It is one matter to identify an objectively defined class structure, but another issue altogether whether people are aware of their class membership and express characteristics of 'groupness', 'behavioural and cultural linkages', and 'transformational capacities', as noted by Pakulski and Waters (1996) above. A class 'for itself' refers to the subjective dimension of the lived reality of class in the form of social groups of people who share class consciousness and collective social identity, and may engage in political action to promote social change. While the objective dimension of class remains as stark as ever, evidenced by the increasing gap between rich and poor, the subjective dimension of class as the basis of individual identity is less clear cut and at the very least intersects with, and may have been overtaken by, group distinctions based on gender, 'race', ethnicity, and other social movements. This has led to the usage of the term **social exclusion** to refer to socially disadvantaged groups (Levitas 2005; Pantazis et al. 2006; Abrams et al. 2007). The persistence of class-based patterns of illness and health-related behaviour suggests that both the objective and subjective dimensions of class are central to any analysis of health inequality.

SOCIAL EXCLUSION
A broad term used to encompass individuals and groups who experience persistent social disadvantage from a range of causes (poverty, unemployment, poor housing, social isolation etc.), preventing participation in social institutions and political processes.

Class and health inequality

If we accept that we should aim to live in a society that has an equality of health outcomes—that is, without health inequalities based on group membership such as class—then by current standards there is considerable room for improvement. Studies of morbidity (illness) and mortality (death) have consistently shown that the poor have the highest rates of illness and the shortest life expectancy. Health inequality was a key focus of early **public health** efforts in the nineteenth century, particularly through the work of Friedrich Engels, Edwin Chadwick, and Rudolf Virchow (Engels 1845/1958; Rosen 1993; Porter 1997). Despite these early efforts, it was not until 1980 and the publication of *Inequalities in Health* (DHSS) in the UK—commonly referred to as *The Black Report* after its chairman Sir Douglas Black—that interest in health inequality was renewed (see also Townsend & Davidson 1982; Whitehead 1987; Townsend et al. 1992). A further UK report, the *Independent Inquiry into Inequalities in Health* (Acheson 1998), reaffirmed the issue and resulted in dedicated government actions.

While a number of small Australian studies in the 1980s had found links between manual occupations and/or low SES and poor health, the most comprehensive evidence of health inequality was first presented in the government report *Enough to Make You Sick: How Income and Environment Affect Health* (NHS 1992). In a detailed review of existing Australian research on health inequality, *Socioeconomic Determinants of Health*, Gavin Turrell and colleagues (1999) state conclusively that 'socioeconomic differences in health are evident for both females and males at every stage of the life-course (birth, infancy, childhood and adolescence, and adulthood) and the relationship exists irrespective of how SES and health are measured' (Turrell et al. 1999, p. 33). Since then, the most up-to-date Australian health inequality data has come from the *National Health Survey 2001* (see ABS 2002; AIHW 2003; 2004; Draper et al. 2004; O'Brien 2005; Turrell et al. 2006), which found that the most disadvantaged groups have higher mortality and morbidity rates, higher rates of sedentary behaviour, smoking, overweight, and obesity, and make the least use of preventive health services—most likely due to an inability to afford such services.

THEORYLINK
See Chapter 1 for more on early public health efforts.

PUBLIC HEALTH INFRASTRUCTURE
Public policies and infrastructure to prevent the onset and transmission of disease among the population, with a particular focus on sanitation and hygiene such as clean air, water and food, and immunisation. Public health infrastructure refers specifically to the buildings, installations, and equipment necessary to ensure healthy living conditions for the population.

Explaining health inequality

The most common explanations of health inequality, as previously mentioned, can be grouped into five main categories:

1 artefact explanations
2 natural/social selection explanations
3 cultural/behavioural explanations
4 materialist/structural explanations, and
5 psycho-social/social capital explanations of the **social gradient of health**.

The first four were initially introduced in *The Black Report* (DHSS 1980) in the UK and were also discussed in the Australian report *Enough to Make You Sick* (NHS 1992). The fifth explanation is the most recent and has been influenced by the work of Michael Marmot and Richard Wilkinson (see Wilkinson 1996; 2005; Marmot 2004; 2006; Marmot & Wilkinson 2006; for good reviews of explanations of health inequality, see Cockerham 2013; Bartley 2004; and Macintyre 1997).

SOCIAL GRADIENT OF HEALTH
A continuum of health inequality in most countries from high to low, where the poorest group of people have the worst health status, and each group above it has progressively better health, with the most socio-economically advantaged group having the best health status.

ARTEFACT EXPLANATIONS

The artefact explanation suggests that links between class and health are artificial and are the result of statistical anomalies or the inability to measure social phenomena accurately. This viewpoint is easily disputed by the vast amount of evidence based on various methods and classificatory schemes that have clearly found proof that health inequality exists. While *The Black Report* (DHSS 1980) dismissed the artefact explanation as being without basis, it highlighted the need to examine the assumptions underpinning the way class and health are measured in social research, as different methods can influence the size of health inequality that is found—a point that has often been overlooked (Macintyre 1997).

SOCIAL DARWINISM
The incorrect application of Charles Darwin's theory of animal evolution to explain social inequality by transferring his idea of 'survival of the fittest' among animals to 'explain' human inequality.

NATURAL/SOCIAL SELECTION EXPLANATIONS

The Black Report (DHSS 1980) also briefly discussed **social Darwinist** explanations suggesting that social and health inequality were due to biological inferiority. This viewpoint acknowledges the relationship between class and health, but explains it by assuming that inequality is 'natural' and thus inevitable, meaning nothing can or should be done about it. Such a viewpoint has been effectively dismissed by social science research, but Sally Macintyre (1997) suggests there is a 'soft' version (her term) of this explanation that is still commonly ascribed to and has some explanatory power. The soft version suggests that social selection can play a part in social and health inequality, in that poor health early in life results in poor educational performance and occupational achievement. The central idea here is that people's health disadvantage (for example, disability) causes social disadvantage such as poverty. Most studies that have examined the social selection explanation have consistently found it can only account for a small percentage of people in groups who suffer health inequality. Furthermore, such an explanation neglects the structural causes of ill-health—for example, being born into a family already in poverty—which then leads to ill-health and a cycle of disadvantage (such as that found among many Indigenous groups).

VICTIM-BLAMING
The process whereby social inequality is explained in terms of individuals being solely responsible for what happens to them in relation to the choices they make and their assumed psychological, cultural, and/or biological inferiority.

THEORYLINK
See Chapter 1 for more on illness-inducing factors outside of an individual's control.

CULTURAL/BEHAVIOURAL EXPLANATIONS

Cultural/behavioural explanations focus on the individual to explain health inequality in the form of risk-taking or illness-related behaviour—such as smoking, drug-taking, excess alcohol consumption, and poor dietary intake—as the primary causes of ill-health. Such accounts have rightly been criticised for their **victim-blaming** and overly simplistic account of inequality. As Wilkinson (1996), among others, has forcefully argued, such views are unhelpful because:

> the underlying flaw in the system is not put right ... even when it comes to tackling the individual risk factors, it may sometimes be more effective to tackle them at a societal level ... to tackle the environment that establishes levels of exposure to risk. (pp. 21–2)

A focus on changing the behaviour of individuals assumes they exist in a social vacuum, ignoring the social context, social relations, and social processes that affect their lives. There are, however, illness-inducing factors that lie outside of an individual's control, such as stressful work environments. The concept of the **risk society** (Beck 1992) epitomises the social basis of risk-imposing environments that impact on people's health and influence health-related behaviours. Therefore, a focus on the individual as the cause and cure of illness, particularly

RISK SOCIETY
A term coined by Ulrich Beck to describe the centrality of risk calculations in people's lives in Western society, whereby the key social problems today are unanticipated hazards, such as the risks of pollution, food poisoning, and environmental degradation.

through behaviour modification (which has often been the prescription of much medical, **epidemiological**, and psychological research), will have limited success and also assumes that individuals have the time, resources, and motivation to change their lifestyle.

Macintyre (1997, p. 728) argues that *The Black Report* did discuss a 'more socially (rather than individually) based model of health-related behaviours'. For example, the report states that behaviour can also be viewed as 'embedded more within social structures; as illustrative of socially distinguishable styles of life, associated with, and reinforced by, class' (Townsend et al. 1992, p. 100). It is indeed true that the working class has higher rates of some health-damaging behaviour, such as smoking, and that working-class people use preventive services less. The question of why there are class differences in health-related behaviour remains an issue that has received scant attention in sociological literature until recently. As Box 5.1 shows, research on lay perspectives of health inequality indicates the complex interrelationship between culture, social structure, and behaviour; finding that many disadvantaged people adopt a victim-blaming stance and deny a link between class and ill-health (Blaxter 1993; 1997; Popay et al. 2003).

EPIDEMIOLOGY/ SOCIAL EPIDEMIOLOGY
The statistical study of patterns of disease in the population. Originally focused on epidemics, or infectious diseases, it now covers non-infectious conditions such as stroke and cancer. Social epidemiology is a sub-field aligned with sociology that focuses on the social determinants of illness.

BOX 5.1
DOING HEALTH SOCIOLOGY: LAY UNDERSTANDINGS OF HEALTH INEQUALITY

In her review of research on lay conceptions of health and illness, Mildred Blaxter (1997) concluded that many disadvantaged people adopted individualistic explanations rather than linking poor living and working conditions to illness. According to Blaxter (1997, p. 754), '[t]o acknowledge "inequality" would be to admit an inferior moral status for oneself and one's peers: hence, perhaps, the emphasis on "not giving in to illness," which can be seen as a claim to moral equality even in the face of clear economic inequality'. Research by Jennie Popay and colleagues (2003, p. 22) reports similar findings, and suggests that 'strength of character and personal control are emphasised' in the face of social disadvantage, so that 'the way the individual responds to these will determine whether health is damaged'. Such views make sense in a culture based on individualism and the moral imperative of self-responsibility for health. Furthermore, as Popay and colleagues (2003, p. 22) state, 'the means to avoid ill health (framed in terms of individual resilience and strength of character) are, potentially at least, within an individual's control ... It is difficult to envisage what an effective individual response would be to any direct causal relationship between structural factors ... and ill health'. Therefore, disadvantaged people's tendency to deny the social origins of health inequality represents a rational response that avoids fatalism and offers the hope of self-determination.

MATERIALIST/STRUCTURAL EXPLANATIONS

Materialist/structural explanations concern the role of social, economic, and political factors in determining the social distribution of health and illness. The basis of this view has been a focus on how poor living and working conditions—particularly poverty, discrimination, lack of educational and employment opportunities, and inadequate nutrition and housing—directly influence illness. Materialist/structural explanations have been particularly addressed

THEORYLINK
See Chapter 2 for a discussion of Marxism and Weberianism.

by Marxist and Weberian perspectives (see Waitzkin 1983; 2000; Connell 1988), which direct attention away from individualistic and victim-blaming accounts towards the basic class structure of society.

THEORYLINK
See Chapter 6 for more on workplace health.

The value of class analysis is evident when examining the role played by employment and unemployment in understanding and addressing health inequality. For those who are employed, work can also be hazardous to health. For example, those employed in the mining industry have the highest occupational mortality and morbidity rates, followed by agriculture, manufacturing, construction, and transport and communication (Driscoll & Mayhew 1999). A growing literature has also documented the health consequences of unemployment, finding higher rates of chronic illness among the unemployed (see Mathers & Schofield 1998; Bartley et al. 1999).

There is continuing debate in this literature over whether unemployment leads to a deterioration of a person's health status or whether poor health status leads to unemployment, echoing the debate over social selection discussed above. Much of the literature on unemployment and health has been influenced by psychological perspectives, which tend to downplay economic insecurity in favour of psycho-social factors such as the impact of unemployment on social isolation, loss of identity, and anxiety, which allegedly increase illness-related behaviour. While these factors are without doubt important, a sociological analysis focuses on the underlying structural basis of unemployment and ill-health, whereby low-income groups (Indigenous populations, recent migrants, and unskilled workers) are over-represented among the unemployed and have the poorest health status. According to Colin Mathers and Deborah Schofield (1998, p. 181), there is clear evidence from a range of studies to show that the actual experience of unemployment 'has a direct effect on health over and above the effects of socioeconomic status, poverty, risk factors, or prior ill-health'.

Macintyre (1997, p. 740) notes that in the wider literature since the publication of *The Black Report* (DHSS 1980), the four explanations of health inequality discussed above have often been viewed as mutually exclusive, establishing false debates between 'artefact versus real differences', 'selection versus causation', and 'behaviour versus material circumstances'. Such 'either/or' debates have been unhelpful, and Macintyre makes a clear case that even though the authors of *The Black Report* favoured the structural explanation, they still acknowledged the minor role of social selection and the role of cultural and behavioural factors. The focus on structural approaches and class analysis leads to policy prescriptions based on **social justice**, such as welfare measures to address poverty, improve workplace safety, and promote health-inducing work and public spaces (such as smoke-free environments). Class analysis has been less successful in explaining the continued difference in health-related behaviour among the poor. A more recent explanation has pointed to psycho-social factors and the lack of **social capital** as the basis for the persistence of health inequality in developed countries.

SOCIAL JUSTICE
A belief system that gives high priority to the interests of the least advantaged.

SOCIAL CAPITAL
Social relations, networks, norms, trust, and reciprocity between individuals that facilitate cooperation for mutual benefit.

PSYCHO-SOCIAL/SOCIAL CAPITAL EXPLANATIONS: THE SOCIAL GRADIENT OF HEALTH

An alternative explanation of health inequality has arisen from the work of social epidemiologists Marmot and Wilkinson (see Wilkinson 1996; 2005; Wilkinson & Marmot 1998; 2003; Marmot 2004; 2006; Marmot & Wilkinson 2006). While concerned with the social origins of illness, they have turned attention away from class analysis to a narrower focus on income inequality and psycho-social factors. Marmot and Wilkinson suggest that the widening income inequality accompanied by work intensification and unemployment has led to increased levels of stress, anxiety, insecurity, anger, and depression in the community, and that these psycho-social factors negatively impact on health not only among the poor, but also among those who experience relative inequality.

Marmot has been the principal researcher in what have become known as the Whitehall studies, which have examined the health of British civil servants since the 1960s (see Marmot et al. 1978; Marmot et al. 1991; Marmot et al. 1997; Marmot et al. 1999). The first study found a 'social gradient' in the mortality rate, whereby life expectancy increased for each employment level up to the top of the public service hierarchy. Participants in the initial study (all men) were grouped into four employment grades, with those in the bottom two grades found to have a life expectancy 4.4 years shorter than those in the top two grades (Marmot et al. 1978). Furthermore, the social gradient applied to a range of conditions such as stroke, cancer, and gastrointestinal disease (Marmot 2000).

There are two sociologically significant aspects to the findings arising from the Whitehall studies. First, the social gradient of health continued along the whole occupational hierarchy, suggesting that health inequality did not only affect those in poverty, but also existed among relatively well-paid, white-collar workers. While the health gap is greatest between the wealthy and the poor, there is a linear, gradated relationship between health and each step up the socio-economic hierarchy, so that health gradually improves the higher up you go until you reach the top. Second, **risk factors** only accounted for a small percentage of the social gradient. Risk factors—such as being overweight, smoking, excessive alcohol consumption, and not exercising—could not explain the health inequality between the occupational grades of the civil servants in the study (see Marmot et al. 1997; Marmot et al. 1999; Marmot 2000). In an attempt to discover what other determinants might be involved, the Whitehall II study (which included women) focused on the impact of stress on employee health, examining the extent of employee control and variety at work, and the role played by social support. The Whitehall II study also found a social gradient for morbidity among women as well as men, and its major conclusion was that those with less control over work had higher rates of heart disease, depression, and other health problems (see Marmot et al. 1991; Marmot et al. 1997; Marmot et al. 1999; Marmot 2000; 2004).

RISK FACTORS
Behaviours or circumstances that are known to increase people's likelihood of injury or illness.

In *Unhealthy Societies*, Richard Wilkinson (1996) presents empirical evidence to support a thesis that societies with lower levels of income inequality have the highest life expectancy. His argument is that once a country reaches a certain amount of wealth determined by **gross domestic product (GDP)** per capita (per head of population) and undergoes the 'epidemiologic transition' from infectious disease to chronic disease as the major cause of mortality, increases in national wealth have little impact on population health. For example, he notes that even though the GDP per head in the US is almost twice that of Greece, life expectancy in Greece is higher (Wilkinson 1999; see also Wilkinson 1992; Wilkinson & Pickett 2006; 2007; 2009). Therefore, for developed countries, Wilkinson argues that it is not the total wealth of a society that is important, but rather the distribution of that wealth—the more egalitarian a society is, the better the life expectancy and hence the less likelihood of health inequality: there is a 'strong relationship between income distribution and national mortality rates. In the developed world, it is not the richest countries which have the best health, but the most egalitarian' (Wilkinson 1996, p. 3).

GROSS DOMESTIC PRODUCT (GDP)
The market value of all goods and services that have been sold during a year.

Wilkinson's work has spawned a significant literature debating the merits of his study and its conclusions. While some studies have supported his findings (see Kaplan et al. 1996; Kennedy et al. 1996), others have cast doubt on the accuracy and strength of his claims. For example, in a significant study by Ken Judge and colleagues (1998), statistical associations between income inequality and population health were found to be small, posing 'a serious challenge to those who believe that the relationship is a very powerful one' (p. 578).

The work of Marmot and Wilkinson extends the health inequality debate beyond a focus on the most socio-economically disadvantaged groups. Instead, they highlight that a social gradient or continuum of health inequality exists, whereby health gradually worsens as you move down the social hierarchy, so that each social group has worse health than the one above it. For these authors, relative inequality is linked to poorer health, even for employed white-collar workers, who by definition are not poor or exposed to hazardous work environments. Therefore, it is not only the working class or the poor who experience health inequality, but groups along the whole social hierarchy. Though these findings are yet to be confirmed in Australia, they suggest that materialist/structural explanations offer an incomplete account of health inequality. Subsequently, a range of authors spearheaded by Marmot and Wilkinson has focused on psycho-social factors as the main explanation of health inequality.

The psycho-social/social capital thesis: an evaluation

The 'psycho-social thesis' is a neo-functionalist perspective that proposes societies with greater income inequality have less social capital. The idea of social capital is a reworking of Émile Durkheim's (1893/1984; 1897/1951) concept of social solidarity. More recently the concept of social capital has been advanced in the work of Pierre Bourdieu (1986), Jonathon Coleman (1988), and Robert Putnam (1993) and has been popularised in Australia by Eva Cox (1995) and Fran Baum (Baum et al. 2000; Bush & Baum 2001; Baum 2002).

Social capital refers to social relations and networks that exist among social groups and communities, and that provide access to resources and opportunities for mutual benefit. Social capital depends on a high level of community participation, altruism, trust, and an expectation of reciprocity. It has been suggested that the lack of social capital explains why certain social groups adopt health-damaging behaviour. The assumption is that access to social capital will lead to improved health outcomes by lowering stress, and providing outlets for social interaction and opportunities for enhancing control over one's life through democratic participation in community life (Winter 2000a; 2000b).

Putnam (1993) and Cox (1995) envisage social capital as a collective property of specific communities or society as a whole, rather than an attribute or trait possessed by individuals. For Cox (1995, p. 46), social capital involves an 'interplay of state and community', and has been a useful concept for counteracting the negative effects of economic rationalism, which she claims has undermined communities by fostering insecurity and anxiety. High levels of social capital are reflected in altruistic activities such as volunteer work that contributes to the welfare of others. Putnam (2000, p. 331) goes so far as to claim that 'if you belong to no groups but decide to join one, you cut your risk of dying over the next year by half'.

Michael Woolcock (1998, p. 195), while supportive of the social capital thesis, suggests that it is often used in an uncritical and imprecise way, resulting in a handy catch-all concept that 'risks trying to explain too much with too little'. The vague nature of the concept and its intangible qualities (trust, reciprocity) have allowed it to be used by both progressive and conservative political groups, notably the World Bank, a key proponent of the concept (Kawachi & Berkman 2000). Conservative commentators (see Coleman 1988) conceptualise social capital as property of individuals, whereby social disadvantage is viewed as being overcome by individuals engaging in volunteer work, joining associations, and making the most of their own support networks. In this formulation, social capital becomes a code word for mutual obligation and individual responsibility. Therefore, social capital can be used to support **economic rationalist** policies of cutting public expenditure on the **social wage** and public health by placing an increased emphasis on community and family responsibility, and voluntary work.

ECONOMIC RATIONALISM/ ECONOMIC LIBERALISM
A political philosophy based on small-government and market-oriented policies, such as deregulation, privatisation, reduced government spending, and lower taxation.

SOCIAL WAGE
Government spending on health, social security, education, and housing (often referred to as welfare spending).

It is interesting to note that working-class examples of social capital, such as collective action through union involvement, tend to be ignored and are rarely taken into account as evidence of social cohesion and democratic participation in community life by psycho-social proponents (Muntaner & Lynch 1999). Advocates of the social capital thesis also downplay the possibility that it can have negative implications, whereby communities and membership of certain clubs and associations can be used for the social exclusion of others such as ethnic minorities. It is even possible to view the close-knit and mutually supportive nature of criminal gangs as exhibiting strong social capital—a particularly unhealthy scenario (Muntaner et al. 2001).

THEORYLINK
See Chapter 2 for a discussion of functionalism.

Much of the literature on social capital resembles the community development approaches advocated in the 1970s, and fits well with current health promotion efforts that advocate empowering individuals to participate in community activities (Baum et al. 2000); however, these efforts have often met with limited success because they ignored the important role that economic resources and public policies play in facilitating social capital and community development (Winter 2000b; Muntaner et al. 2001; Szreter & Woolcock 2004). High rates of poverty and unemployment in a community are unlikely to support social cohesion. As Putnam states (1993, p. 42), '[s]ocial capital is not a substitute for effective public policy but rather a prerequisite for it and, in part, a consequence of it'. Public policies that facilitate employment opportunities, social services, and access to social institutions, such as education, set the conditions for social capital and health-enhancing environments.

BRINGING CLASS ANALYSIS BACK IN: THE STRUCTURE–AGENCY DEBATE AND HEALTH BEHAVIOUR

The benefit of the psycho-social/social capital approach is its engagement with the **structure-agency debate**. Theories of health inequality have tended to be vague on the issue of class patterns of health-related behaviour, particularly the so-called 'poor behaviour of the poor'. There has been little detailed examination of the processes through which social structure shapes individuals' health-related behaviour (Macintyre 1997; Cockerham 2005; 2013). The psycho-social/social capital explanation provides some insights into the dynamic relationship between structure and agency, establishing pathways between the experience of inequality and health-damaging behaviour (see Marmot & Siegrist 2004).

STRUCTURE–AGENCY DEBATE
A key debate in sociology over the extent to which human behaviour is determined by social structure.

THEORYLINK
See Chapter 1 for more on the structure–agency debate.

Even though Marmot and Wilkinson (2006) acknowledge the need to address structural issues such as poverty, unemployment, and income redistribution, their preferred policy prescriptions have focused on facilitating social cohesion (trust, reciprocity, cooperation, and community participation), rather than political and economic change, downplaying the class relations that create income inequality in the first place (Muntaner & Lynch 1999; Coburn 2000; Lynch 2000). As David Coburn (2000) argues, there is an implicit assumption that wider reform—such as income redistribution to decrease inequality—is beyond reach. Instead, attention is focused on psycho-social factors at the level of the individual and the community in which people live, rather than wider structural factors such as the social and economic policies pursued by governments. By marginalising the role of public policy in both undermining and creating social capital, there is the potential to fall into the trap of a 'community-level version of "blaming the victim"' (Muntaner & Lynch 1999, p. 59). For example, issues of work intensification and occupational health and safety are sidelined in the discussion of psycho-social factors such as stress, anxiety, and depression. Furthermore, it is likely that social capital is more extensive in middle-class and upper-class communities, where individuals have the time and resources to contribute to and participate in community life. Therefore, social capital may be important for psycho-social health, but the lack of a class analysis in the social capital literature undermines its value as an explanatory concept.

Conclusion: towards health equity or health equality?

The link between the working class and high rates of morbidity and mortality is now undisputed, but it remains fair to say that aside from poverty and work-related conditions, the reasons for class-based health inequality—particularly health-damaging behaviours—remain unclear. The social patterning of behaviour clearly indicates that it is not simply an outcome of individual choice: there are social processes at work. Individual behaviour occurs in a social context of living and working conditions that create exposure to health-enhancing or health-damaging environments.

In much of the health-inequality literature, the five explanations discussed here have often been contrasted as either/or propositions—considerable effort has gone into supporting or refuting a particular theory over all others. While no single theory has offered an adequate explanation, a way forward is offered by a multifactorial approach that addresses structural, cultural, and psycho-social factors (see Vågerö & Illsley 1995; Macintyre 1997; Graham 2007; Bambra et al. 2010; Friel & Marmot 2011; Marmot et al. 2012; Mackenbach 2012; Cockerham 2013). Only such theoretical pluralism can effectively deal with the range of social and psychological determinants of health inequality.

At this point it is important to make a distinction between health inequality and health inequity (Whitehead 1990; 1992; Harris et al. 1999; Baggott 2000). While the terms 'inequality' and 'inequity' are often used interchangeably, '[n]ot all inequalities are necessarily inequitable' (Baggott 2000, p. 221). For example, some people can run faster than others or are more industrious at their work. Such inequalities would rarely be seen as unfair or inequitable. In the same vein, health inequality is inevitable given genetic variation, lifestyle choices, and socio-economic differences among the population. Therefore, health inequality refers to the different health statuses associated with various social groups, particularly in terms of class, gender, age, ethnicity, and indigeneity. Health inequity refers to whether such inequality is unfair and avoidable. In other words, health inequity concerns whether health outcomes are the result of everyone having equal opportunity to be optimally healthy, or whether they are due to inadequate income, education, food, and health care. Given that there is no universally accepted understanding of what is equitable or fair, there remains considerable debate as to appropriate goals and interventions to address health inequality.

Margaret Whitehead (1995; 2007) suggests there are four 'policy levels' at which interventions to address health inequality can occur:

1 strengthening individuals through health education to encourage health-enhancing behaviour;
2 strengthening communities by facilitating social cohesion to enable collective action to address health hazards and establish health-conducive environments;
3 improving living and working conditions through better access to safer workplaces, nutritious food, affordable recreation facilities, and preventive services;
4 encouraging macro-economic and cultural change through income maintenance for those in poverty; education and training to prevent long-term poverty; and income redistribution through welfare and taxation policies to reduce overall rates of inequality.

Whitehead (1995) acknowledges that all policy levels are necessary to ensure a comprehensive approach to addressing health inequalities; however, she cautions against an over-reliance on health education and suggests that it is often the lack of time and resources available to the poor that prevents them from adopting healthier lifestyles—something that can be addressed by the other three levels of policy intervention. Health interventions should be guided by a social justice imperative so that the ultimate goal is the maximisation of the health status of the most disadvantaged (Rawls 1970; Connell 1988). Until this aspect of the social structure is addressed, it is likely that little will change in respect of class-based health inequality.

SUMMARY OF MAIN POINTS

- Although class is a major form of social inequality, there are other important intersecting structures of inequality based on gender, 'race', ethnicity, and other social factors, such as youth and age. While there is disagreement in the wider literature between objective (class 'in itself') and subjective (class 'for itself') notions of class, with some suggesting class in subjective terms 'is dead', class is still strongly associated with health status.
- Numerous studies using different research methods and forms of measurement have consistently found that the working class (or low-SES groups) have higher rates of mortality and morbidity.
- Studies have also exposed a social gradient of health, whereby a continuum of health inequality exists from top to bottom of the occupational and income hierarchy.
- There are five main explanations of health inequality: artefact; natural/social selection; cultural/behavioural; materialist/structural; and psycho-social/social capital.
- Health inequality can be reduced through social justice strategies that address class inequality through structural change in the economy, the workplace, and the community.

SOCIOLOGICAL REFLECTION

ADDRESSING CLASS-BASED HEALTH INEQUALITY

Whitehead (1995) suggests there are four 'policy levels' through which health inequality can be addressed:

1 strengthening individuals;

2 strengthening communities;

3 improving access to essential facilities and services;

4 encouraging macroeconomic and cultural change.

What do you think needs to be done to minimise class differences in health status? Think of examples for each of the four policy levels and reflect on how effective these might be. Why might some levels of intervention be focused on more than others?

DISCUSSION QUESTIONS

1 What class do you belong to? Do you believe class has influenced your beliefs, lifestyle, and life chances?

2 In what ways might the upper class in Australia also be considered a ruling class? Think of some real-life examples in your response.

3 In what ways can class analysis shed light on why health inequality exists? What are the limits of class analysis?

4 What is meant by the social gradient of health? What are the benefits and limitations of psycho-social/social capital explanations of health inequality, particularly given the existence of the social gradient?

5 Why do members of the working class exhibit higher rates of health-damaging behaviour?

6 Given that there are social patterns of health-related behaviour, to what extent are individuals responsible for their health?

FURTHER INVESTIGATION

1 Research the latest evidence on the social gradient of health and evaluate the competing explanations.

2 Equal access to health care does not lead to equal health outcomes. Discuss.

3 Compare and contrast the neo-functionalist approach of psycho-social/social capital explanations of health inequality with the neo-Marxist approach. Which provides the best fit in explaining health inequality in Australia?

4 Health education as a policy response to addressing health inequality individualises the social origins of illness. Discuss.

5 'Not all inequalities are necessarily inequitable' (Baggott 2000, p. 221). Discuss with reference to class-based health inequality.

FURTHER READING

Australian Bureau of Statistics (ABS) 2011, *Household Wealth and Wealth Distribution, 2009–10*, Cat. no. 6554.0, ABS, Canberra: <www.abs.gov.au/AUSSTATS/abs@.nsf/DetailsPage/6554.02009-10?OpenDocument>.

Bambra, C., Gibson, M., Sowden, A., Wright, K., Whitehead, M. & Petticrew, M. 2010, 'Tackling the wider social determinants of health and health inequalities: evidence from systematic reviews', *Journal of Epidemiology & Community Health*, vol. 64, no. 4, pp. 284–91.

Bartley, M. 2004, *Health Inequality: An Introduction to Theories, Concepts and Methods*, Polity, Cambridge.

Cockerham, W.C. 2013, *Social Causes of Health and Disease*, 2nd edn, Polity Press, Cambridge.

Friel, S. & Marmot, M.G. 2011, 'Action on the social determinants of health and health inequities goes global', *Annual Review of Public Health*, vol. 32, pp. 225–36.

Graham, H. 2007, *Unequal Lives: Health and Socioeconomic Inequality*, Open University Press, Maidenhead.

Habibis, D. & Walter, M. 2009, *Social Inequality in Australia: Discourses, Realities & Futures*, Oxford University Press, Melbourne.

Mackenbach, J.P. 2012, 'The persistence of health inequalities in modern welfare states: the explanation of a paradox', *Social Science & Medicine*, vol. 75, no. 4, pp. 761–9.

Marmot, M. 2004, *Status Syndrome: How your Social Standing Directly Affects your Health and Life Expectancy*, Bloomsbury, Oxford.

Marmot, M. 2006, 'Health in an unequal world', *Lancet*, vol. 368, no. 9552, pp. 2081–94: <www.who.int/social_determinants/publications/health_in_an_unequal_world_marmott_lancet.pdf>.

Marmot, M. & Siegrist, J. (eds) 2004, 'Health inequalities and the psychosocial environment', *Social Science & Medicine*, special issue, vol. 58, no. 8, pp. 1461–74.

Marmot, M., Allen, J., Bell, R., Bloomer, E. & Goldblatt, P. 2012, 'WHO European review of social determinants of health and the health divide', *The Lancet*, vol. 380, no. 9846, pp. 1011–29.

Savage, M., Devine, F., Cunningham, N., Taylor, M., Li, Y., Hjellbrekke, J., Le Roux, B., Friedman, S. & Miles, A. 2013, 'A new model of social class? Findings from the BBC's Great British Class Survey experiment', *Sociology*, vol. 47, no. 2, pp. 219–50: <http://soc.sagepub.com/content/47/2/219.full.pdf+html>.

Turrell, G., Stanley, L., de Looper, M. & Oldenburg, B. 2006, *Health Inequalities in Australia: Morbidity, Health Behaviours, Risk Factors and Health Service Use*, Health Inequalities Monitoring Series no. 2, AIHW Cat. no. PHE 72, Queensland University of Technology and AIHW, Canberra: <www.aihw.gov.au/publication-detail/?id=6442467837>.

Wilkinson, R.G. & Pickett, K. 2009, *The Spirit Level: Why More Equal Societies Almost Always Do Better*, Allen Lane, London.

WEB RESOURCES

European Portal for Action on Health Inequalities: <www.health-inequalities.eu/HEALTHEQUITY/EN/about_hi/health_inequalities>.

The Great British Class Survey: Results: <www.bbc.co.uk/science/0/21970879>.

International Society for Equity in Health (ISEqH): <www.iseqh.org>. NATSEM: National Centre for Social and Economic Modelling: <www.natsem.canberra.edu.au>.

UCL Institute of Health Equity: <www.instituteofhealthequity.org>.

Whitehall II study: <www.ucl.ac.uk/whitehallII>.

WHO: Social Determinants of Health: <www.who.int/social_determinants/en>.

DOCUMENTARIES/FILMS

The Castle (1997): 85 minutes.

Motion picture, directed by Rob Sitch, Working Dog Productions. An Australian comedy that examines the working-class lives of the fictional Kerrigan family.

People like Us: Social Class in America (2001): 124 minutes.

A documentary depicting people's experiences of class in everyday life.

REFERENCES

Abrams, D., Christian, J. & Gordon, D. (eds) 2007, *Multidisciplinary Handbook of Social Exclusion Research*, John Wiley & Sons, Chichester.

Acheson, D. 1998, *Independent Inquiry into Inequalities in Health*, Stationery Office, London.

Australian Bureau of Statistics (ABS) 2002, *National Health Survey 2001: Summary of Results*, Cat. no. 4364.0, ABS, Canberra.

Australian Bureau of Statistics (ABS) 2011, *Household Wealth and Wealth Distribution, 2009–10*, Cat. no. 6554.0, ABS, Canberra: <www.abs.gov.au/AUSSTATS/abs@.nsf/DetailsPage/6554.02009-10?OpenDocument>.

Australian Institute of Health and Welfare (AIHW) 2003, *Indicators of Health Risk Factors: The AIHW View*, AIHW Cat. no. PHE 47, AIHW, Canberra.

Australian Institute of Health and Welfare (AIHW) 2004, *Australia's Health 2004*, AIHW, Canberra.

Baggott, R. 2000, *Public Health: Policy and Politics*, Palgrave, Basingstoke.

Bambra, C., Gibson, M., Sowden, A., Wright, K., Whitehead, M. & Petticrew, M. 2010, 'Tackling the wider social determinants of health and health inequalities: evidence from systematic reviews', *Journal of Epidemiology & Community Health*, vol. 64, no. 4, pp. 284–91.

Bartley, M. 2004, *Health Inequality: An Introduction to Theories, Concepts and Methods*, Polity, Cambridge.

Bartley, M., Ferrie, J. & Scott, S.M. 1999, 'Living in a high-unemployment economy: understanding the health consequences', in M. Marmot & R. G. Wilkinson (eds), *Social Determinants of Health*, Oxford University Press, Oxford, pp. 81–104.

Baum, F. 2002, *The New Public Health*, 2nd edn, Oxford University Press, Melbourne.

Baum, F., Palmer, C., Modra, C., Murray, C. & Bush, R. 2000, 'Families, social capital and health', in I. Winter (ed.), *Social Capital and Public Policy in Australia*, Australian Institute of Family Studies, Melbourne, pp. 250–75.

Baxter, J., Emmison, M. & Western, M. 1991, *Class Analysis and Contemporary Australia*, Macmillan, Melbourne.

Beck, U. 1992, *Risk Society: Towards a New Modernity*, Sage, London.

Blaxter, M. 1993, 'Why do victims blame themselves?', in A. Radley (ed.), *Worlds of Illness: Biographical and Cultural Perspectives of Health and Disease*, Routledge, London, pp. 124–42.

Blaxter, M. 1997, 'Whose fault is it? People's own conceptions of the reasons for health inequalities', *Social Science & Medicine*, vol. 44, no. 6, pp. 747–56.

Bourdieu, P. 1986, 'The forms of capital', in J. Richardson (ed.), *Handbook of Theory and Research for the Sociology of Education*, Greenwood Press, New York, pp. 241–58.

Bush, R. & Baum, F. 2001, 'Health inequities, community and social capital', in R. Eckersley, J. Dixon & J. Douglas (eds), *The Social Origins of Health and Well-being*, Cambridge University Press, Melbourne, pp. 189–204.

Business Review Weekly (BRW) 2012, 'Rich 200', 24 May – 27 June.

Capgemini 2012, *World Wealth Report 2012 from Capgemini and RBC Wealth Management*: <www.capgemini.com/wwr12>.

Coburn, D. 2000, 'Income Inequality, social cohesion and the health status of populations: the role of neo-liberalism', *Social Science & Medicine*, vol. 51, no. 1, pp. 135–46.

Cockerham, W.C. 2005, 'Health lifestyle theory and the convergence of agency and structure', *Journal of Health and Social Behavior*, vol. 46, no. 1, pp. 51–67.

Cockerham, W.C. 2013, *Social Causes of Health and Disease*, 2nd edn, Polity Press, Cambridge.

Coleman, J. 1988, 'social capital in the creation of human capital', *American Journal of Sociology*, vol. 94, supplement, pp. S95–S120.

Connell, R.W. 1977, *Ruling Class, Ruling Culture*, Cambridge University Press, Cambridge.

Connell, R.W. 1983, *Which Way is Up? Essays on Sex, Class and Culture*, Allen & Unwin, Sydney.

Connell, R.W. 1988, 'Class inequalities and "just health"', *Community Health Studies*, vol. 12, no. 2, pp. 212–17.

Connell, R.W. & Irving, T.H. 1992, *Class Structure in Australian History: Poverty and Progress*, 2nd edn, Longman Cheshire, Melbourne.

Cox, E. 1995, *A Truly Civic Society: Boyer Lectures 1995*, ABC Books, Sydney.

Crompton, R. 1998, *Class and Stratification: An Introduction to Current Debates*, 2nd edn, Polity Press, Cambridge.

Crompton, R., Devine, F., Savage, M. & Scott, J. (eds) 2000, *Renewing Class Analysis*, Blackwell, Oxford.

Department of Health and Social Security (DHSS) 1980, *Inequalities in Health (The Black Report)*, Report of a Working Group Chaired by Sir Douglas Black, DHSS, London.

Draper, G., Turrell, G. & Oldenburg, B. 2004, *Health Inequalities in Australia: Mortality*, Health Inequalities Monitoring Series no. 1, Australian Institute of Health and Welfare (AIHW) Cat. no. PHE 55, Queensland University of Technology and AIHW, Canberra.

Driscoll, T. & Mayhew, C. 1999, 'Extent and cost of occupational injury and illness', in C. Mayhew & C.L. Peterson (eds), *Occupational Health and Safety in Australia*, Allen & Unwin, Sydney, pp. 28–51.

Durkheim, É. 1893/1984, *The Division of Labor in Society*, trans. W. Halls, Free Press, New York.

Durkheim, É. 1897/1951, *Suicide*, Free Press, New York.

Eder, K. 1993, *The New Politics of Class: Social Movements and Cultural Dynamics in Advanced Societies*, Sage, London.

Engels, F. 1845/1958, *The Condition of the Working Class in England*, trans. W.O. Henderson & W.H. Chaloner, Basil Blackwell, Oxford.

Friel, S. & Marmot, M.G. 2011, 'Action on the social determinants of health and health inequities goes global', *Annual Review of Public Health*, vol. 32, pp. 225–36.

Goldthorpe, J. 1996, 'Class and politics in advanced industrial societies', in D.J. Lee & B.S. Turner (eds), *Conflicts About Class*, Longman, London.

Graham, H. 2007, *Unequal Lives: Health and Socioeconomic Inequality*, Open University Press, Maidenhead.

Harris, E., Sainsbury, P. & Nutbeam, D. (eds) 1999, *Perspectives on Health Inequity*, Australian Centre for Health Promotion, University of Sydney, Sydney.

Judge, K., Mulligan, J. & Benzenval, M. 1998, 'Income inequality and population health', *Social Science & Medicine*, vol. 46, nos 4–5, pp. 567–79.

Kaplan, G.A., Pamuk, E., Lynch, J.W., Cohen, R.D. & Balfour, J.L. 1996, 'Income inequality and mortality in the United States: analysis of mortality and potential pathways', *British Medical Journal*, vol. 312, no. 7037, pp. 999–1003.

Kawachi, I. & Berkman, L. 2000, 'Social cohesion, social capital, and health', in L.F. Berkman & I. Kawachi (eds), *Social Epidemiology*, Oxford University Press, New York, pp. 174–90.

Kennedy, B.P., Kawachi, I. & Prothrow-Stith, D. 1996, 'Income distribution and mortality: cross-sectional ecological study of the Robin Hood Index in the United States', *British Medical Journal*, vol. 312, no. 7037, pp. 1004–7.

Levitas, R. 2005, *The Inclusive Society? Social Exclusion and New Labour*, Palgrave Macmillan, Basingstoke.

Lynch, J. 2000, 'Income inequality and health: expanding the debate', *Social Science & Medicine*, vol. 51, no. 3, pp. 1001–5.

Macintyre, S. 1997, '*The Black Report* and beyond: what are the issues?', *Social Science & Medicine*, vol. 44, no. 6, pp. 723–45.

Mackenbach, J.P. 2012, 'The persistence of health inequalities in modern welfare states: the explanation of a paradox', *Social Science & Medicine*, vol. 75, no. 4, pp. 761–9.

Marmot, M.G. 2000, 'Social determinants of health: from observation to policy', *Medical Journal of Australia*, vol. 172, no. 8, 17 April, pp. 379–82.

Marmot, M.G. 2004, *Status Syndrome: How your Social Standing Directly Affects your Health and Life Expectancy*, Bloomsbury, Oxford.

Marmot, M.G. 2006, 'Health in an unequal world', *The Lancet*, vol. 368, no. 9552, pp. 2081–94: < www.thelancet.com/journals/lancet/article/PIIS0140-6736(06)69746-8/fulltext>

Marmot, M.G. & Siegrist, J. (eds) 2004, 'Health inequalities and the psychosocial environment', *Social Science & Medicine*, special issue, vol. 58, no. 8, pp. 1461–574: <www.sciencedirect.com/science/journal/02779536/58/8>.

Marmot, M.G. & Wilkinson, R. (eds) 2006, *Social Determinants of Health*, 2nd edn, Oxford University Press, Oxford.

Marmot, M.G., Allen, J., Bell, R., Bloomer, E. & Goldblatt, P. 2012, 'WHO European review of social determinants of health and the health divide', *The Lancet*, vol. 380, no. 9846, pp. 1011–29.

Marmot, M.G., Bosma, H., Hemingway, H., Brunner, E. & Stansfeld, S. 1997, 'Contribution of job control and other risk factors to social variations in coronary heart disease incidence', *The Lancet*, vol. 350, no. 9073, pp. 235–9.

Marmot, M.G., Davey Smith, G., Stansfield, S., Patel, C., North, F., Head, J., White, I., Brunner, E. & Feeney, A. 1991, 'Health inequalities among British civil servants: the Whitehall II Study', *The Lancet*, vol. 337, no. 8754, pp. 1387–93.

Marmot, M.G., Rose, G., Shipley, M. & Hamilton, P.J.S. 1978, 'Employment grade and coronary heart disease in British civil servants', *Journal of Epidemiology and Community Health*, vol. 32, no. 4, pp. 244–9.

Marmot, M.G., Siegrist, J., Theorell, T. & Feeney, A. 1999, 'Health and the psychosocial environment at work', in M.G. Marmot & R.G. Wilkinson (eds), *Social Determinants of Health*, Oxford University Press, Oxford.

Mathers, C.D. & Schofield, D. 1998, 'The health consequences of unemployment: the evidence', *Medical Journal of Australia*, vol. 168, no. 4, pp. 178–82.

Muntaner, C. & Lynch, J. 1999, 'Income inequality, social cohesion, and class relations: a critique of Wilkinson's Neo-Durkheimian research program', *International Journal of Health Services*, vol. 29, no. 1, pp. 59–81.

Muntaner, C., Lynch, J. & Davey Smith, G. 2001, 'Social capital, disorganized communities and the third way: understanding the retreat from structural inequalities in epidemiology and public health', *International Journal of Health Services*, vol. 31, no. 2, pp. 213–37.

National Health Strategy (NHS) 1992, *Enough to Make You Sick: How Income and Environment Affect Health*, AGPS, Canberra.

O'Brien, K. 2005, *Living Dangerously: Australians with Multiple Risk Factors for Cardio-vascular Disease*, Bulletin no. 24, Australian Institute of Health and Welfare (AIHW) Cat. no. AUS 57, AIHW, Canberra.

Pakulski, J. 2005, *Globalising Inequalities: New Patterns of Social Privilege and Disadvantage*, Allen & Unwin, Sydney.

Pakulski, J. & Waters, M. 1996, *The Death of Class*, Sage, London.

Pantazis, C., Gordon, D. & Levitas, R. (eds.) 2006, *Poverty and Social Exclusion in Britain: The Millennium Survey*, Policy Press, Bristol.

Popay, J., Bennett, S., Thomas, C., Williams, G., Gatrell, A. & Bostock, L. 2003, 'Beyond "beer, fags, egg and chips"? Exploring lay understandings of social inequalities in health', *Sociology of Health & Illness*, vol. 25, no. 1, pp. 1–23.

Porter, R. 1997, *The Greatest Benefit to Mankind: A Medical History of Humanity from Antiquity to the Present*, HarperCollins, London.

Putnam, R. 1993, *Making Democracy Work: Civic Traditions in Modern Italy*, Princeton University Press, Princeton.

Putnam, R. 2000, *Bowling Alone: The Collapse and Revival of American Community*, Simon & Schuster, New York.

Rawls, J. 1970, *A Theory of Justice*, Clarendon Press, Oxford.

Rosen, G. 1993, *A History of Public Health*, Johns Hopkins University Press, New York.

Savage, M., Devine, F., Cunningham, N., Taylor, M., Li, Y., Hjellbrekke, J., Le Roux, B., Friedman, S. & Miles, A. 2013, 'A new model of social class? Findings from the BBC's Great British Class Survey experiment',

Sociology, vol. 72, no. 2, pp. 219–50: <http://soc.sagepub.com/content/47/2/219.full.pdf+html>.

Szreter, S. & Woolcock, M. 2004, 'Health by association? Social capital, social theory, and the political economy of public health', *International Journal of Epidemiology*, vol. 33, no. 4, pp. 650–67.

Townsend, P. & Davidson, N. (eds) 1982, *Inequalities in Health: The Black Report*, Penguin, Harmondsworth.

Townsend, P., Davidson, N. & Whitehead, M. (eds) 1992, *Inequalities in Health: The Black Report and the Health Divide*, Penguin, London.

Turrell, G., Oldenburg, B., McGuffog, I. & Dent, R. 1999, *Socioeconomic Determinants of Health: Towards a National Research Program and a Policy and Intervention Agenda*, Centre for Public Health Research, School of Public Health, Queensland University of Technology, Brisbane.

Turrell, G., Stanley, L., de Looper, M. & Oldenburg, B. 2006, *Health Inequalities in Australia: Morbidity, Health Behaviours, Risk Factors and Health Service Use*, Health Inequalities Monitoring Series no. 2, Australian Institute of Health and Welfare (AIHW) Cat. no. PHE 72, Queensland University of Technology and AIHW, Canberra.

Vågerö, D. & Illsley, R. 1995, 'Explaining health inequalities: beyond Black and Barker', *European Sociological Review*, vol. 11, no. 3, pp. 219–41.

Waitzkin, H. 1983, *The Second Sickness: Contradictions of Capitalist Health Care*, Free Press, New York.

Waitzkin, H. 2000, *The Second Sickness: Contradictions of Capitalist Health Care*, 2nd edn, Rowman & Littlefield, Lanham.

Westergaard, J. 1995, *Who Gets What? The Hardening of Class Inequality in the Late Twentieth Century*, Polity Press, Cambridge.

Western, M. 2000, 'Class in Australia in the 1980s and 1990s', in J.M. Najman & J.S. Western (eds), *A Sociology of Australian Society*, 3rd edn, Macmillan, Melbourne, pp. 68–88.

Western, M. & Baxter, J. 2007, 'Class and inequality in Australia', in J. Germov & M. Poole (eds), *Public Sociology: An Introduction to Australian Society*, Allen & Unwin, Sydney, pp. 214–36.

Western, M. & Baxter, J. 2011, 'Class and inequality in Australia', in J. Germov & M. Poole (eds), *Public Sociology: An Introduction to Australian Society*, 2nd edn, Allen & Unwin, Sydney, pp. 206–29.

Whitehead, M. 1987, *The Health Divide: Inequalities in Health in the 1980s*, Health Education Council, London.

Whitehead, M. 1990, *The Concepts and Principles of Equity and Health*, World Health Organization (WHO) Regional Office for Europe, Copenhagen.

Whitehead, M. 1992, 'The concepts and principles of equity and health', *International Journal of Health Services*, vol. 22, no. 3, pp. 429–45.

Whitehead, M. 1995, 'Tackling inequalities: a review of policy initiatives', in M. Benzeval, K. Judge & M. Whitehead (eds), *Tackling Inequalities in Health: An Agenda or Action*, King's Fund, London.

Whitehead, M. 2007, 'A typology of actions to tackle social inequalities in health', *Journal of Epidemiology and Community Health*, vol. 61, no. 6, pp. 473–8.

Wilkinson, R.G. 1992, 'Income distribution and life expectancy', *British Medical Journal*, vol. 304, no. 6820, pp. 165–8.

Wilkinson, R.G. 1996, *Unhealthy Societies: The Afflictions of Inequality*, Routledge, London.

Wilkinson, R.G. 1999, 'Putting the picture together: prosperity, redistribution, health, and welfare', in M. Marmot & R.G. Wilkinson (eds), *Social Determinants of Health*, Oxford University Press, Oxford, pp. 256–74.

Wilkinson, R.G. 2005, *The Impact of Inequality: How to Make Sick Societies Healthier*, The New Press, New York.

Wilkinson, R.G. & Marmot, M.G. (eds) 1998, *The Solid Facts: Social Determinants of Health*, World Health Organization (WHO), Copenhagen.

Wilkinson, R.G. & Marmot, M.G. (eds) 2003, *The Solid Facts: Social Determinants of Health*, 2nd edn, World Health Organization (WHO), Copenhagen.

Wilkinson, R.G. & Pickett, K.E. 2006, 'Income inequality and population health: a review and explanation of the evidence', *Social Science & Medicine*, vol. 62, no. 7, pp. 1768–84.

Wilkinson, R.G. & Pickett, K.E. 2007, 'The problems of relative deprivation: why some societies do better than others', *Social Science & Medicine*, vol. 65, no. 9, pp. 1965–78.

Wilkinson, R.G. & Pickett, K.E. 2009, *The Spirit Level: Why More Equal Societies Almost Always do Better*, Allen Lane, London.

Winter, I. (ed.) 2000a, *Social Capital and Public Policy in Australia*, Australian Institute of Family Studies, Melbourne.

Winter, I. 2000b, 'Major themes and debates in the social capital literature: the Australian connection', in I. Winter (ed.), *Social Capital and Public Policy in Australia*, Australian Institute of Family Studies, Melbourne, pp. 7–42.

Woolcock, M. 1998, 'Social capital and economic development: toward a theoretical synthesis and policy framework', *Theory and Society*, vol. 27, no. 2, pp. 151–208.

Wright, E.O. 1997, *Class Counts: Comparative Studies in Class Analysis*, Cambridge University Press, Cambridge.

Wright, E.O. (ed.) 2005, *Approaches to Class Analysis*, Cambridge University Press, Cambridge.

Housing and Neighbourhood

Objectives

By the end of your study of this chapter, you should be able to

- distinguish between housing and neighbourhood effects on health;
- understand how and why urban design and the built environment influence health outcomes;
- appreciate how public policies and government programs modify the health effects of housing and neighbourhood variables.

> Where people live affects their health and chances of leading flourishing lives. Communities and neighbourhoods that ensure access to basic goods, that are socially cohesive, that are designed to promote good physical and psychological well-being, and that are protective of the natural environment are essential for health equity. (Closing the gap in a generation, CSDH, 2008)

Synopsis

Chapter 9 reviews the impact of housing quality and homelessness on health, before turning to a discussion of healthy and unhealthy neighbourhood characteristics. Policy implications for improving population health, including healthy urban design and housing policy, complete the chapter.

Homes and Health

Being appropriately housed is an obvious determinant of good health. Appropriate housing—homes with good ventilation, well-regulated heating and cooling, low-density occupancy, ample and well-designed food storage, and adequate toilets and washing facilities—supports the health of the occupants.

Bad housing is associated with a host of ill-health effects. Poor ventilation, especially if combined with heating or cooking with wood- or coal-burning appliances (or smoking indoors), contributes significantly to respiratory diseases ranging from asthma in children to chronic bronchitis in adults to risk of lung cancer in older adults. Poor ventilation is also associated with poor control of humidity. High-humidity levels foster the growth of harmful moulds, mildews, and bacteria, which in turn increase risk of respiratory disease. Overcrowding in housing, particularly if combined with inadequate garbage disposal and toilet facilities, increases the risk of communicable disease, especially the risk of respiratory and food-borne illnesses. Overcrowding also fosters, as Engels pointed out 150 years ago, stress, depression, family violence, and substance abuse.

Housing may also be dangerous in other ways. Low-income housing often does not meet safety standards. Smoke detectors and hand railings may be missing or damaged. Wiring might be unsafe. Consequently, the preponderance of home injuries and fatalities from house fires, children falling on stairs, from balconies, or other causes occur in low-income contexts.

Inadequate food storage and refuse disposal create insect and animal vectors for disease, such as cockroaches and rodents. Additionally, improper food storage and waste disposal can lead directly to food poisoning. Environmental hazards in older houses, such as lead paint and asbestos fibre, pose serious health threats to occupants, particularly toddlers and young children who are most often indoors and most likely to ingest substances like paint residues.

Lead-based paints were used until the 1970s. Degraded paint yields chips and dust heavily contaminated with lead. Lead poisoning irreversibly damages the brain, and small children can suffer large effects at low doses. An estimated 310,000 mostly poor, inner-city American children between the ages of 1 and 5, in consequence of lead paint in older homes, have elevated blood-lead levels (Jacobs et al., 2002). Almost 35 per cent of all low-cost housing in the United States is contaminated with lead.

Inadequate regulation of heating and cooling can literally kill people, as happens both in hot spells and cold snaps to the homebound disabled. "Fuel poverty", the inability of poorer people to pay for adequate electricity, gas, or oil fuel to heat their homes, is a significant health risk. Cold housing is associated with stress and mental illness, especially among children. It is also associated with elevated incidence of viral infection and with exacerbation of symptoms of arthritis. In the UK, up to 27,000 additional deaths each winter are associated with fuel poverty (BBC, 2011). Death rates in the summertime in the US are 42 per cent lower among people whose houses are air conditioned (Rogot, Sorlie, and Backlund, 1992).

Homelessness and Health

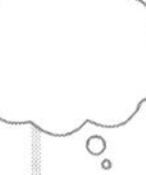

Pause and Reflect* ● *Causal Pathways and Homelessness

A disproportionate number of homeless people have a health problem such as a mental disorder or an addiction. Does homelessness lead to those health problems or, alternatively, do the health problems lead to homelessness?

Homelessness would be expected to negatively affect health, but the relationship between ill health and homelessness is complicated by the fact that people who are not well, especially those with substance abuse or mental health issues, are most at risk of becoming homeless. Poor health, substance abuse, or disability may lead to low income which in turn leads to homelessness. But it is also true that being without a home creates stress, disrupts the person's capacity to lead a stable life, and thus leads to mental illness, especially depression and anxiety. It is also true that being on the street, partly through stress and partly through exposure to "street culture," can lead to substance abuse. It can also lead to becoming a victim of violence.

Table 9.1 Variables Associated with Homelessness

Individual	Societal
Lack of job skills	Income inequality
Low educational attainment	Economy/unemployment
Mental illness	High housing costs
Substance abuse	Lack of social assistance and income support
Family breakdown	Discrimination
Adverse childhood experience (abuse)	
Chronic illness or disability	

It is wrong to think that people are homeless because of pre-existing mental illness or substance abuse. Surveys show that a larger proportion of the homeless than the general population have serious mental illness such as schizophrenia, but the seriously mentally ill still make up only 6 per cent of the total homeless population in Canada (Frankish, Hwang, and Quantz, 2005).

For obvious reasons, homeless people have significantly worse health than the general population. Mortality rates in Canada are approximately eight times higher for homeless men and 30 times higher for homeless women than for their housed counterparts. In the US, being homeless will reduce life expectancy by 20 years. The situation is worse in Britain; the average life expectancy of a homeless person in the United Kingdom is 42 years.

Exposure to the elements can lead to heat stroke or hypothermia and frostbite. The lack of a secure place to stay also makes homeless people victims of violence. In Canada, approximately 40 per cent of homeless people are assaulted each and every year and 25 per cent of homeless women report being raped (Hwang, 2001). Homeless shelters are often unsafe and overcrowded. Prolonged walking and sitting on the pavement, combined with inadequate hygiene, lead to foot infections and pressure ulcers.

The stress of living on the street contributes to high rates of smoking and alcohol and drug abuse. Poor nutrition, elevated stress, lack of sleep, and alcohol abuse compromise immune status, making homeless people more susceptible to infectious diseases such as TB. Moreover, homeless people face substantial barriers in accessing health and social services and, when they do, frequently fail to comply with treatment. Life on the streets is not conducive to following a treatment plan. Homeless people are also barred from use of food banks; only people with a fixed address may seek support from food bank charities.

Scope of the Problem of Homelessness

Homelessness is not a trivial health problem in wealthy countries such as Canada, the United States, and the United Kingdom. An estimated 250,000 people experience homelessness each year in Canada; approximately 30,000 Canadians are homeless on any given night. About 3.5 million people, 1.35 million of them children, are estimated to experience homelessness every year in the United States. Rates of homelessness for families and women have been steadily rising (National Coalition for the Homeless, 2011).

A significant factor driving up rates of homelessness is the housing boom—rapidly rising housing prices and associated increases in rent. In the United Kingdom, rents have soared in recent years—up 67 per cent between 1997 and 2007. In the short term, increases in welfare spending and rises in the housing benefit prevented homelessness from soaring along with rents. However, the emergency budget in June 2011 cut £1.8 billion from housing benefits and a further £7 billion cut is now being applied to welfare spending. Crisis (2011), a coalition dealing with the homeless in the UK, estimates that over 62,000 people will be made homeless by the changes. A further 1 million households will face housing and food insecurity. Meanwhile, the number of people in England depending on the food charity FairShare for free food has risen from 29,500 to 35,000 within 12 months (Rayner, 2011). The situation in Canada is not much better. Vacancy rates have been steadily falling and now average around 2 per cent. (They are substantially lower in the "hot property" markets of Calgary and Vancouver.) Assuming a person was lucky enough to find one, the rent he or she would pay for an average two-bedroom apartment rose from $860 to $883 between 2010 and 2011 (CMHC, 2011).

Neighbourhood and Health

In general, the patterning of health status in a population is determined, in part, by the contexts, places, and locations where people spend their lives. Extensive systematic review of high quality research literature found consistent effects of places on human health, independent of individual level attributes (Pickett and Pearl, 2001). Area level socio-economic variables are strongly associated with individual level health outcomes and strong associations have been demonstrated between area of residence, health behaviour, and self-rated health (Blaxter, 1990). Differential access to services and amenities afforded by neighbourhoods affect health behaviour, mental-health status, body size and shape, and activity level (Ellaway and Macintyre, 1996, 1997; Robert and Reither, 2004; Seliske, Pickett and Janssen, 2012). The degree of social cohesion in a neighbourhood is predictive of rates of schizophrenia (Van Os, et al., 2000). Collective efficacy, community capacity, and social cohesion affect health outcomes and the developmental trajectories of children (Kawachi, Kennedy and Glass, 1999; Hertzman and Power, 2006). Hertzman and Power (2006) showed that neighbourhood characteristics influence child readiness for school and a range of child-development outcomes independently of family of origin variables (although those remain the most important). Kohen et al. (2002) showed that safer and more cohesive neighbourhoods have better child-development outcomes. Neighbourhood-level measures of deprivation are predictive of both the rates of uptake of smoking and the amount of tobacco smoked (Duncan, Jones and Moon, 1996). There is more than a three-fold difference in coronary heart disease between rich and poor neighbourhoods after controlling for individual-level income (Diez-Roux et al., 2001).

In many ways, it is not surprising that characteristics of neighbourhoods can exert strong influence on health. Neighbourhoods differ in the degree of personal security and sense of safety, the quality of housing, access to good quality shops, the availability of transportation, the proximity and character of green spaces, parks and recreational facilities, access to social services and health care, and the quality of schools and other services.

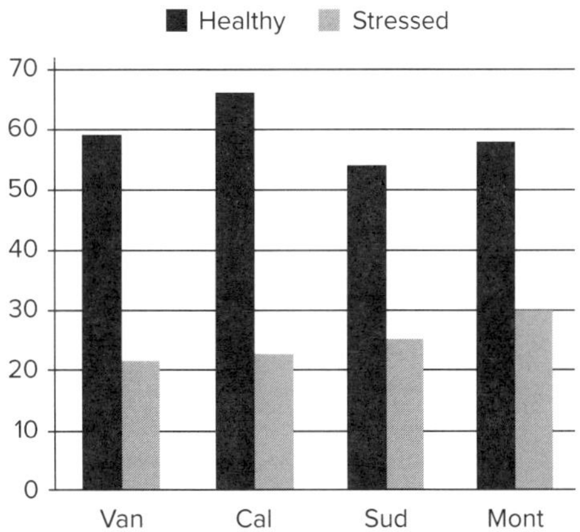

Figure 9.1 Self-Reported Health and Stress Levels by Select Canadian Cities (Per Cent)

Source: Based on Gandhi, 2006.

Neighbourhoods, Community Resources, and Opportunity Structures

From a materialist perspective, most neighbourhood characteristics can be regarded as resources or opportunities for the residents.The range of shops and what they stock at what price point, amenities like parks, recreation facilities, and public libraries, schools and health care, public transit, and so on are all part of the opportunity structure afforded by the neighbourhood. Those opportunity structures follow a pattern of **deprivation amplification** (Macintyre and Ellaway, 2000), meaning that there is generally a direct relationship between the opportunities a community has on offer and the income and education of its residents. Poorer and less-educated people, in other words, end up, not by choice but by necessity, living in neighbourhoods with impoverished opportunity structures whereas those already privileged end up in neighbourhoods with rich amenities. Hence we find the amplification effect.

A well-known example is the so-called food desert. Poor people, particularly in the United States (which has significant neighbourhood segregation by income and race), end up in neighbourhoods where there aren't any quality grocery stores offering reasonably priced fruit and vegetables nor any readily accessible and affordable transit to stores that do. Poor neighbourhoods are riddled with convenience stores, tobacco shops, liquor stores, and fast food outlets, but are wastelands when it comes to vendors of healthy foods. Products such as fresh food, when they can be found, are paradoxically more expensive than the same products in more affluent areas. The reasons for this are not fully understood but likely include lack of competition, a "captive market" due to the lack of ready access to affordable transportation, the lower educational level of the clientele, and straightforward exploitation of vulnerable people.

The pattern of what shops are available, what they offer for sale, and what they charge shapes the choices residents make regarding their purchases. That is not only true for food but for other health-relevant choices as well. For example, Frohlich et al. (2002) explored opportunity structures for smoking in Quebec. The researchers sought out community variables which might facilitate or discourage smoking, such as locations where tobacco was sold. They found that 51 per cent of smoking behaviour in Quebec could be attributed to community-level variables. Alcohol consumption has also been shown to vary depending on the number of bars and liquor retail outlets within a neighbourhood.

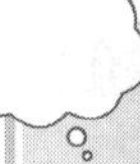

Pause and Reflect ● *Effect on Poorer People of Living in Richer Neighbourhood*

Poorer parents sometimes move from low income to higher income neighbourhoods, believing their children will have better opportunities and consequently do better over their life course. Often, lower-class children face discrimination, teasing, and bullying because they do not have the latest clothes, bikes, gadgets, etc. Overall, do you think parents who move into more affluent neighbourhoods are doing something positive or negative for their children? Why?

We know more affluent neighbourhoods, in terms of median income, generate better health outcomes for both their rich and their less-rich inhabitants whereas the opposite is true for less-affluent neighbourhoods. The lower the degree of neighbourhood segregation, the more mixing there is at the neighbourhood level of richer and poorer people, the greater the health of the average resident. This appears to be a key reason why Canada has a better overall health profile than the United States. It also helps explain why income inequality in Canada does not have the same devastating health effects typically found in the United States (Ross et al., 2000; Ross, 2004).

Merkin and colleagues (2009) established that Americans living in poorer neighbourhoods, regardless of their personal incomes, suffered adverse health effects. The negative health results of living in a deprived neighbourhood are worse for blacks than for Hispanics and whites, illustrating the cumulative effects of social segregation and negative neighbourhood characteristics and the ability of those population-level effects to amplify individual-level impacts such as personal income.

Comparing Canada to the US offers an interesting test of the psychosocial hypothesis. Based on psychosocial thinking, one might assume a neighbourhood made up of people all of similar income level might have a better health profile than a more mixed neighbourhood. Certainly the stress of everyday interpersonal comparisons of status would be reduced by mixing only with people with a similar socio-economic status. But recent research shows exactly the opposite is true (Hou and Miles, 2005). Poorer people do better when mixed with richer ones, presumably because they benefit from an improved opportunity structure at the neighbourhood level—better schools, better shops, better public services, and so on. Poorer people are well aware of this and many try to move to better neighbourhoods precisely so their children might benefit from better schools or so that they may feel safer.

A worrying recent trend is the growing segregation within Canadian cities. From a situation just 35 years ago when Canadian cities were quite homogeneous, with few rich or poor enclaves, cities are polarizing. The once ubiquitous "middle-class neighbourhood" comprised of mixed incomes is disappearing (McMartin, 2012). The outcome is called "socio-spatial income polarization" (Ley and Lynch, 2012) and marks a potentially dangerous divide between income and racial groups. Should the trend continue, the large health disparities associated with US cities are likely to emerge in Canada.

Neighbourhood Order, Disorder, and Stress

Ross et al. (2000) ranked US and Canadian neighbourhoods based on order/disorder. People in **disordered neighbourhoods**—defined as having poorly functioning public services, graffiti, and crime—feel powerless to enact positive change, experience elevated stress, and engage in more risky behaviour (Brody et al., 2001). Klinenburg (2002) added to Ross's findings of stress and powerlessness the idea of "**dangerous ecology**." Disordered neighbourhoods are less likely settings for individuals to be watchful over the vulnerable (children, the elderly, the disabled) or to offer assistance to those in need. Thus we find deaths of the elderly during heat waves or cold snaps to be much more common in disordered neighbourhoods. The observed effects stem from disorder, not poverty. Even in poor neighbourhoods, those that are less disordered (vibrant ethnic enclaves, for example) have higher levels of health and safety, largely due to better social integration.

Box 9.1

Case Study ○ The Urban Environment and Health

Urban health is complex because the solutions to health challenges in towns and cities do not lie with the health sector alone but with decisions made by others: in local government, education, urban planners, engineers, and those who determine physical infrastructure to social and health services. These professionals have to face the challenges of overloaded water and sanitation systems, polluting traffic and factories, lack of space to walk or cycle, inadequate waste disposal, crime, and injury.

Nevertheless, solutions exist to tackle the root causes of urban health challenges. Urban planning can promote healthy behaviour and safety through investment in active transport, designing areas to promote physical activity and passing regulatory controls on tobacco and food safety. Improving urban living conditions in the areas of housing, water, and sanitation will go a long way to mitigating health risks. Building green, inclusive cities that are accessible and age-friendly benefits all urban residents and their health. The Healthy Cities movement emphasizes the need for community participation in the decisions that affect people's lives.

World Health Organization, 2011. Urban Health at http://www.euro.who.int/en/what-we-do/health-topics/environment-and-health/urban-health.

How might the characteristics of the urban environment impact health? Given your analysis, why is it a common finding that residents living in or near the city centre enjoy better health and fitness than residents with a similar income living in the suburbs? What message(s) should that send to municipal planners and local governments?

There are some important psychosocial health effects of neighbourhood characteristics in addition to the materialist ones just discussed. Stress over personal safety has been linked to emotional disorders and destructive heath behaviours such as overeating. Access to green spaces and parks has been shown to reduce stress, blood pressure, anxiety, and depression. High levels of neighbourhood stability provide a buffer to the otherwise damaging effects of excess stress (Boardman, 2004). Neighbourhoods can also provide psychosocial benefits in terms of personal identity and sense of belonging (Omariba, 2010).

Urban Design, the Built Environment, and Physical Activity

Access to recreational facilities, parks, and urban design features such as bike paths, sidewalks, and adequate lighting at night deeply influence the physical activity level of people living in the area. So do transport policies such as rules for road use and availability and affordability of public transportation (Heath et al., 2012). The installation of fitness equipment in outdoor parks, now fairly commonplace in British Columbian communities (and standard practice in countries as diverse as China and Turkey for decades), increases the activity levels among children, adults, and the elderly (Cohen et al., 2012). Heath et al. (2006) showed, for Canada and the US, that road patterns, whether grid or cul-de-sac, influenced walking, jogging, and cycling. *Ciclovia* ("open streets"), the practice of closing streets to motor vehicles, has been a feature of life in Bogota, Colombia since 1976. Every Sunday, streets are closed to cars and trucks from 8:00 a.m. to 2:00 p.m., not only in Bogata, but also in Cali and Medellin. Some Canadian cities have conducted limited experiments in creating space for pedestrians and cyclists, notably Winnipeg, Calgary, Vancouver, Hamilton, and Ottawa.

Inactivity and Health

Much of the current interest in urban design is focused on increasing the activity level of the population, based on the premise that better health will inevitably follow. Inactivity is associated with a number of adverse health outcomes, whereas regular physical activity is associated with lower incidence of heart disease, diabetes, hypertension, and obesity (Lee et al., 2012). However, the relationship between population-level inactivity and population-level health outcomes is imperfect, to say the least. Consider Table 9.2 below.

Japan is the healthiest of the countries listed and has an obesity rate of only 3.2 per cent in spite of having one of world's least active populations. France, a middle ranking country in terms of activity levels, has excellent health and a relatively low rate of obesity (9 per cent). The UK and the US , have high rates of obesity (23 per cent and 30 per cent respectively), as well as high rates of heart disease and diabetes, but the (more inactive) British have better health than the (heavier and sicker but much more active) Americans. Obesity and health, then, do not track well with activity levels, demonstrating that diet and other factors are overall of greater import than physical activity. Nevertheless, physical activity is an important determinant of health and it, like eating patterns and food choices, is heavily influenced by characteristics of the community in which a person resides.

Table 9.2 Per Cent of Population Inactive* By Gender and Country (2012)

Country	Men and Women	Men	Women
Argentina	68.3	65.8	70.9
United Kingdom	63.3	58	68.6
Japan	60.2	58.9	61.6
United States	40.5	33.5	47.4
Australia	37.9	35.9	39.9
Canada	33.9	32.3	35.4
France	32.5	27.7	37.2
Netherlands	18.2	21.3	15.2

* inactivity is defined as not meeting any of the following criteria: 1. 5 X 30 minutes of moderate intensity exercise per week; 2. 3 X 20 minutes vigorous intensity exercise per week; 3. a combination of 1 and 2 achieving 600 metabolic equivalent minutes per week.

Source: Adapted from Guardian Datablog, 2012, "Which are the laziest countries on earth?" www.theguardian.com/news/datablog/2012/jul/18/physical-inactivity-country-laziest.

Housing Policy and Health

We learned earlier that housing is a significant determinant of health. The quality of housing refers to ventilation, heating and cooling, food storage and preparation capabilities, presence of toxins, washing and toilet facilities, and the number of rooms/amount of space for the number of occupants. Quality of housing also refers to neighbourhood variables, the opportunity structure of the area, security, and the standard of living of neighbours.

The cost of housing—its affordability—is also important. From the point of view of family budgets, housing is a relatively fixed cost and people must pay the rent or mortgage before they pay for other things. Otherwise they will be homeless. If reasonable quality housing is relatively expensive, downward pressure is put on other discretionary family budget items, especially food, causing food insecurity, another important contributor to poor health. Lower-income families may be confronted with poor-quality housing, in bad neighbourhoods that is nevertheless expensive and thus crowds out other health-related budget items.

After the Second World War, governments in Canada, the United States, the United Kingdom, and Australia all busied themselves with funding affordable housing. This had much to do with their experience earlier with demobilization of millions of armed forces personnel after the First World War. Governments failed to ensure that housing and jobs were available in 1918 at the end of hostilities leading to a period of riots, social unrest, and potential civil insurrection by ex-military personnel. No one wanted a repeat of that in 1945.

By 1975 several things had changed. First, Anglo-American economies faced the first post-war credit crunch. Second, government deficits soared to record peacetime levels. Third, the economic slowdown reduced government revenues. In short, there was something of a perfect storm. As noted earlier, Keynesian economics was a victim of these remarkable circumstances. Related to this was government's withdrawal from the housing market. First came a cutback on funding for social housing, then a transfer of responsibilities for backing mortgages from government to quasi-private agencies, and then, in the 1980s, an effort to sell off public housing and return it to the private property market. In short, after 1975, housing in the Anglo-American world was increasingly turned over to private market forces.

Private property developers and house builders share an interest in building large homes packed with as many luxury items as possible because those properties generate the most profit, just as big luxury cars are far more profitable to manufacturers and dealers than basic small cars. In the absence of regulation through building codes and local government zoning, the market will increasingly skew toward more expensive, larger houses even as average family size decreases. Rising prices in the new-build sub-sector will put upward pressure on prices of existing houses. That in turn creates incentives to renovate and render more modern and luxurious old housing stock, especially when the location is desirable. By and large, governments are supportive of those trends because a lot of money and jobs are generated through the supply chain from forestry to mills, home improvement stores, to the construction trades, furniture making to furniture and appliance retailing.

But the unfettered housing-market forces up all housing prices. Along with higher costs of buying homes, the process both reduces the number of places to rent (because it is more profitable to renovate and sell than have tenants) and increases the cost of rent (because the alternative for landlords, selling, becomes more lucrative). Also, areas of modest housing become "gentrified" and put out of the reach of modest income earners, but areas with very poor housing—bad locations or bad reputations—are ignored by developers, becoming blighted yet increasingly the only places low-income people can afford.

Middle- and low-income earners are thus confronted with fewer housing choices and higher prices. Some are driven into poor quality neighbourhoods, others into homelessness. All of this was made worse by deregulation, which lessened tenants' rights and reduced the obligations on developers to produce low-cost and multiple-family residences in addition to the lucrative single-family luxury houses and condominiums they prefer to build.

Once housing costs comprise more than 30 per cent of a household's disposable income, that household is both housing and food insecure—in other words, at risk of not being able to maintain their home and unable to afford adequate amounts of healthy food. Rising housing costs, for lower-income people, are thus a serious threat to their health.

The collapse of the housing boom in 2007 may bring some reason back into housing markets and may lead governments back into more regulation of the sector. The response by government to the banking crisis, however, suggests faint hope. Rather, Anglo-American governments appear to be waiting, hoping things will go back to the way they were in the early 2000s.

Some municipalities, however, have shown leadership in terms of support for social housing, a more aggressive stance with developers on multiple family and affordable housing, stricter zoning and better town planning. Portland, Oregon, stands out with its robust effort to house homeless people through a "housing first" initiative, which recognizes a person is unlikely to get control over his or her life or find secure work unless they are safely and appropriated housed. The approach was pioneered by Dr Tsemberis at the New York University School of Medicine in the 1990s and has been thoroughly evaluated since (Larimer et al., 2009). Seattle, Washington, and Vancouver, along with many other American and Canadian cities, and British local authorities have adopted "housing first" with promising results. Not only have clients' lives been stabilized by being housed, but their health and social function has also significantly improved.

Theoretical Considerations

Chapter 9 once again demonstrates the importance and power of multi-level analysis. At the individual level, risks to health arise from housing conditions; at the community level, the neighbourhood and the built environment support or undermine the health of residents. As Boardman (2004) showed, neighbourhood attributes can mediate and moderate (or amplify) effects arising from individual-level variables. Bad housing in a bad neighbourhood, the usual case, is substantially worse for health than bad housing in a good neighbourhood. Contrariwise, a good neighbourhood amplifies the positive effects of good housing. These effects have been empirically demonstrated in studies of childhood development, infectious disease, chronic disease, coronary heart disease, health behaviour, and mental health.

Summary

The quality of housing and the capacity to heat and cool residential accommodation are significant determinants of health, especially for infants, children, and the frail elderly. Housing quality is primarily a function of income. Exposure to poor indoor-air quality, inadequate food storage, mould, poor ventilation, overcrowding, indoor contaminants such as lead, asbestos, and radon gas, all rise as income falls. This is a key reason why respiratory disease tracks so closely with income.

Very low income, in the absence of robust social assistance and social housing, results in homelessness. Homelessness is associated with infectious and chronic disease, elevated stress, anxiety and depression, exposure to violence, substance abuse, and premature death.

Rising house prices in the context of flat or declining earnings among the lower-middle and lower classes decreases the quality of housing available to less well-off people and pushes up rates of homelessness.

Characteristics of residential neighbourhoods have profound health effects ranging from conditioning the type and amount of exercise undertaken by residents, to influencing the type and amounts of food consumed, to the levels of stress or emotional well-being experienced by residents. Neighbourhood characteristics also shape social networks and health behaviour, ranging from the amount people smoke or drink to the degree people engage in risky behaviour such as criminal activity or unsafe sex.

Urban design and the built environment heavily influence how people use spaces. Sidewalks and bicycle paths can encourage non-vehicular travel. Parks and green spaces can encourage active recreation. Road design and public transport can influence automobile use. All of these may have health impacts.

Some key policy directions emerging from Chapter 9 are listed below.

- We need enhanced co-operation amongst all levels of government to fund an appropriate level of social housing.
- Local governments and citizen coalitions must work together to ensure that municipal planning, approvals for property development and zoning by-laws are consistent with the principles of population health.
- National and sub-national levels of government must act in co-operation with local authorities in support of affordable housing, healthy neighbourhoods, and housing the homeless.
- National governments need to regulate credit and mortgage lending as well as tax law respecting capital gains to prevent property speculation, profiteering and housing market "bubbles."

Critical Thinking Questions

1. In what ways did your housing situation and neighbourhood influence your childhood development, health, and overall well-being? Which factors do you consider most significant?

2. Examining your current housing situation, how might your home influence your health?
3. Examining your current neighbourhood, how might the built environment and "opportunity structure" influence your health and well-being?

Annotated Suggested Readings

An excellent resource on the topic of neighbourhoods and health is I. Kawachi and L. Berkman (eds.) *Neighborhood and Health* (New York: Oxford University Press, 2003). The chapter by Sally Macintyre and Anne Ellaway, "Neighbourhoods and Health, An Overview" (pp. 20–42) is clear and comprehensive. The chapter "Multi-level Methods for Public Health Research" (S. Subramanin, K. Jones and C. Duncan, pp. 65–112) provides an accessible overview of the theoretical importance of multi-level research.

Elesevier publishes the excellent academic journal *Health and Place.* The journal includes a wide range of international articles ranging from obesity and the local environment to alcohol consumption and the location of retail sales outlets.

A lot of attention has gone into planning for healthier cities, especially in Europe. *Healthy Urban Planning in Practice: Experience of European Cities* (World Health Organization) outlines European experience in planning urban spaces that will improve population health. The electronic book (available at www.euro.who.int/__data/assets/pdf_file/0003/98400/E82657.pdf) discusses how we may best promote healthy exercise, social cohesion, equity, and environmental, economic and social sustainability.

In 2001, Ana Diez Roux published what is now a classic in the field: "Investigating Neighborhood and Area Effects in Health," available at www.ncbi.nlm.nih.gov/pmc/articles/PMC1446876/. The article summarizes the literature to date, and explores the conceptual, theoretical, and methodological issues that arise.

Annotated Websites

The Robert Wood Johnson Foundation developed two excellent briefing papers on housing and neighbourhoods, available at the link below. While the analysis and data is American, the principles and policy considerations transfer well to Canada, the UK, and Australia. www.rwjf.org/content/dam/farm/reports/issue_briefs/2011/rwjf70451

Canada Research Chair David Ley heads a project on neighbourhood change and building inclusive cities. A wealth of resources for Vancouver can be found on the project's website neighbourhoodchange.ca/cities/vancouver/

The World Health Organization hosts a portal into urban health and healthy cities. A large number of policy-related resources may be found at www.euro.who.int/en/health-topics/environment-and-health/urban-health/activities/healthy-cities